Movement Disorders

Disorders

SOURCEBOOK

Third Edition

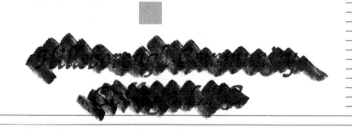

Health Reference Series

Third Edition

Movement Disorders SOURCEBOOK

*Basic Consumer Health Information about the
Symptoms and Causes of Movement Disorders, Including
Parkinson Disease, Amyotrophic Lateral Sclerosis, Cerebral
Palsy, Muscular Dystrophy, Multiple Sclerosis, Myasthenia,
Myoclonus, Spina Bifida, Dystonia, Essential Tremor,
Choreatic Disorders, Huntington Disease, Tourette
Syndrome, and Other Disorders That Cause Slowed,
Absent, or Excessive Movements*

*Along with Information about Surgical and
Nonsurgical Interventions, Physical Therapies,
Strategies for Independent Living, Clinical Trials, a
Glossary of Related Terms, and a Directory of
Resources for Additional Help and Information*

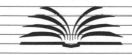

OMNIGRAPHICS

615 Griswold, Ste. 901, Detroit, MI 48226

Bibliographic Note
Because this page cannot legibly accommodate all the copyright notices, the Bibliographic Note portion of the Preface constitutes an extension of the copyright notice.

* * *

OMNIGRAPHICS
Greg Mullin, *Managing Editor*
***

Copyright © 2018 Omnigraphics

ISBN 978-0-7808-1609-1
E-ISBN 978-0-7808-1610-7

Library of Congress Cataloging-in-Publication Data

Names: Omnigraphics, Inc., issuing body.

Title: Movement disorders sourcebook: basic consumer health information about the symptoms and causes of movement disorders, including parkinson disease, amyotrophic lateral sclerosis, cerebral palsy, muscular dystrophy, multiple sclerosis, myasthenia, myoclonus, spina bifida, dystonia, essential tremor, choreatic disorders, huntington disease, tourette syndrome, and other disorders that cause slowed, absent, or excessive movements; along with information about surgical and nonsurgical interventions, physical therapies, strategies for independent living, a glossary of related terms, and a directory of resources for additional help and information.

Description: Third edition. | Detroit, MI: Omnigraphics, [2018] | Series: Health reference series | Includes bibliographical references and index.

Identifiers: LCCN 2017056199 (print) | LCCN 2017057181 (ebook) | ISBN 9780780816107 (eBook) | ISBN 9780780816091 (hardcover: alk. paper)

Subjects: LCSH: Movement disorders--Popular works.

Classification: LCC RC376.5 (ebook) | LCC RC376.5.M693 2018 (print) | DDC 616.8/3--dc23

LC record available at https://lccn.loc.gov/2017056199

Table of Contents

Part III: Other Hypokinetic Movement Disorders: Slowed or Absent Movements

Part IV: Hyperkinetic Movement Disorders: Excessive or Unwanted Movements

Part V: Diagnosis and Treatment of Movement Disorders

Part VI: Living with Movement Disorders

Part VII: Clinical Trials and Research on Movement Disorders

Part VIII: Additional Help and Information

Preface

About This Book

Every year millions of Americans experience the slowed, stiff, jerky, or excessive motions that characterize the neurological conditions known as movement disorders. For many, movement disorders cause chronic pain, weakness, and disability and make employment and independent living difficult or impossible. Although most movement disorders cannot be cured, patients who get timely diagnoses and educate themselves about medications, surgeries, and therapies may find relief of painful symptoms and face fewer limitations.

Movement Disorders Sourcebook, *Third Edition* provides information about the common types and symptoms of movement disorders in children and adults. This book details the causes and treatments of Parkinson disease and provides information on other hypokinetic movement disorders, such as amyotrophic lateral sclerosis, cerebral palsy, muscular dystrophy, multiple sclerosis, myasthenia, myoclonus, spina bifida, and spinal cord injury. Basic facts about hyperkinetic movement disorders, including dystonia, essential tremor, choreatic disorders, Huntington disease, movement disorders during sleep, and Tourette syndrome, are provided. In addition, the book offers information about surgical and nonsurgical treatments, physical therapies, strategies for independent living, and tips for spouses, caregivers, and parents of people with movement disorders, as well as clinical trials and research on various movement disorders. The volume concludes with a glossary of related terms and a directory of resources.

How to Use This Book

This book is divided into parts and chapters. Parts focus on broad areas of interest. Chapters are devoted to single topics within a part.

Part I: Introduction to Movement Disorders provides general information about how the brain, bones, muscles, and joints contribute to the body's movement. This part also offers an overview of some of the most common types of movement disorders and their related symptoms, including ataxia, spasticity, stiffness, cramps, twitching, and tremor.

Part II: Parkinson Disease offers detailed facts on the causes, symptoms, and progression of this well-known movement disorder and its related syndromes. Information on PD therapies and treatments, such as deep brain stimulation, as well as strategies for coping with pain, nutrition, relationships, and employment concerns are also discussed.

Part III: Other Hypokinetic Movement Disorders: Slowed or Absent Movements identifies the symptoms and treatments for hypokinetic movement disorders, including amyotrophic lateral sclerosis, cerebellar or spinocerebellar degeneration, cerebral palsy, muscular dystrophy, multiple sclerosis, myasthenia, myoclonus, spina bifida, and spinal cord injury.

Part IV: Hyperkinetic Movement Disorders: Excessive or Unwanted Movements explains the basics of hyperkinetic disorders, such as dystonia, tremor disorders, chorea, Huntington disease, restless legs syndrome and periodic limb movement disorders, neuroacanthocytosis and neurodegeneration, spastic paraplegia, and Tourette syndrome.

Part V: Diagnosis and Treatment of Movement Disorders highlights specific tests and procedures used to diagnose movement disorders and offers patients advice on assembling a trusted healthcare team. Current therapies used to treat the symptoms of movement disorders — including surgical options, medications, and physical therapy — are also discussed, as is the future potential of stem cell therapy for reducing the pain and disability associated with movement disorders.

Part VI: Living with Movement Disorders identifies the everyday concerns of people with movement disorders and their caregivers. Tips on assembling legal documents, dressing, driving, working independently, coping with chronic illness, and supporting and parenting a loved one with a movement disorder are all included in this part.

Part VII: Clinical Trials and Research on Movement Disorders focuses on various clinical trials and research being carried out on various movement disorders such as Parkinson disease, Huntington disease, cerebral palsy, multiple sclerosis, and muscular dystrophy.

Part VIII: Additional Help and Information includes a glossary of important terms and a directory of organizations for patients with movement disorders and their families.

Bibliographic Note

This volume contains documents and excerpts from publications issued by the following government agencies: Centers for Disease Control and Prevention (CDC); *Eunice Kennedy Shriver* National Institute of Child Health and Human Development (NICHD); Genetic and Rare Diseases Information Center (GARD); Genetics Home Reference (GHR); National Center for Biotechnology Information (NCBI); National Center for Complementary and Alternative Medicine (NCCAM); National Eye Institute (NEI); National Guideline Clearinghouse (NGC); National Heart, Lung, and Blood Institute (NHLBI); National Highway Traffic Safety Administration (NHTSA); National Human Genome Research Institute (NHGRI); National Institute of Arthritis and Musculoskeletal and Skin Diseases (NIAMS); National Institute of Environmental Health Sciences (NIEHS); National Institute of Mental Health (NIMH); National Institute of Neurological Disorders and Stroke (NINDS); National Institute on Aging (NIA); National Institute on Deafness and Other Communication Disorders (NIDCD); National Institutes of Health (NIH); *NIH News in Health*; Office of Disability Employment Policy (ODEP); Office of Disease Prevention and Health Promotion (ODPHP); Surveillance, Epidemiology and End Results Program (SEER); U.S. Department of Health and Human Services (HHS); U.S. Department of Justice (DOJ); U.S. Department of Veterans Affairs (VA); U.S. Food and Drug Administration (FDA); U.S. National Library of Medicine (NLM); U.S. Small Business Administration (SBA); and the U.S. Social Security Administration (SSA).

It may also contain original material produced by Omnigraphics and reviewed by medical consultants.

About the Health Reference Series

The *Health Reference Series* is designed to provide basic medical information for patients, families, caregivers, and the general public. Each volume takes a particular topic and provides comprehensive coverage. This is especially important for people who may be dealing with a newly diagnosed disease or a chronic disorder in themselves or in a family member. People looking for preventive guidance, information about disease warning signs, medical statistics, and risk factors for health problems will also find answers to their questions in the *Health Reference Series*. The *Series*, however, is not intended to serve as a tool for diagnosing illness, in prescribing treatments, or as a substitute for the physician/patient relationship. All people concerned about medical symptoms or the possibility of disease are encouraged to seek professional care from an appropriate healthcare provider.

A Note about Spelling and Style

Health Reference Series editors use *Stedman's Medical Dictionary* as an authority for questions related to the spelling of medical terms and the *Chicago Manual of Style* for questions related to grammatical structures, punctuation, and other editorial concerns. Consistent adherence is not always possible, however, because the individual volumes within the *Series* include many documents from a wide variety of different producers, and the editor's primary goal is to present material from each source as accurately as is possible. This sometimes means that information in different chapters or sections may follow other guidelines and alternate spelling authorities. For example, occasionally a copyright holder may require that eponymous terms be shown in possessive forms (Crohn's disease vs. Crohn disease) or that British spelling norms be retained (leukaemia vs. leukemia).

Medical Review

Omnigraphics contracts with a team of qualified, senior medical professionals who serve as medical consultants for the *Health Reference Series*. As necessary, medical consultants review reprinted and originally written material for currency and accuracy. Citations including the phrase, "Reviewed (month, year)" indicate material reviewed by this team. Medical consultation services are provided to the *Health Reference Series* editors by:

Dr. Vijayalakshmi, MBBS, DGO, MD
Dr. Senthil Selvan, MBBS, DCH, MD
Dr. K. Sivanandham MBBS, DCH, MS (Research), PhD

Our Advisory Board

We would like to thank the following board members for providing initial guidance on the development of this series:

- Dr. Lynda Baker, Associate Professor of Library and Information Science, Wayne State University, Detroit, MI

- Nancy Bulgarelli, William Beaumont Hospital Library, Royal Oak, MI

- Karen Imarisio, Bloomfield Township Public Library, Bloomfield Township, MI

- Karen Morgan, Mardigian Library, University of Michigan-Dearborn, Dearborn, MI

- Rosemary Orlando, St. Clair Shores Public Library, St. Clair Shores, MI

Health Reference Series *Update Policy*

The inaugural book in the *Health Reference Series* was the first edition of *Cancer Sourcebook* published in 1989. Since then, the *Series* has been enthusiastically received by librarians and in the medical community. In order to maintain the standard of providing high-quality health information for the layperson the editorial staff at Omnigraphics felt it was necessary to implement a policy of updating volumes when warranted.

Medical researchers have been making tremendous strides, and it is the purpose of the *Health Reference Series* to stay current with the most recent advances. Each decision to update a volume is made on an individual basis. Some of the considerations include how much new information is available and the feedback we receive from people who use the books. If there is a topic you would like to see added to the update list, or an area of medical concern you feel has not been adequately addressed, please write to:

Managing Editor
Health Reference Series
Omnigraphics
615 Griswold, Ste. 901
Detroit, MI 48226

Part One

Introduction to Movement Disorders

Chapter 1

Anatomy of the Brain: How the Brain Controls the Body's Movements

Anatomy and Function Areas of the Brain and Central Nervous System (CNS)

The CNS consists of the brain and spinal cord, which are located in the dorsal body cavity. The brain is surrounded by the cranium, and the spinal cord is protected by the vertebrae. The brain is continuous with the spinal cord at the foramen magnum. In addition to bone, the CNS is surrounded by connective tissue membranes, called meninges, and by cerebrospinal fluid. The following are the major components of the brain and CNS.

- Neurons and Glial Cells

- Brain

- Meninges

- Spinal Cord

This chapter includes text excerpted from "Brain and CNS Tumors—Anatomy," Surveillance, Epidemiology and End Results Program (SEER), National Cancer Institute (NCI), September 8, 2016.

- Cranial Nerves
- Pineal and Pituitary Glands

Neurons and Glial Cells

Neurons

Neurons are the conducting cells of the nervous system. A typical neuron consists of a cell body, containing the nucleus and the surrounding cytoplasm; several short radiating processes (called dendrites); and one long process (called the axon), which terminates in twig like branches and may have branches projecting along its course.

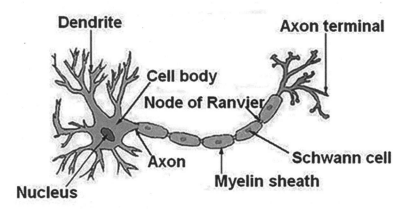

Figure 1.1. *Structure of a Typical Neuron*

Cell Body

In many ways, the cell body is similar to other types of cells. It has a nucleus with at least one nucleolus and contains many of the typical cytoplasmic organelles. It lacks centrioles, however. Because centrioles function in cell division, the fact that neurons lack these organelles is consistent with the amitotic nature of the cell.

Dendrites and Axons

An axon is a long, hair-like extension of a nerve cell that carries a message to another nerve cell.

Dendrites are thread like extensions of the cytoplasm of a neuron that receive signals from other neurons. Typically, as in multipolar neurons, dendrites branch into treelike processes, but in unipolar and bipolar neurons, dendrites resemble axons.

Glial Cells

Glial (neuroglial) cells do not conduct nerve impulses, but instead, support, nourish, and protect the neurons. Glial cells are far more numerous than neurons and, unlike neurons, are capable of mitosis.

Brain

Cerebrum

The cerebrum is the part of the brain that receives and processes conscious sensation, generates thought, and controls conscious activity. It is the uppermost and largest part of the brain and is divided into left and right hemispheres, which are joined by and communicated through the corpus callosum.

Each cerebral hemisphere is divided into five lobes, four of which have the same name as the bone over them: the frontal lobe, the parietal lobe, the occipital lobe, and the temporal lobe. A fifth lobe, the insula or Island of Reil, lies deep within the lateral sulcus.

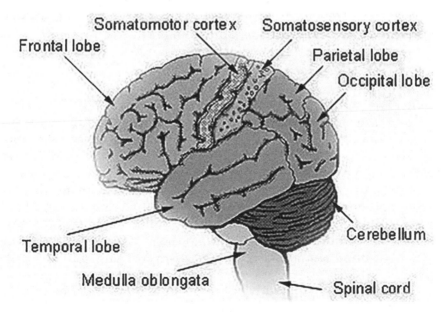

Figure 1.2. *Lobes of the Cerebrum*

Cerebellum

The cerebellum is a cauliflower shaped section of the brain located in the hindbrain, at the bottom rear of the head, directly behind the pons. The cerebellum is a complex system mostly dedicated to the intricate coordination of voluntary movement, including walking and balance. Damage to the cerebellum leaves the sufferer with a gait that appears drunken and is difficult to control.

Ventricles and Cerebrospinal Fluid

A series of interconnected, fluid filled cavities called ventricles lie within the brain. The fluid is cerebrospinal fluid (CSF), which also circulates over the outside of the brain and spinal cord.

Brainstem

The brainstem is the part of the brain continuous with the spinal cord and comprising the medulla oblongata, pons, midbrain, and parts of the hypothalamus.

Tentorium

The tentorium is a fold of the dura mater, which separates the cerebellum from the cerebrum, and often encloses a process or plate of the skull called the bony tentorium.

Meninges

There are three layers of meninges around the brain and spinal cord. The outer layer, the dura mater, is tough, white fibrous connective tissue. The middle layer of meninges is arachnoid, a thin layer resembling a cobweb with numerous thread like strands attaching it to the innermost layer. The space under the arachnoid, the subarachnoid space, is filled with cerebrospinal fluid and contains blood vessels. The pia mater is the innermost layer of meninges. This thin, delicate membrane is tightly bound to the surface of the brain and spinal cord and cannot be dissected away without damaging the surface.

Meningiomas are tumors of the nerve tissue covering the brain and spinal cord. Although meningiomas are unlikely to spread, physicians often treat them as though they were malignant because symptoms may develop when a tumor applies pressure to the brain.

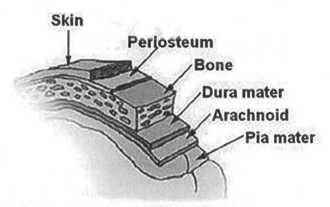

Skin
Periosteum
Bone
Dura mater
Arachnoid
Pia mater

Dura mater -- outer layer lining skull
Arachnoid (mater) -- contains blood vessels
Subarachnoid space -- filled with CSF
Pia mater -- covers brain

Figure 1.3. *Meninges*

Spinal Cord

The spinal cord extends from the foramen magnum at the base of the skull to the level of the first lumbar vertebra. The cord is continuous with the medulla oblongata at the foramen magnum. Like the brain, the spinal cord is surrounded by bone, meninges, and cerebrospinal fluid.

The spinal cord is divided into 31 segments, with each segment giving rise to a pair of spinal nerves. At the distal end of the cord, many spinal nerves extend beyond the conus medullaris to form a collection that resembles a horse's tail. This is the cauda equina. In cross section, the spinal cord appears oval in shape.

Cranial Nerves

The cranial nerves are composed of 12 pairs of nerves that emanate from the nervous tissue of the brain. In order to reach their targets they must ultimately exit/enter the cranium through openings in the skull. Hence, their name is derived from their association with the cranium. The following are the list of cranial nerves, their functions, and tumor examples:

Table 1.1. Cranial Nerves and Their Functions

Name	Function	Tumor Example
Olfactory	The olfactory nerve carries impulses for the sense of smell.	Esthesioneuronblastoma
Optic	The optic nerve carries impulses for the sense of sight.	Optic nerve glioma
Occulomotor	The occulomotor nerve is responsible for motor enervation of upper eyelid muscle, extraocular muscle and pupillary muscle.	Schwannoma
Trochlear	The trochlear nerve controls an extraocular muscle.	Schwannoma
Trigeminal	The trigeminal nerve is responsible for sensory enervation of the face and motor enervation to muscles of mastication (chewing).	Malignant peripheral nerve sheath tumor (MPNST)
Abducent	The abducent nerve enervates a muscle, which moves the eyeball.	Schwannoma
Facial	The facial nerve enervates the muscles of the face (facial expression).	Schwannoma (rare)
Vestibulocochlear	The vestibulocochlear nerve is responsible for the sense of hearing and balance (body position sense).	Vestibular Schwannoma
Glossopharyngeal	The glossopharyngeal nerve enervates muscles involved in swallowing and taste. Lesions of the ninth nerve result in difficulty swallowing and disturbance of taste.	Glomus tumor
Vagus	The vagus nerve enervates the gut (gastrointestinal tract), heart and larynx.	MPNST, paraganglioma

Table 1.1. Continued

Name	Function	Tumor Example
Accessory	The accessory nerve enervates the sternocleidomastoid muscles and the trapezius muscles.	Schwannoma
Hypoglossal	The hypoglossal nerve enervates the muscles of the tongue.	Schwannoma

Pineal and Pituitary Glands

The pineal gland is a small endocrine gland in the brain, situated beneath the back part of the corpus callosum, and secretes melatonin. The pituitary gland is located at the base of the brain that secretes hormones and regulates and controls other hormone secreting glands and many body processes, including reproduction.

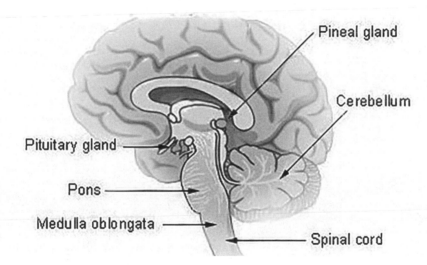

Figure 1.4. *Pituitary and Pineal Glands*

Chapter 2

Bones, Muscles, and Joints: What They Do and How They Move

What You Know about Your Bones

Bones support your body and allow you to move. They protect your brain, heart, and other organs from injury.

Bone is a living, growing tissue. It is made mostly of two materials: collagen, a protein that provides a soft framework; and calcium, a mineral that adds strength and hardness. This combination makes bone strong and flexible enough to hold up under stress.

Bone releases calcium and other minerals into the body when you need them for other uses.

This chapter contains text excerpted from the following sources: Text under the heading "What You Know about Your Bones" is excerpted from "Healthy Bones Matter," National Institute of Arthritis and Musculoskeletal and Skin Diseases (NIAMS), April 12, 2017; Text under the heading "Basic Facts about Muscles" is excerpted from "Healthy Muscles Matter," National Institute of Arthritis and Musculoskeletal and Skin Diseases (NIAMS), March 9, 2017; Text under the heading "What Exactly Is a Joint?" is excerpted from "Healthy Joints Matter," National Institute of Arthritis and Musculoskeletal and Skin Diseases (NIAMS), April 12, 2017.

How Bones Grow

Think of your bones as a "bank" where you "deposit" and "withdraw" bone tissue. During your childhood and teenage years, new bone is added (or deposited) to the skeleton faster than old bone is removed (or withdrawn). As a result, your bones become larger, heavier, and denser.

For most people, bone formation continues at a faster pace than removal until sometime after age 20. After age 30, bone withdrawals can begin to go faster than deposits. If your bone deposits don't keep up with withdrawals, you can get osteoporosis when you get older. Osteoporosis is a disease in which the bones become weak and more likely to break (fracture). People with osteoporosis most often break bones in the hip, spine, and wrist.

What You Need to Do Now—and Why

If you want to be able to make "deposits" of bone tissue and reach your greatest possible peak bone mass, you need to get enough calcium, vitamin D, and physical activity—important factors in building bone. If you want the strongest bones possible, the best time to build up your "account" is during your childhood and teenage years.

Why Should I Care about This Now?

You may know some older people who worry about their bones getting weak. You might even know someone who has trouble getting around because they have broken a bone because of osteoporosis. You might think that this is something that only older people need to worry about.

BUT—you can take action right now to help make sure that as you get older your bones are as healthy as they can be. Eating a balanced diet that includes calcium and vitamin D, getting plenty of physical activity, and having good health habits now can help keep your bones healthy for your whole life.

Basic Facts about Muscles

Did you know you have more than 600 muscles in your body? These muscles help you move, lift things, pump blood through your body, and even help you breathe.

When you think about your muscles, you probably think most about the ones you can control. These are your voluntary muscles, which means you can control their movements. They are also called skeletal muscles, because they attach to your bones and work together with your bones to help you walk, run, pick up things, play an instrument, throw a baseball, kick a soccer ball, push a lawnmower, or ride a bicycle. The muscles of your mouth and throat even help you talk!

Keeping your muscles healthy will help you to be able to walk, run, jump, lift things, play sports, and do all the other things you love to do. Exercising, getting enough rest, and eating a balanced diet will help to keep your muscles healthy for life.

Why Healthy Muscles Matter to You

Healthy muscles let you move freely and keep your body strong. They help you to enjoy playing sports, dancing, walking the dog, swimming, and other fun activities. And they help you do those other (not so fun) things that you have to do, like making the bed, vacuuming the carpet, or mowing the lawn.

Strong muscles also help to keep your joints in good shape. If the muscles around your knee, for example, get weak, you may be more likely to injure that knee. Strong muscles also help you keep your balance, so you are less likely to slip or fall.

And remember—the activities that make your skeletal muscles strong will also help to keep your heart muscle strong!

Different Kinds of Muscles Have Different Jobs

- **Skeletal** muscles are connected to your bones by tough cords of tissue called tendons. As the muscle contracts, it pulls on the tendon, which moves the bone. Bones are connected to other bones by ligaments, which are like tendons and help hold your skeleton together.

- **Smooth** muscles are also called involuntary muscles since you have no control over them. Smooth muscles work in your digestive system to move food along and push waste out of your body. They also help keep your eyes focused without your having to think about it.

- **Cardiac** muscle. Did you know your heart is also a muscle? It is a specialized type of involuntary muscle. It pumps blood through your body, changing its speed to keep up with the demands you put on it. It pumps more slowly when you're sitting or lying down, and faster when you're running or playing sports and your skeletal muscles need more blood to help them do their work.

What Can Go Wrong?

Injuries

Almost everyone has had sore muscles after exercising or working too much. Some soreness can be a normal part of healthy exercise. But, in other cases, muscles can become strained. Muscle strain can be mild (the muscle has just been stretched too much) to severe (the muscle actually tears). Maybe you lifted something that was too heavy and the muscles in your arms were stretched too far. Lifting heavy things in the wrong way can also strain the muscles in your back. This can be very painful and can even cause an injury that will last a long time and make it hard to do everyday things.

The tendons that connect the muscles to the bones can also be strained if they are pulled or stretched too much. If ligaments (remember, they connect bones to bones) are stretched or pulled too much, the injury is called a sprain. Most people are familiar with the pain of a sprained ankle.

What Exactly Is a Joint?

A joint is where two or more bones are joined together. Joints can be rigid, like the joints between the bones in your skull, or movable, like knees, hips, and shoulders. Many joints have cartilage on the ends of the bones where they come together. Healthy cartilage helps you move by allowing bones to glide over one another. It also protects bones by preventing them from rubbing against each other.

Keeping your joints healthy will allow you to run, walk, jump, play sports, and do the other things you like to do. Physical activity, a balanced diet, avoiding injuries, and getting plenty of sleep will help you stay healthy and keep your joints healthy too.

What Can Go Wrong

Some people get arthritis. The term arthritis is often used to refer to any disorder that affects the joints. Although you might think arthritis affects only older people, it can affect young people, too. There are many different forms of arthritis:

- **Osteoarthritis** is the most common type of arthritis and is seen especially among older people. In osteoarthritis, the surface cartilage in the joints breaks down and wears away, allowing the bones to rub together. This causes pain, swelling, and loss of motion in the joint. Sometimes, it can be triggered by an injury to a joint, such as a knee injury that damages the cartilage.

- **Rheumatoid arthritis** is known as an autoimmune disease, because the immune system attacks the tissues of the joints as if they were disease causing germs. This results in pain, swelling, stiffness, and loss of function in the joints. People with rheumatoid arthritis may also feel tired and sick, and they sometimes get fevers. It can cause permanent damage to the joints and sometimes affects the heart, lungs, or other organs.

- **Gout** is a form of arthritis that is caused by a buildup of uric acid crystals in the joints, most commonly in the big toe. It can be extremely painful. There are several effective treatments for gout that can reduce disability and pain.

- **Juvenile arthritis** is a term often used to describe arthritis in children. Children can develop almost all types of arthritis that affect adults, but the most common type that affects children is juvenile idiopathic arthritis (JIA).

- **Other forms of arthritis** may be associated with diseases like lupus, fibromyalgia, psoriasis, or certain infections. In addition, other diseases might affect the bones or muscles around a joint, causing problems in that joint.

Chapter 3

Types of Movement Disorders

Imagine if parts of your body moved when you didn't want them to. If you have a movement disorder, you experience these kinds of impaired movements. Dyskinesia is abnormal uncontrolled movement and is a common symptom of many movement disorders. Tremors are a type of dyskinesia.

Nerve diseases cause many movement disorders, such as Parkinson disease. Other causes include injuries, autoimmune diseases, infections and certain medicines. Many movement disorders are inherited, which means they run in families.

Treatment varies by disorder. Medicine can cure some disorders. Others get better when an underlying disease is treated. Often,

---

This chapter contains text excerpted from the following sources: Text in this chapter begins with excerpts from "Movement Disorders," MedlinePlus, National Institutes of Health (NIH), November 4, 2016; Text under the heading "Dystonia" is excerpted from "Dystonias Fact Sheet," National Institute of Neurological Disorders and Stroke (NINDS), January 2012. Reviewed January 2018; Text under the heading "Friedreich Ataxia" is excerpted from "Friedreich's Ataxia Information Page," National Institute of Neurological Disorders and Stroke (NINDS), December 21, 2016; Text under the heading "Essential Tremor" is excerpted from "Essential Tremor," National Institute of Neurological Disorders and Stroke (NINDS), May 5, 2017; Text under the heading "Huntington Disease" is excerpted from "Huntington's Disease Information Page," National Institute of Neurological Disorders and Stroke (NINDS), January 30, 2016; Text under the heading "Multiple System Atrophy" is excerpted from "Multiple System Atrophy Information Page," National Institute of Neurological Disorders and Stroke (NINDS), November 15, 2014. Reviewed January 2018;

however, there is no cure. In that case, the goal of treatment is to improve symptoms and relieve pain.

Dystonia

Dystonia is a disorder characterized by involuntary muscle contractions that cause slow repetitive movements or abnormal postures. The movements may be painful, and some individuals with dystonia may have a tremor or other neurologic features. There are several different forms of dystonia that may affect only one muscle, groups of muscles, or muscles throughout the body. Some forms of dystonia are genetic but the cause for the majority of cases is not known.

Friedreich Ataxia

Friedreich ataxia (FA) is a rare inherited disease that causes progressive damage to the nervous system and movement problems. Neurological symptoms include awkward, unsteady movements, impaired sensory function, speech problems, and vision and hearing loss. Thinking and reasoning abilities are not affected. Impaired muscle coordination (ataxia) results from the degeneration of nerve tissue in the spinal cord and of nerves that control muscle movement in the arms and legs. Symptoms usually begin between the ages of 5 and 15 but can appear in adulthood or later. The first symptom is usually difficulty in walking. The ataxia gradually worsens and slowly spreads to the arms and then the trunk. People lave loss of sensation in the arms and legs, which may spread to other parts of the body. Many people with Friedreich ataxia develop scoliosis (a curving of the spine to one side), which, if severe, may impair breathing. Other

---

Text under the heading "Parkinson Disease" is excerpted from "Parkinson's Disease Information Page," National Institute of Neurological Disorders and Stroke (NINDS), December 19, 2016; Text under the heading "Progressive Supranuclear Palsy" is excerpted from "Progressive Supranuclear Palsy Fact Sheet," National Institute of Neurological Disorders and Stroke (NINDS), September 2015; Text under the heading "Rett Syndrome" is excerpted from "Rett Syndrome," *Eunice Kennedy Shriver* National Institute of Child Health and Human Development (NICHD), December 1, 2016; Text under the heading "Spasticity" is excerpted from "Spasticity Information Page," National Institute of Neurological Disorders and Stroke (NINDS), August 19, 2017; Text under the heading "Tourette Syndrome" is excerpted from "Facts About Tourette Syndrome," Centers for Disease Control and Prevention (CDC), May 11, 2017; Text under the heading "Wilson Disease" is excerpted from "Wilson Disease Information Page," Centers for Disease Control and Prevention (CDC), October 6, 2011. Reviewed January 2018.

symptoms include chest pain, shortness of breath, and heart problems. Some individuals may develop diabetes. Doctors diagnose Friedreich ataxia by performing a careful clinical examination, which includes a medical history and a thorough physical examination. Several tests may be performed, including electromyogram (EMG, which measures the electrical activity of cells) and genetic testing.

Essential Tremor

Essential tremor is an incurable, degenerative brain disorder that results in increasingly debilitating tremor, and afflicts an estimated 7 million people in the United States. In one study, 25 percent of essential tremor patients were forced to change jobs or take early retirement because of tremor. Essential tremor is directly linked to progressive functional impairment, social embarrassment, and even depression. The tremor associated with essential tremor is typically slow, involves the hands (and sometimes the head and voice), worsens with intentional movements, and is insidiously progressive over many years. Deep brain stimulation has emerged as a highly effective treatment for intractable, debilitating essential tremor. However, since the intention tremor of essential tremor is typically intermittent, and commonly absent at rest, the currently available continuous deep brain stimulation may be delivering unnecessary current to the brain that increases undesirable side effects such as slurred speech and walking difficulty, and hastens the depletion of device batteries, necessitating more frequent surgical procedures to replace spent pulse generators. The overall objective of this early feasibility study is to provide preliminary data on the safety and efficacy of "closed-loop" deep brain stimulation for intention tremor using novel deep brain stimulation devices capable of continuously sensing brain activity and delivering therapeutic stimulation only when necessary to suppress tremor.

Huntington Disease

Huntington disease (HD) is an inherited disorder that causes degeneration of brain cells, called neurons, in motor control regions of the brain, as well as other areas. Symptoms of the disease, which gets progressively worse, include uncontrolled movements (called chorea), abnormal body postures, and changes in behavior, emotion, judgment, and cognition. People with HD also develop impaired coordination, slurred speech, and difficulty feeding and swallowing. HD typically begins between ages 30 and 50. An earlier onset form called juvenile

HD, occurs under age 20. Symptoms of juvenile HD differ somewhat from adult onset HD and include unsteadiness, rigidity, difficulty at school, and seizures. More than 30,000 Americans have HD.

Huntington disease is caused by a mutation in the gene for a protein called huntingtin. The defect causes the cytosine, adenine, and guanine (CAG) building blocks of DNA to repeat many more times than is normal. Each child of a parent with HD has a 50–50 chance of inheriting the HD gene. If a child does not inherit the HD gene, he or she will not develop the disease and generally cannot pass it to subsequent generations. There is a small risk that someone who has a parent with the mutated gene but who did not inherit the HD gene may pass a possibly harmful genetic sequence to her/his children. A person who inherits the HD gene will eventually develop the disease. A genetic test, coupled with a complete medical history and neurological and laboratory tests, helps physicians diagnose HD.

Multiple System Atrophy

Multiple system atrophy (MSA) is a progressive neurodegenerative disorder characterized by symptoms of autonomic nervous system failure such as fainting spells and bladder control problems, combined with motor control symptoms such as tremor, rigidity, and loss of muscle coordination. MSA affects both men and women primarily in their 50s. Although what causes MSA is unknown, the disorder's symptoms reflect the loss of nerve cells in several different areas in the brain and spinal cord that control the autonomic nervous system and coordinate muscle movements. The loss of nerve cells may be due to the buildup of a protein called alpha-synuclein in the cells that support nerve cells in the brain.

Parkinson Disease

Parkinson disease (PD) belongs to a group of conditions called motor system disorders, which are the result of the loss of dopamine-producing brain cells. The four primary symptoms of PD are tremor, or trembling in hands, arms, legs, jaw, and face; rigidity, or stiffness of the limbs and trunk; bradykinesia, or slowness of movement; and postural instability, or impaired balance and coordination. As these symptoms become more pronounced, patients may have difficulty walking, talking, or completing other simple tasks. PD usually affects people over the age of 60. Early symptoms of PD are subtle and occur gradually. In some people the disease progresses more quickly than in others.

As the disease progresses, the shaking, or tremor, which affects the majority of people with PD may begin to interfere with daily activities. Other symptoms may include depression and other emotional changes; difficulty in swallowing, chewing, and speaking; urinary problems or constipation; skin problems; and sleep disruptions. There are currently no blood or laboratory tests that have been proven to help in diagnosing sporadic PD. Therefore the diagnosis is based on medical history and a neurological examination. The disease can be difficult to diagnose accurately. Doctors may sometimes request brain scans or laboratory tests in order to rule out other diseases.

Progressive Supranuclear Palsy

Progressive supranuclear palsy (PSP) is an uncommon brain disorder that affects movement, control of walking (gait) and balance, speech, swallowing, vision, mood and behavior, and thinking. The disease results from damage to nerve cells in the brain. The disorder's long name indicates that the disease worsens (progressive) and causes weakness (palsy) by damaging certain parts of the brain above nerve cell clusters called nuclei (supranuclear). These nuclei particularly control eye movements. One of the classic signs of the disease is an inability to aim and move the eyes properly, which individuals may experience as blurring of vision.

Estimates vary, but only about three to six in every 100,000 people worldwide, or approximately 20,000 Americans, have PSP—making it much less common than Parkinson disease (another movement disorder in which an estimated 50,000 Americans are diagnosed each year). Symptoms of PSP begin on average after age 60, but may occur earlier. Men are affected more often than women.

Rett Syndrome

Rett syndrome (RS) is a neurological and developmental genetic disorder that occurs mostly in females. Infants with Rett syndrome seem to grow and develop normally at first, but then they stop developing and even lose skills in different stages of the disease over a lifetime.

Spasticity

Spasticity is a condition in which there is an abnormal increase in muscle tone or stiffness of muscle, which might interfere with movement, speech, or be associated with discomfort or pain. Spasticity is usually caused by damage to nerve pathways within the brain or spinal cord that control muscle movement. It may occur in association with spinal cord injury, multiple sclerosis, cerebral palsy, stroke, brain or head trauma, amyotrophic lateral sclerosis, hereditary spastic paraplegias, and metabolic diseases such as adrenoleukodystrophy, phenylketonuria, and Krabbe disease. Symptoms may include hypertonicity (increased muscle tone), clonus (a series of rapid muscle contractions), exaggerated deep tendon reflexes, muscle spasms, scissoring (involuntary crossing of the legs), and fixed joints (contractures). The degree of spasticity varies from mild muscle stiffness to severe, painful, and uncontrollable muscle spasms. Spasticity can interfere with rehabilitation in patients with certain disorders, and often interferes with daily activities.

Tourette Syndrome

Tourette syndrome (TS) is a condition of the *nervous system*. TS causes people to have "tics."

Tics are sudden twitches, movements, or sounds that people do repeatedly. People who have tics cannot stop their body from doing these things. For example, a person might keep blinking over and over again. Or, a person might make a grunting sound unwillingly.

Having tics is a little bit like having hiccups. Even though you might not want to hiccup, your body does it anyway. Sometimes people can stop themselves from doing a certain tic for awhile, but it's hard. Eventually the person has to do the tic.

Wilson Disease

Wilson disease (WD) is a rare inherited disorder of copper metabolism in which excessive amounts of copper accumulate in the body. The buildup of copper leads to damage in the liver, brain, and eyes. Although copper accumulation begins at birth, symptoms of the disorder only appear later in life. The most characteristic sign of WD is the Kayser-Fleisher ring—a rusty brown ring around the cornea of the eye that can best be viewed using an ophthalmologist's slit lamp. The primary consequence for most individuals with WD is liver disease, appearing in late childhood or early adolescence as acute hepatitis, liver failure, or progressive chronic liver disease in the form of chronic active hepatitis or cirrhosis of the liver. In others, the first symptoms are neurological, occur later in adulthood, and commonly include slurred speech (dysarthria), difficulty swallowing (dysphagia), and drooling. Other symptoms may include tremor of the head, arms, or legs; impaired muscle tone, and sustained muscle contractions that produce abnormal postures, twisting, and repetitive movements (dystonia); and slowness of movements (bradykinesia). Individuals may also experience clumsiness (ataxia) and loss of fine motor skills. One-third of individuals with WD will also experience psychiatric symptoms such as an abrupt personality change, bizarre and inappropriate behavior, depression accompanied by suicidal thoughts, neurosis, or psychosis. WD is diagnosed with tests that measure the amount of copper in the blood, urine, and liver.

Chapter 4

Common Symptoms of Movement Disorders

Chapter Contents

Section 4.1

Ataxia

This section contains text excerpted from the following sources: Text in this section begins with excerpts from "Ataxias and Cerebellar or Spinocerebellar Degeneration Information Page," National Institute of Neurological Disorders and Stroke (NINDS), January 5, 2018; Text beginning with the heading "Treatment" is excerpted from "Spinocerebellar Ataxia," Genetic and Rare Diseases Information Center (GARD), National Center for Advancing Translational Sciences (NCATS), January 19, 2017.

Ataxia often occurs when parts of the nervous system that control movement are damaged. People with ataxia experience a failure of muscle control in their arms and legs, resulting in a lack of balance and coordination or a disturbance of gait. While the term ataxia is primarily used to describe this set of symptoms, it is sometimes also used to refer to a family of disorders. It is not, however, a specific diagnosis.

Most disorders that result in ataxia cause cells in the part of the brain called the cerebellum to degenerate, or atrophy. Sometimes the spine is also affected. The phrases *cerebellar degeneration* and *spinocerebellar degeneration* are used to describe changes that have taken place in a person's nervous system; neither term constitutes a specific diagnosis. Cerebellar and spinocerebellar degeneration have many different causes. The age of onset of the resulting ataxia varies depending on the underlying cause of the degeneration.

Many ataxias are hereditary and are classified by chromosomal location and pattern of inheritance: *autosomal dominant*, in which the affected person inherits a normal gene from one parent and a faulty gene from the other parent; and *autosomal recessive*, in which both parents pass on a copy of the faulty gene. Among the more common inherited ataxias are *Friedreich ataxia (FA)* and *Machado-Joseph disease (MJD)*. Sporadic ataxias can also occur in families with no prior history.

Ataxia can also be acquired. Conditions that can cause acquired ataxia include stroke, multiple sclerosis, tumors, alcoholism, peripheral neuropathy, metabolic disorders, and vitamin deficiencies.

Treatment

There is no known cure for spinocerebellar ataxia (SCA). The best treatment options for SCA vary by type and often depend on the signs and symptoms present in each person. The most common symptom of SCA is ataxia (a condition in which coordination and balance are affected). Physical therapy can help strengthen muscles, while special devices (e.g., cane, crutches, walker, or wheelchair) can assist in mobility and other activities of daily life. Many people with SCA have other symptoms in addition to the ataxia such as tremors, stiffness, muscle spasms, and sleep disorders; medications or other therapies may be suggested for some of these symptoms. One report described some improvement in the symptoms with zolpidem 10 mg in four out of five family members with SCA type 2, and a trial of 20 patients with SCA3 found that varenicline led to improvement in some, but not all of the symptoms.

Prognosis

The long-term outlook for people with spinocerebellar ataxia (SCA) varies. Disease progression and severity often depend on the type of SCA.

Most available information on the prognosis of SCA is based on the four most common types: SCA1, SCA2, SCA3, and SCA6. People affected by one of these types of SCA usually require a wheelchair by 10–15 years after the onset of symptoms. Many will eventually need assistance to perform daily tasks.

Section 4.2

Spasticity

This section includes text excerpted from "Spasticity Information Page," National Institute of Neurological Disorders and Stroke (NINDS), August 19, 2017.

About Spasticity

Spasticity is a condition in which there is an abnormal increase in muscle tone or stiffness of muscle, which might interfere with movement, speech, or be associated with discomfort or pain. Spasticity is usually caused by damage to nerve pathways within the brain or spinal cord that control muscle movement. It may occur in association with spinal cord injury, multiple sclerosis, cerebral palsy, stroke, brain or head trauma, amyotrophic lateral sclerosis, hereditary spastic paraplegias, and metabolic diseases such as adrenoleukodystrophy, phenylketonuria, and Krabbe disease. Symptoms may include hypertonicity (increased muscle tone), clonus (a series of rapid muscle contractions), exaggerated deep tendon reflexes, muscle spasms, scissoring (involuntary crossing of the legs), and fixed joints (contractures). The degree of spasticity varies from mild muscle stiffness to severe, painful, and uncontrollable muscle spasms. Spasticity can interfere with rehabilitation in patients with certain disorders, and often interferes with daily activities.

Treatment

Treatment may include such medications as baclofen, diazepam, tizanidine, or clonazepam. Physical therapy regimens may include muscle stretching and range of motion exercises to help prevent shrinkage or shortening of muscles and to reduce the severity of symptoms. Targeted injection of botulinum toxin into muscles with the most tome can help to selectively weaken these muscles to improve range-of-motion and function. Surgery may be recommended for tendon release or to sever the nerve-muscle pathway.

Prognosis

The prognosis for those with spasticity depends on the severity of the spasticity and the associated disorder(s).

Section 4.3

Stiffness, Cramps, and Twitching

"Stiffness, Cramps, and Twitching," © 2018 Omnigraphics.
Reviewed January 2018.

Stiffness, cramps, or twitching can happen when muscles contract abnormally. These can be symptoms of muscle weakness or neuromuscular disease. Muscle contractions can be painful, annoying, or crippling. While they are common and mostly do not indicate any serious medical condition, there are various methods by which the stiffness, cramps, or twitching can be managed.

Muscle Cramps

A muscle cramp is a sudden and involuntary contraction of the muscle. While such cramps can happen in any muscle and can cause severe pain, most cramps occur in the leg muscles. These contractions are caused by abnormal nerve activity rather than muscle activity. A muscle cramp has a sudden onset with a sharp pain and can be relieved by stretching the muscle passively. Muscle cramps are harmless; however, it may be impossible to use the affected muscle during the cramp.

Types of Cramps

Two major types of cramps include:

1. **Exercise-induced cramps:** Mostly common in legs, especially hamstrings and calves. Exercise-induced cramps are often triggered due to overheat and fatigue and are quiet intense and painful. They predominantly occur in athletes.

2. **Night cramps:** Similar to exercise-induced cramps but they occur without exercise. Causes for night cramps include drug side effects, iron deficiency, and other health conditions. They affect the thighs, calves, and foot arches.

Causes of Cramps

There are several causes for muscle cramps; but, for certain cramps, causes are unknown. Some of the known causes are discussed below:

- **General causes:** Some general causes such as dehydration, overuse of muscles, muscle strain, or staying in a particular position for a long time can cause muscle cramps.

- **Nerve compression:** If a nerve is compressed in the spine region (lumbar stenosis), it can cause cramp-like pain in the legs. The pain increases when the person keeps walking. If the walk is done in a slightly flexed position, chances of delaying the cramps are possible.

- **Mineral depletion:** Cramps in the legs can also be caused due to lessening of potassium, calcium, and magnesium in the diet. Certain medications recommended for high blood pressure can also deplete the minerals and cause cramps.

- **Inadequate blood supply:** When arteries that supply blood to the legs narrow, it can cause cramp-like pain in the legs and feet while exercising. The cramps go away once exercising is stopped.

- **Other risk factors:** The risk of muscle cramps can also be increased due to factors such as age, pregnancy, or other medical conditions.

Muscle Stiffness

Muscle stiffness is when the muscles get tight and the condition makes it difficult for the muscle to be moved, even after rest. Along with stiffness, there can be pain, cramps, and discomfort. The condition is different from muscle rigidity and spasticity and goes away on its own. Regular exercise and stretching can bring some relief to stiff muscles. If the condition persists, the healthcare provider may recommend a specific treatment based on the cause; also, anti-inflammatory medications can reduce pain and discomfort.

Causes for Muscle Stiffness

There are many causes of muscle stiffness, and they usually occur after exercise, hard physical labor, or lifting weights. Sprains and strains are the most common causes for muscle stiffness. When a sprain or strain happens from certain activities they cause pain, swelling, bruising, redness, and limited movement. Other common conditions that can cause muscle stiffness are anesthesia or medication, injury from extreme heat or cold, infection, or insect bite.

Muscle Twitch or Fasciculation

Muscle twitches are brief, repetitive muscle contractions that are caused by abnormal nerve activity. Damage or stimulation to a nerve causes the muscle fiber to twitch because muscles are made of fibers that the nerves control. They affect a small portion of the muscle and are not painful. Stress, lack of sleep, and caffeine can aggravate twitches. Even healthy people get fasciculation—eyelid twitching is an example that is common. However, this condition is mostly seen in people with amyotrophic lateral sclerosis (ALS), spinal bulbar muscular atrophy, and X-linked SMA (spinal muscular atrophy) and SMA type 1. Though treatment is not necessary for muscle twitching, serious conditions do require medical attention.

Causes for Muscle Twitch

Causes for muscle twitch can be minor and major. Minor twitches are the results of a less serious cause. Severe twitches can indicate serious health conditions.

Minor causes include:

- Stress and anxiety that can affect any muscle and are called "nervous ticks."

- Dehydration can cause twitching that affects the legs, arms, and torso.

- After physical activity, twitching can occur as lactic acid accumulates in the muscle during exercise.

- Caffeine and other stimulants are also major contributors to twitching.

- Reactions to certain drugs such as corticosteroids and estrogen pills can cause twitches and spasms.

- Nutritional deficiencies of vitamin D, vitamin B, and calcium deficiencies can cause twitches and spasms in eyelids, calves, and hands.

Major causes include:

- Lou Gehrig disease or amyotrophic lateral sclerosis (ALS) that causes nerve cells to die.

- Isaac syndrome results in frequent muscle twitching and affects the nerves.

- Muscular dystrophies weaken and damage muscles over time; they are inherited.

- Spinal muscular atrophy affects the motor nerve cells in the spinal cord. This condition affects muscle movement and it can cause the tongue to twitch.

References

1. "Simply Stated: Stiffness, Cramps and Twitching," The Muscular Dystrophy Association (MDA), June 1, 2000.

2. Ingraham, Paul. "Cramps, Spasms, Tremors & Twitches," Pain Science, July 11, 2017.

3. "Muscle Cramp," Mayo Clinic, August 8, 2017.

4. Holloway, Beth. "What Causes Muscle Stiffness?" Healthline, September 19, 2016.

5. Allen, Suzanne; Cirino, Erica. "What Causes Muscle Twitch?" Healthline, April 15, 2016.

Section 4.4

Tremor

This section contains text excerpted from the following sources: Text in this section begins with excerpts from "Tremor Information Page," National Institute of Neurological Disorders and Stroke (NINDS), May 2017; Text under the heading "Cause of Tremors" is excerpted from "Tremor," MedlinePlus, National Institutes of Health (NIH), September 9, 2016.

Tremor is an unintentional, rhythmic, muscle movement involving to-and-fro movements of one or more parts of the body. Most tremors occur in the hands, although they can also affect the arms, head, face, voice, torso, and legs. Generally, tremor is caused by a problem in the deep parts of the brain that control movements. Some forms of tremor are inherited and run in families, while others have no known cause. Sometimes tremor is a symptom of another neurological disorder or a side effect of certain drugs, but the most common form occurs in otherwise healthy people. Excessive alcohol consumption or alcohol withdrawal can kill certain nerve cells, resulting in tremor, especially in the hand. Other causes include an overactive thyroid and the use of certain drugs. Tremor may occur at any age but is most common in middle-aged and older adults. There are several types of tremor, one of the most common of which is essential tremor (sometimes called benign essential tremor). The hands are most often affected but the head, voice, tongue, legs, and trunk may also be involved. Head tremor may be seen as a "yes-yes" or "no-no" motion. Onset is most common after age 40, although symptoms can appear at any age. Parkinsonian tremor is caused by damage to structures within the brain that control movement. The tremor is classically seen as a "pill-rolling" action of the hands but may also affect the chin, face, lips, and legs. Dystonic tremor occurs in individuals of all ages who are affected by dystonia, a movement disorder which causes muscles to be over-active, resulting in abnormal postures or sustained, unwanted movements.

Cause of Tremors

The cause of tremors is a problem in the parts of the brain that control muscles in the body or in specific parts of the body, such as the hands. They commonly occur in otherwise healthy people. They may also be caused by problems such as

- Parkinson disease
- Dystonia
- Multiple sclerosis
- Stroke
- Traumatic brain injury
- Alcohol abuse and withdrawal
- Certain medicines

Some forms are inherited and run in families. Others have no known cause.

There is no cure for most tremors. Treatment to relieve them depends on their cause. In many cases, medicines and sometimes surgical procedures can reduce or stop tremors and improve muscle control. Tremors are not life threatening. However, they can be embarrassing and make it hard to perform daily tasks.

Chapter 5

Drugs for Movement Disorders

Parkinson Disease (PD) Medications

Carbidopa / Levodopa

Carbidopa

- decarboxylase inhibitor (prevents breakdown of levodopa in extra-cerebral tissues)

- does not cross the blood brain barrier and therefore does not affect the central nervous system (CNS) metabolism of levodopa

- decreases the amount of levodopa required to produce a response by 75 percent and increases the plasma half life of levodopa from 50–90 minutes

Levodopa

- amino acid that becomes dopamine by removal of a carboxyl group

---

This chapter includes text excerpted from "Drugs in Movement Disorders— Truths, Myths and More," U.S. Department of Veterans Affairs (VA), November 2015.

Formulations

- c/l 10/100 (IR)
- c/l 25/100 (IR)
- c/l 25/250 (IR)
- c/l CR/SA 25/100
- c/l CR/SA 50/200

Parcopa

- Orally disintegrating tablets—not really a true "sublingual" preparation as it is still absorbed in the lower gastrointestinal (GI) tract and not through the oral mucosa
- Similar pharmacokinetics to IR c/l with a slightly shorter time to Tmax
- Inactive ingredients include aspartame, phenylalanine, and citric acid

Rytary

- Combination of IR and SA forms
- Inactive ingredients include talc and gelatin
- Initial peak at 1 hour
- Plasma concentrations are maintained for 4–5 hours before declining
- Bioavailability of levodopa from Rytary is approximately 70 percent relative to IR c/l (dose conversion can be tricky)
- Caution in patients with cardiac history
- Placebo controlled study in patients with early PD—percent who reported ischemic CV adverse reactions:
  - 2.4 percent (7/289) Rytary treated patients
  - 1.1 percent (1/92) placebo treated patients
- Active controlled study in patients with advanced PD—percent who reported ischemia CV adverse reactions
  - 0.7 percent (3/450) Rytary treated patients
  - 0 percent (0/471) of oral IR c/l treated patients

Duopa

- Enteral suspension of c/l (4.63 mg c/20 mg l pcr mL)

  - Maximum recommended dose is 2000 mg of levodopa over 16 hours (1 cassette)

  - Prior to initiating duopa, patients must be converted to IR c/l from all other forms of levodopa

  - Administered through a PEG-J tube (can be given short term through an NG tube if needed)

  - Peak plasma levels reached in 2.5 hours

  - Must be stored in freezer ($-20°C$) and thawed in refrigerator ($2-8°C$) prior to dispensing (12 week expiration after thawing)

  - Gastric emptying rate does not influence the absorption of duopa as it is administered by continuous intestinal infusion

Dopamine Agonist

- Ropinirole (Requip)

  - Agonist at D2 and D3 receptors, stimulates postsynaptic D2 receptors in basal ganglia

  - Rapidly absorbed, peak concentration in 1–2 hours with a half life of 6 hours

  - Inactive ingredient: anhydrous lactose

- Pramipexole (Mirapex)

  - Same mechanism of action as above

  - Peak concentration in 2 hours, half life 8–12 hours (12 hours in elderly population)

- Rotigotine (Neupro)

  - Same mechanism of action as above

  - Patch form, continuous 24 hour delivery of medication

  - Contains sodium metabisulfite — can cause allergic reactions in patients with sulfite sensitivity

- Apomorphine

  - Injectable form (subcutaneous)

- Rapid absorption, peak concentration in 4–12 minutes, half life of 30 minutes

- Need to used in conjunction with antiemetic—trimethoben- zamide (Tigan)

- Cannot use with ondansetron—several reports of profound hypotension and LOC

- Caution in patients with sulfite sensitivity—contains sodium metabisulfate

- Pergolide, bromocriptine (rarely used)

MAO-B Inhibitor

- Rasagiline (azilect)

  - Irreversibly inhibits the action of MAO-B enzyme—decreases the breakdown of dopamine in the brain and inhibits the reuptake of dopamine at the presynaptic receptor

  - 5 times more potent than selegiline

- Selegiline

  - Amphetamine metabolite—can have a stimulant effect caus- ing insomnia, anxiety and hallucinations

COMT Inhibitor

- Entacapone/Tolcapone

  - Reversible, peripherally acting COMT inhibition—decreases the breakdown of dopamine

  - Increases the half life of levodopa by 30–50 percent (from 1.5–2.5 hours)

  - Rapidly absorbed, Tmax of 1 hour. Bioavailability not affected by food

  - Used mostly for patients with "wearing off" prior to next dose

  - Not used alone must be given with levodopa

  - Can cause increased dyskinesias, diarrhea, abdominal pain

Anticholinergics

- May be of benefit for "tremor predominant" PD
- Trihexyphenadyl (Artane), benztropine (Cogentin)
- Side effects.
    - Dry mouth
    - Blurred vision
    - Constipation
    - Urinary issues
    - Memory issues/confusion
    - Hallucinations

Amantadine

- Antiviral drug originally developed to prevent influenza but was found to improve mild motor symptoms in PD patients
- May help to reduce dyskinesias secondary to levodopa use, but benefit if transient
- Side effects:
    - Hallucinations
    - Confusion
    - LE edema
    - Livedo reticularis

Droxidopa

- Synthetic amino acid precursor which acts as a prodrug to norepinephrine
- Unlike NE, droxidopa can cross the BBB
- Used for neurogenic orthostatic hypotension
- Used in Asia since 1989, U.S. Food and Drug Administration (FDA) approved here in February 2014
- Inactive ingredient: gelatin

- Caution when used in combination with other agents that increase blood pressure (BP) (midodrine, triptans)
- Caution in patients with pre-existing CHF, ischemic heart disease, or arrhythmias

New Drugs in Development

- New COMT inhibitors
- New MAO-B inhibitor
- New dopamine agonists
- Adenosine A (2A) receptor antagonists (proposed to block unwanted activity of receptors in the BG)
- Alpha-adrenergic receptor antagonists (proposed to help balance the GABA activity in the BG)
- Serotonergic agonists (proposed to enhance the transmission of serotonin)
- Neuroprotective medications
- Pioglitozone (DM drug)
- Isradipine
- Glutathione
- Growth Factor Neurturin

Essential Tremor Medications

Topiramate

- Exact mechanism of action unknown for tremor control but blocks voltage-dependent sodium channels, augments GABA activity and antagonizes glutamate
- Rapid absorption, peak plasma concentration within 2 hours
- Not extensively metabolized, 70 percent is excreted unchanged in the urine
- Inactive ingredient: lactose monohydrate

Primidone

- Exact mechanism of action unknown for tremor control

- Metabolized to phenobarbitol which acts as a GABAa receptor agonist and antagonist at some subtypes of glutamate receptors
- Phenobarbitol is metabolized by the liver and induces many P450 isozymes (especially CYP2B6)
- Inactive ingredients: lactose monohydrate, sodium lauryl sulfate, talc

Propranolol

- Nonselective beta-adrenergic receptor blocking agent
- Rapidly absorbed with peak plasma concentration from 1–4 hours after oral dose
- High first pass metabolism by the liver (P450 system), only approximately 25 percent of propranolol reaches the systemic circulation
- Inactive ingredient: gelatin

What Common Side Effects or Interactions Can Occur?

PD

- There is no "correct" starting medication—this will vary by providers and depending on patient profile
- Often use dopamine agonists first for younger patients
- Need to take into account comorbidities and side effects

Side Effects/Interactions

Carbidopa / Levodopa

- Nausea
- Mood/behavioral changes
- Daytime somnolence
- Orthostatic hypotension
- Dark urine or sweat due to increased urinary excretion of dopamine (more commonly seen in patients also taking entacapone)

- High protein diet may delay the absorption of levodopa due to competition for binding as both are transported across the small intestine by the same amino acid transport system

- Excessive stomach acidity may also delay the absorption of levodopa due to a delay in stomach emptying into the small intestine

- Iron salts (often a part of a multivitamin) also may reduce the amount of levodopa available to the body by forming chelates with the carbidopa and levodopa

- Good initial choice for:

  - "Older" patients with suspected PD

  - Patients with significant mood disorder (other than depression or anxiety)

Dopamine Agonists

- Mood/behavioral changes (more common in DA than with levodopa)

  - obsessions, compulsions, impulse control disorders—sexual, gambling, shopping

  - hallucinations

- Daytime somnolence (sleep attacks)

- Leg edema

- Orthostatic hypotension

- Ropinirole is metabolized by P450 enzyme system (CYP1A2)

  - Drug level altered by enzyme inducers (smoking, omeprazole) and inhibitors (ciprofloxacin, verapamil, grapefruit juice, cumin, tumeric)

  - Hormone replacement therapy also reduces clearance (estrogen effect)

- Pramipexole is not metabolized by P450 enzymes (90% of drug excreted in urine unchanged)

  - For renal impairment:

  - Cr clearance 30–50 mL/min—maximum dose is 0.75 mg tid

  - Cr clearance 15–30 mL/min—maximum dose is 1.5 mg daily

- Rotigotine patch has aluminum backing—must be removed before cardioversion or MRI
- Heat may increase drug absorption—avoid direct heat source (heating pads, electric blankets, heat lamps, hot tubs, hair dryers, prolonged direct sunlight)
- Good initial choice for:
  - "younger" patients with PD symptoms
  - Patient with mild PD symptoms
  - Patient with restless legs syndrome

Topiramate

- Cognitive slowing
- Numbness and tingling of fingers and toes
- Weight loss (average of 5 lbs—mechanism unclear)
- Metallic taste with drinking "dark sodas"
- Decreased sweating and hyperthermia
- Reduce dose in patients with renal impairment (Cr clearance <70 mL/min)
- Risk of secondary angle closure glaucoma (myopia, eye pain, ocular redness) and visual field deficits
- Risk for metabolic acidosis—caused by renal bicarbonate loss:
  - Caution in conditions which would predispose patients to acidosis—renal disease, severe respiratory disorders, diarrhea, ketogenic diet, some drugs—metformin— can lead to fatigue, renal stones, altered mental status, weakness.
- Kidney stones (occurs in approximately 1.5 percent of patients)—suspected due to inhibition of carbonic anhydrase which reduces urinary citrate excretion and increases urinary pH

Primidone

- Sedation
- Ataxia

- Vertigo
- Use with caution in patients on other sedative drugs (muscle relaxants, benzodiazepines, opiates) or with chronic ETOH use
- Phenobarbitol is metabolized by the liver and induces many P450 isozymes (especially CYP2B6) therefore dosage adjustments need to be made for patients with hepatic failure
- **Note:** Notify other providers when starting this medication as it may alter the levels of other medications (statins, mental health medications)

Propranolol

- Fatigue
- Bradycardia
- Hypotension
- Worsening of depression
- Worsening of asthma
- Use with caution in diabetics on insulin (may mask symptoms of hypoglycemia)
- SJS
- SLE-like reaction
- Chronic renal failure has been associated with a decrease in propranolol metabolism via downregulation of P450 activity resulting in a lower "firstpass" clearance = higher peak plasma levels in patients with renal failure as well as in patients with hepatic failure
- P450 inhibitors increase plasma levels of propranolol (amiodarone, cimetidine, fluoxetine, paroxetine, ciprofloxacin, fluconazole)
- P450 inducers decrease plasma levels of propranolol (phenytoin, phenobarbitol, cigarette smoking)

Other Interesting Facts

Glaucoma

- Levodopa therapy is contraindicated in patients with narrow/closed angle glaucoma

- While levodopa primarily is a dopaminergic agent, there may be cross-over onto cholinergic receptors.
- These receptors are generally responsible for pupil dilation which can cause narrowing of the angle which can increase eye pressure.

Melanoma

- Overall risk for cancer in patients with PD is lower but risk for malignant melanoma is higher (4x increased risk)
- Unclear etiology—initially suspected due to relationship between dopamine and melanin (dopamine is precursor of melanin), but more complex than that—new genetic studies going on as studies finding early PD patients with melanoma (not treated with levodopa)
- From the current literature there is:
  - Consistent data supporting an association between cutaneous melanoma and PD
  - A possible association between nonmelanoma skin cancers and PD
  - Insufficient data to conclude on the association between L-dopa and melanoma in PD patients
  - Insufficient data to conclude on the association between MAO-B inhibitors, DA or other anti-parkinsonian drugs and melanoma or other skin cancers in PD patients
  - Insufficient data about the risk factors for skin cancer in PD patients and therefore no EBM recommendations regarding the need for periodic dermatological screening
- Carbidopa/levodopa
  - Pyridoxine (B6) may reverse the effects of levodopa by increasing the rate of decarboxylation, but carbidopa inhibits this action.
- To eat or not to eat:
  - Protein competes with levodopa for transport across the small intestine and can decrease its absorption/plasma concentration

- Protein rich foods increase the bioavailability of propranolol by about 50 percent

- Patients who take levodopa on an empty stomach will often complain of nausea, can add additional carbidopa 25 mg to each dose or instruct patients to take with carbohydrate meal

- Can these medications be stopped abruptly or do they need to be tapered?

  - There is a risk of neuroleptic malignant syndrome with abrupt discontinuation of sinemet or a dopamine agonist, but this is rare

  - Primidone must be tapered off as metabolite is phenobarbitol—increased risk of seizures with abrupt discontinuation

  - Propranolol must be tapered off due to risk of rebound hypertension if abruptly stopped

Conclusions

- Variability in medication and dosing regimen between providers

- No "one correct" starting medication for all patients

- New medication trials currently underway

- Providers need to be aware of side effects, inactive ingredients and pharmacology/pharmacokinetics of medications

Part Two

Parkinson Disease

Chapter 6

Understanding Parkinson Disease (PD)

Parkinson disease (PD) is a brain disorder that leads to shaking, stiffness, and difficulty with walking, balance, and coordination.

Parkinson symptoms usually begin gradually and get worse over time. As the disease progresses, people may have difficulty walking and talking. They may also have mental and behavioral changes, sleep problems, depression, memory difficulties, and fatigue.

Both men and women can have Parkinson disease. However, the disease affects about 50 percent more men than women.

One clear risk factor for Parkinson is age. Although most people with Parkinson first develop the disease at about age 60, about 5–10 percent of people with Parkinson have "early-onset" disease, which begins before the age of 50. Early-onset forms of Parkinson are often, but not always, inherited, and some forms have been linked to specific gene mutations.

What Causes Parkinson Disease?

Parkinson disease occurs when nerve cells, or neurons, in an area of the brain that controls movement become impaired and/or die. Normally, these neurons produce an important brain chemical known as

This chapter includes text excerpted from "Parkinson's Disease," National Institute on Aging (NIA), National Institutes of Health (NIH), May 16, 2017.

dopamine. When the neurons die or become impaired, they produce less dopamine, which causes the movement problems of Parkinson. Scientists still do not know what causes cells that produce dopamine to die.

People with Parkinson also lose the nerve endings that produce norepinephrine, the main chemical messenger of the sympathetic nervous system, which controls many automatic functions of the body, such as heart rate and blood pressure. The loss of norepinephrine might help explain some of the nonmovement features of Parkinson, such as fatigue, irregular blood pressure, decreased movement of food through the digestive tract, and sudden drop in blood pressure when a person stands up from a sitting or lying-down position.

Many brain cells of people with Parkinson contain Lewy bodies, unusual clumps of the protein alpha-synuclein. Scientists are trying to better understand the normal and abnormal functions of alpha-synuclein and its relationship to genetic mutations that impact Parkinson disease and Lewy body dementia.

Although some cases of Parkinson appear to be hereditary, and a few can be traced to specific genetic mutations, in most cases the disease occurs randomly and does not seem to run in families. Many researchers now believe that Parkinson disease results from a combination of genetic factors and environmental factors such as exposure to toxins.

Symptoms of Parkinson Disease

Parkinson disease has four main symptoms:

1. Tremor (trembling) in hands, arms, legs, jaw, or head

2. Stiffness of the limbs and trunk

3. Slowness of movement

4. Impaired balance and coordination, sometimes leading to falls

Other symptoms may include depression and other emotional changes; difficulty swallowing, chewing, and speaking; urinary problems or constipation; skin problems; and sleep disruptions.

Symptoms of Parkinson and the rate of progression differ among individuals. Sometimes people dismiss early symptoms of Parkinson as the effects of normal aging. In most cases, there are no medical tests to definitively detect the disease, so it can be difficult to diagnose accurately.

Early symptoms of Parkinson disease are subtle and occur gradually. For example, affected people may feel mild tremors or have difficulty getting out of a chair. They may notice that they speak too softly, or that their handwriting is slow and looks cramped or small. Friends or family members may be the first to notice changes in someone with early Parkinson. They may see that the person's face lacks expression and animation, or that the person does not move an arm or leg normally.

People with Parkinson often develop a parkinsonian gait that includes a tendency to lean forward, small quick steps as if hurrying forward, and reduced swinging of the arms. They also may have trouble initiating or continuing movement.

Symptoms often begin on one side of the body or even in one limb on one side of the body. As the disease progresses, it eventually affects both sides. However, the symptoms may still be more severe on one side than on the other.

Many people with Parkinson note that prior to experiencing stiffness and tremor, they had sleep problems, constipation, decreased ability to smell, and restless legs.

Diagnosis of Parkinson Disease

A number of disorders can cause symptoms similar to those of Parkinson disease. People with Parkinson-like symptoms that result from other causes are sometimes said to have parkinsonism. While these disorders initially may be misdiagnosed as Parkinson, certain medical tests, as well as response to drug treatment, may help to distinguish them from Parkinson. Since many other diseases have similar features but require different treatments, it is important to make an exact diagnosis as soon as possible.

There are currently no blood or laboratory tests to diagnose nongenetic cases of Parkinson disease. Diagnosis is based on a person's medical history and a neurological examination. Improvement after initiating medication is another important hallmark of Parkinson disease.

Treatment of Parkinson Disease

Although there is no cure for Parkinson disease, medicines, surgical treatment, and other therapies can often relieve some symptoms.

Medicines for Parkinson Disease

Medicines prescribed for Parkinson include:

- Drugs that increase the level of dopamine in the brain

- Drugs that affect other brain chemicals in the body

- Drugs that help control nonmotor symptoms

The main therapy for Parkinson is levodopa, also called L-dopa. Nerve cells use levodopa to make dopamine to replenish the brain's dwindling supply. Usually, people take levodopa along with another medication called carbidopa. Carbidopa prevents or reduces some of the side effects of levodopa therapy—such as nausea, vomiting, low blood pressure, and restlessness—and reduces the amount of levodopa needed to improve symptoms.

People with Parkinson should never stop taking levodopa without telling their doctor. Suddenly stopping the drug may have serious side effects, such as being unable to move or having difficulty breathing.

Other medicines used to treat Parkinson symptoms include:

- Dopamine agonists to mimic the role of dopamine in the brain

- MAO-B inhibitors to slow down an enzyme that breaks down dopamine in the brain

- COMT inhibitors to help break down dopamine

- Amantadine, an old antiviral drug, to reduce involuntary movements

- Anticholinergic drugs to reduce tremors and muscle rigidity

Deep Brain Stimulation

For people with Parkinson who do not respond well to medications, deep brain stimulation, or DBS, may be appropriate. DBS is a surgical procedure that surgically implants electrodes into part of the brain and connects them to a small electrical device implanted in the chest. The device and electrodes painlessly stimulate the brain in a way that helps stop many of the movement-related symptoms of Parkinson, such as tremor, slowness of movement, and rigidity.

Other Therapies

Other therapies may be used to help with Parkinson disease symptoms. They include physical, occupational, and speech therapies, which help with gait and voice disorders, tremors and rigidity, and decline in mental functions. Other supportive therapies include a healthy diet and exercises to strengthen muscles and improve balance.

Chapter 7

Sleep Disorders in Parkinson Disease

Sleep disorders manifest in diverse presentations, and are often interrelated in complex ways. For these purposes, researchers deconstruct sleep symptoms to a core of symptomatic presentations: insomnia, excessive daytime sleepiness (EDS), sleep fragmentation, circadian rhythm disorders, restless legs syndrome (RLS) and periodic limb movements in sleep (PLMS), rapid eye movement (REM) behavior disorder (RBD), and obstructive sleep apnea (OSA).

The inability to initiate or maintain sleep is one of the more commonly encountered symptoms in patients. Insomnia is more frequently seen as Parkinson disease (PD) progresses, where increased nocturnal symptoms of rigidity, motor fluctuations, and pain can disrupt sleep. Medications are a common cause for insomnia, where dopaminergic therapy, selegiline, amantadine, and anticholinergic therapy have all been implicated. Of particular importance is the relationship between insomnia and mood disorders such as depression, which have been found to be correlated in the PD population.

EDS is also frequently encountered in PD, and can be a common side effect of dopaminergic therapy. Differentiating true daytime sleepiness from feelings of fatigue is important, as it may guide clinical

---

This chapter includes text excerpted from "Sleep Dysfunction and Its Management in Parkinson's Disease," U.S. Department of Health and Human Services (HHS), August 1, 2015.

decision making for activities of daily living (ADLs) such as driving, and need for further sleep assessments. Screening for EDS with an Epworth sleepiness scale (ESS) is fast and reliable.

Sleep fragmentation may be the most common sleep complaint in PD. In addition to PD symptoms and medication, nocturia is frequently implicated and should always be considered with this presentation. Hallucinations and altered dream phenomena may also contribute to fragmented sleep. Of clinical concern, poor sleep efficiency predicts worsening scores of attention and executive function.

RLS is the most frequent movement disorder in the general population, and has an even higher incidence among PD patients, with an estimated prevalence as high as 12 percent, perhaps owing to a suspected common pathophysiology of dopamine and iron dysfunction. The relationship between iron deficiency and RLS is so strong that ferritin levels should be checked in all symptomatic patients, with iron supplementation generally initiated for ferritin levels less than 50. RLS is strongly correlated with PLMS, and together they can contribute to insomnia, sleep fragmentation, and EDS. The four cardinal features of RLS are an urge to move the legs (with or without uncomfortable sensations) that is worse at night and relieved by movement. Later, a fifth feature is added that specifies that these four cardinal features cannot be solely accounted for as symptoms of other conditions (e.g., RLs mimics). The worsening of symptoms at night may be a manifestation of a circadian influence. RLS symptoms most commonly involve the lower extremities, but may involve the arms or body, particularly in severe cases.

Disruption to circadian rhythms has been described in PD. Accompanying this is a blunting of the amplitude of melatonin secretion, also correlated to symptoms of excessive daytime sleepiness. In addition, PD patients treated with dopaminergic medication were found to have a phase-advanced melatonin onset relative to sleep onset, suggesting that dopamine therapy may play a role in circadian disruption. A phase-advanced circadian rhythm may present as insomnia, particularly as early morning awakenings, or as excessive sleepiness in the early evening. Circadian rhythm dysfunction may also evolve into an irregular sleep—wake cycle, with no clear dominant sleep block and frequent naps throughout the day. As disease progresses, this can be exacerbated by a loss of daytime social cues commonly seen in the elderly and demented.

Since first being described in 1986, RBD, characterized by the lack of typical muscle atonia during REM sleep and subsequent "acting out" of dreams, has morphed from a clinical curiosity to a well-defined feature of PD. While being associated with all alpha-synucleinopathy, RBD is well-known to predate frank symptom onset by several years, though it can occur at any time during the course of PD. Polysomnography demonstrating REM sleep without atonia, along with documented abnormal movements or history of injurious behavior, is required for a diagnosis.

There is controversy regarding whether PD increases the risk of OSA. While some have suggested an association between the two, more recent studies have found no increased risk and that there is little difference between OSA in PD and in the general population. While the possibility of PD increasing the risk for OSA remains unresolved, OSA is a common enough disorder in the typical age of presentation that it should be considered in any patient presenting with sleep fragmentation and daytime sleepiness. Presence of further history and exam findings such as loud snoring, witnessed apneas, elevated body mass index (BMI), and enlarged neck circumference would further support the need for evaluation by polysomnography.

Chapter 8

The Genetics of PD

What Do We Know about Heredity and Parkinson Disease?

Parkinson disease (PD) is a neurological condition that typically causes tremor and/or stiffness in movement. The condition affects about 1–2 percent of people over the age of 60 years and the chance of developing PD increases as we age. Most people affected with PD are not aware of any relatives with the condition but in a number of families, there is a family history. When three or more people are affected in a family, especially if they are diagnosed at an early age (under 50 years), there may be a gene making this family more likely to develop the condition.

Genetics: The Basics

Our genetic material is stored in the center of every cell in our bodies (skin cells, hair cells, blood cells). This genetic material comes in individual units called genes. We all have thousands of genes. Genes carry the information the body needs to make proteins, which are the substances in the body that actually carry out all the functions we need to live and grow. Our genes affect many things about us: our height,

---

This chapter includes text excerpted from "Learning about Parkinson's Disease," National Human Genome Research Institute (NHGRI), March 14, 2014. Reviewed January 2018.

eye color, why we respond to some medications better than others and our likelihood of developing certain conditions. We have two copies of every gene: we inherit one copy, one member of each pair, from our mother and the other from our father. We then pass only one copy of a gene from each pair of genes to the next generation. Whether we pass on the gene we got from our father or the one from our mother is purely by chance, like flipping a coin heads or tails.

We all have genes that don't work properly. In most cases the other copy of the gene makes up for the one that does not work properly and we are healthy. A problem only arises if we meet someone else who has a nonworking copy of the same gene and we have a child who inherits two nonworking copies of that gene. This is called recessive inheritance.

Sometimes if one of our genes is not working properly the other copy of the gene cannot make up for it and that causes a condition or an increased risk of developing a condition. Each time we have a child we randomly pass on one copy of each gene. If the child inherits the copy that doesn't work properly, they too may develop the condition. This is called dominant inheritance.

What Genes Are Linked to Parkinson Disease?

Researchers studied a large family that came from a small town in Southern Italy in which PD was inherited from parent to child (dominant inheritance). They found the gene that caused their inherited PD and it coded for a protein called alpha-synuclein. If one studies the brains of people with PD after they die, one can see tiny little accumulations of protein called Lewy bodies (named after the doctor who first found them). Research has shown that there is a large amount of alpha-synuclein protein in the Lewy bodies of people who have noninherited PD as well as in the brains of people who have inherited PD. This immediately told that alpha-synuclein played an important role in all forms of PD and researchers are still doing a lot of research to better understand this role.

Seven genes that cause some form of Parkinson disease have been identified. Mutations (changes) in three known genes called *SNCA* (*PARK1*), *UCHL1* (*PARK 5*), and *LRRK2* (*PARK8*) and another mapped gene (*PARK3*) have been reported in families with dominant inheritance. Mutations in three known genes, *PARK2* (*PARK2*), *PARK7* (*PARK7*), and *PINK1* (*PARK6*) have been found in affected individuals who had siblings with the condition but whose parents did not have Parkinson disease (recessive inheritance). There is some research to suggest that these genes are also involved in early-onset Parkinson disease (diagnosed before the age of 30) or in dominantly inherited Parkinson disease but it is too early yet to be certain.

Research studies, called genome-wide association studies (GWAS) are an approach that involves rapidly scanning markers across the complete sets of deoxyribonucleic acid (DNA), or genomes, of many people to find genetic variations associated with a particular disease. GWAS have been able to identify genetic variations that contribute to common diseases including Parkinson disease.

What Determines Who Gets Parkinson Disease?

In most cases inheriting a nonworking copy of a single gene will not cause someone to develop Parkinson disease. Researchers believe that many other complicating factors such as additional genes and environmental factors determine who will get the condition, when they get it and how it affects them. In the families they have studied, some people who inherit the gene develop the condition and others live their entire lives without showing any symptoms. There is a lot of research on genes and the environment that is attempting to understand how all these factors interact.

Genetic Testing in Parkinson Disease

Genetic testing has recently become available for the parkin and *PINK1* genes. Parkin is a large gene and testing is difficult. At the last available stage of understanding, testing is likely to give a meaningful result only for people who develop the condition before the age of 30 years. *PINK1* appears to be a rare cause of inherited Parkinson disease. A small percentage (~2 percent) of those developing the condition at an early age appear to carry mutations in the *PINK1* gene. Genetic testing for the *PARK7, SNCA,* and *LRRK2* genes is also available.

Individuals and families who are interested in having genetic testing can learn more about their risk for Parkinson disease and the availability and accuracy of genetic testing for this disease by setting up an appointment with a genetics health professional. Genetic professionals work as members of healthcare teams providing information and support to individuals or families who have genetic disorders or may be at risk for inherited conditions. Genetic professionals can discuss the risks, benefits and limitations of available genetic testing for Parkinson disease.

Chapter 9

Pain in PD

People with Parkinson disease (PD) can experience pain or discomfort during the course of the disease. Pain is a quite common nonmotor symptom of PD but is often unexpected. Around 30–85 percent of patients with PD experience chronic pain.

Causes of Pain in Parkinson Disease (PD)

Some types of discomfort or pain cannot be directly linked to PD. However, there are different types of pain associated with the disease.

- **Musculoskeletal pain:** The pain happens in the muscles and bones and is usually felt as an ache around the arms, legs, and joints. Some people have lower back pain as well. The pain can be due to limited movement, falls, fractures, or postural changes. The pain stagnates in one area and does not move around the body, and it increases as people grow older. Painkillers and regular exercise can help to reduce the pain.

- **Dystonic pain:** This is an involuntary muscle contraction that causes an abnormal posture. The contractions can affect any body part, such as fingers, toes, ankles, or wrists. The pain usually manifests itself by curling or bending the affected body part and makes it go into spasm. Low dopamine levels can also cause dystonic pain. The contractions often happen early in the morning or even late at night. Relaxation techniques can help manage the pain.

- **Central pain:** In PD patients, the sensation and pain process in the brain regions may not work correctly, which leads to a syndrome called "central pain." Approximately 10 percent of people with PD are affected with this pain. The symptoms of central pain vary from person to person and may include a vague gnawing, boring, or deep pain. The pain can be widespread throughout the body or can happen in a particular area. The pain may be an intermittent sharp pain or a burning sensation.

- **Dyskinesia:** A pain that occurs because of abnormal, involuntary movement (dyskinesia). It can happen before or after movement and is not limited to but can occur anywhere in the body. Involuntary movements can be writhing, fidgeting, or wriggling.

- **Muscle stiffness:** The stiffness can occur in any part of the body or a specific region. Rigidity and slowness of movement can result in pain and aches. Sometimes, an uncontrolled tremor can also cause pain.

- **Joint pain:** PD and arthritis are common with aging, and the pain can be difficult to differentiate. People with PD experience severe joint pain.

- **Abdominal pain:** PD patients generally experience constipation or an upset stomach. This causes abdominal pain and can occur even before diagnosis.

How Is Pain Assessed?

When a PD patient experiences pain, the best approach is to talk to a healthcare provider and seek advice. A healthcare professional can assess a nonmotor symptom, including pain. The patient can also provide valuable information to the healthcare provider by writing down symptoms, including:

- Area of pain
- Type of pain
- Frequency of pain
- Intensity of pain

Pain Management in PD

Treating or managing pain in PD is difficult; however, finding the cause of the problem will help in prescribing the proper treatment. Common ways of reducing pain in PD patients include regular gentle exercise, painkillers, or massage. Common types of pain that occur in the shoulders and head can be treated by a healthcare provider. However, involuntary movements and mouth burning will need the attention of a specialist. Some methods of managing pain in PD are listed below:

- The source of the pain needs to be identified and the right kind of treatment should be given. A movement disorder specialist needs to be involved in the diagnosis process to direct the appropriate treatment.

- The inability to control motor symptoms can result in pain. Dyskinesia or dystonia are contributing pain factors; and dopamine medication adjustments are given for reduction of pain.

- Optimizing control of motor symptoms.

- Nonpharmacological methods include meditation techniques, massage therapy, acupuncture, and heat or cold application. They can be followed as per medical advice.

- Exercise is the best and most beneficial form of treatment, though it might be difficult for a patient with PD during the initial phases. However, a personalized regimen that is given by an occupational therapist can help in managing the pain.

- Anti-inflammatories are recommended for musculoskeletal and other pain. For extreme pain, low doses of opioids are prescribed under constant supervision, as opioids can be addictive. Antidepressants can also be administered for central pain when depression is co-present.

References

1. Dolhun, Rachel. "Pain and Parkinson's Disease," The Michael J. Fox Foundation, February 22, 2017.

2. "Pain," Parkinson's Disease Society of the United Kingdom, n.d.

3. Kristin Della Volpe. "Pain in Parkinson's Disease: A Spotlight on Women," Practical Pain Management (PPM), May 16, 2017.

Chapter 10

PD: Treatments and Research

Chapter Contents

Section 10.1

All about PD Treatments and Research Developments

This section includes text excerpted from "Parkinson's Disease: Challenges, Progress, and Promise," National Institute of Neurological Disorders and Stroke (NINDS), September 30, 2015.

Known Genetic Mutations

Inherited PD has been found to be associated with mutations in a number of genes including *SNCA, LRRK2, PARK2, PARK7,* and *PINK1.* Many more genes may yet be identified. Genome-wide association studies have shown that common variants in these genes also play a role in changing the risk for sporadic cases.

Mutations in other types of genes, including *GBA*, the gene in which a mutation causes Gaucher disease, do not cause PD, but appear to modify the risk of developing the condition in some families. There may also be variations in other genes that have not been identified that contribute to the risk of the disease.

Gene for Alpha-Synuclein (SNCA)

In 1997, scientists identified the first genetic mutation *(SNCA)* associated with PD among three unrelated families with several members affected with PD. The *SNCA* gene provides instructions for making the protein alpha-synuclein, which is normally found in the brain as well as other tissues in the body. Finding this mutation led to the discovery that alpha-synuclein aggregates were the primary component of the Lewy body. This is an example of how a disease-causing rare mutation can shed light on the entire disease process.

PD related to *SNCA* gene mutations is autosomal dominant, meaning that just one mutated copy of the gene in each cell is sufficient for a person to be affected. People with this mutation usually have a parent with the disease.

Though more than a dozen mutations in the *SNCA* gene have been linked to PD, these mutations are considered a relatively rare cause of the disease. In some cases, *SNCA* gene mutations are believed to cause the alpha-synuclein protein to misfold. Other *SNCA* mutations create extra copies of the gene, leading to excessive production of the alpha-synuclein protein. Even when no mutation is present, buildup of abnormal synuclein is a hallmark of PD. The NINDS is funding multiple studies aimed at determining how misfolded and excessive levels of alpha-synuclein might contribute to developing PD.

Gene for Leucine-Rich Repeat Kinase 2 (LRRK2)

Mutations of the *LRRK2* gene are the most common genetic cause of autosomal dominant PD. These mutations play a role in about 10 percent of inherited forms of PD and about 4 percent of people who have no family history of the disease. Studies show that one particular *LRRK2* mutation, G2019S, accounts for up to 20 percent of PD in specific groups, such as the Ashkenazi Jewish population.

Researchers are still studying exactly how *LRRK2* gene mutations lead to PD, but it appears these mutations influence both the manufacturing and disposal of unwanted proteins in multiple ways. PD associated with *LRRK2* mutations involves both early- and late-onset forms of the disease. The *LRRK2* gene is a kinase enzyme, a type of protein that tags molecules within cells with chemicals called phosphate groups. This process of tagging, called phosphorylation, regulates protein enzymes by turning them "on" or "off" and it is fundamental to basic nerve cell function and health.

NINDS-supported investigators at the Udall Center at Johns Hopkins University (JHU) have found that *LRRK2* mutations increase the rate at which the gene's protein tags ribosomal proteins, a key component of the protein-making machinery inside cells. This can cause the machinery to manufacture too many proteins, leading to cell death.

LRRK2 gene mutations also are believed to inhibit a waste disposal method called autophagy, the process by which cells break down nutrients, recycle cellular components, and get rid of unusable waste. Autophagy is a critical means for quality control by enabling the cell to eliminate damaged organelles and abnormal proteins.

LRRK2 gene mutations inhibit a type of autophagy called chaperone-mediated autophagy. During this type of autophagy a "chaperone" protein escorts a damaged protein to the lysosome, spherical vesicles within cells that contain acid that help breakdown unwanted molecules. As a result, the *LRRK2* gene mutations may lead to the buildup of alpha-synuclein into toxic aggregates within the cells. Researchers are exploring whether certain compounds might be capable of overriding *LRRK2* gene mutation effects by rebooting the chaperone-mediated disposal system.

Gene for Parkin (PARK2) / Gene for PTEN Induced Putative Kinase 1, or PINK1 (PARK6)

PARK2 mutations are the most common genetic mutations associated with early-onset PD, which first appear at age 50 or younger. *PARK6* gene mutations also are associated with early-onset PD, but they are far more rare. Both types of mutations are associated with autosomal recessive PD, meaning that two mutated copies of the gene are present in each cell and that anyone affected may have unaffected parents who each carried a single copy of the mutated gene.

Findings from a NINDS-funded study suggest that people with *PARK2* mutations tend to have slower disease progression compared with those who do not carry *PARK2* mutations.

The genes *PARK2*, *PARK6*, *PINK1*, along with the protein parkin, are all involved at different points along a pathway that controls the integrity of mitochondria, the powerhouses inside cells that produce energy by regulating quality control processes. Brain cells are especially energetic and dependent upon mitochondrial energy supply. Specifically, parkin and *PINK1* regulate mitochondrial autophagy—a process known as mitophagy. These processes are critical for maintaining a healthy pool of mitochondria by providing a means to eliminate those that no longer function properly.

Much work remains to be done to understand the association of *PARK2* and *PARK6* mutations and mitochondrial dysfunction, as well as to investigate if and how mitochondrial dysfunction leads to PD. Evidence suggests that parkin and *PINK1* function together. When *PINK1* (which is located on mitochondria) senses mitochondrial damage, it recruits parkin to get the process of mitophagy underway.

NINDS researchers are exploring ways to stimulate the *PINK1/* parkin pathway to encourage mitophagy. Scientists hope this will help them develop treatments for people with mitochondrial diseases, including certain forms of PD. Additionally, NINDS researchers are screening chemicals to identify agents that may be able to stimulate the expression of *PINK1*, and looking for other genes that may affect the functions of *PINK1* and parkin.

Evidence suggests that parkin is a factor in several additional pathways leading to PD, including sporadic forms of the disease associated with alpha-synuclein toxicity.

Gene for DJ-1 (PARK7)

The *PARK7* gene encodes for the protein DJ-1. Several mutations in the gene for DJ-1 are associated with some rare, early-onset forms of PD. The function of the DJ-1 gene remains a mystery. However, one theory is it can help protect cells from oxidative stress. Oxidative stress occurs when unstable molecules called free radicals accumulate to levels that can damage or kill cells. Some studies suggest that the DJ-1 gene strengthens the cells' ability to protect against metal toxicity and that this protective function is lost in some DJ-1 mutations. Animal studies suggest DJ-1 plays a role in motor function and helps protect cells against oxidative stress.

Gene for Beta-Glucocerebrosidase (GBA)

Mutations in the gene encoding the lysosomal enzyme beta-glucocerebrosidase (*GBA*) are associated with a lysosomal storage disorder, Gaucher disease. People with Gaucher disease are also more likely to have parkinsonism, a group of nervous disorders with symptoms similar to Parkinson disease. This has spurred investigators to look for a possible link between the two diseases. NIH-funded researchers have conducted studies of individuals with both disorders to assess their brain changes, family histories, and to screen tissues and DNA samples, which have helped confirm this link.

An NIH-led, multicenter study involving more than 10,000 people with and without PD showed that people with PD were more than 5 times more likely to carry a *GBA* mutation than those without the disease. Mutation carriers also were more likely to be diagnosed with PD earlier in their lives and to have a family history of the disease. Scientists have observed that depletion of beta-glucocerebrosidase results in alpha-synuclein accumulation and neurodegeneration.

Further research is needed to understand the association between *GBA* gene mutations and PD. The NINDS supports many lines of research investigating the role of *GBA* gene mutations. Projects are aimed at estimating the risk of PD associated with being a *GBA* carrier and identifying the phenotypic traits.

Studying the genes responsible for inherited cases of PD can help shed light on both inherited and sporadic cases of PD. The same genes and proteins that are altered in inherited cases of PD may play a role in sporadic cases of the disease. In some cases genetic mutations may not directly cause PD but may increase the susceptibility of developing the disease, especially when environmental toxins or other factors are present.

Cellular and Molecular Pathways to PD

What happens in a person's brain that causes him or her to develop PD? To answer this question scientists are working to understand the cellular and molecular pathways that lead to PD.

Mitochondrial Dysfunction

Research suggests that damage to mitochondria plays a major role in the development of PD. Mitochondria are unique parts of the cell that have their own DNA entirely separate from the genes found in the nucleus of every cell.

Mitochondrial dysfunction is a leading source of free radicals—molecules that damage membranes, proteins, DNA, and other parts of the cell. Oxidative stress is the main cause of damage by free radicals. Oxidative stress-related changes, including free radical damage to DNA, proteins, mitochondria, and fats has been detected in the brains of individuals with PD. A number of the genes found to cause PD disturb the process by which damaged mitochondria are disposed of in the neuron (mitophagy).

To learn more about how the process of mitophagy relates to PD, scientists have turned to RNA interference (RNAi), a natural process occurring in cells that helps regulate genes. Scientists are able to use RNAi as a tool to turn off genes of interest to investigate their function in cultured cells or animal models of PD. A technique known as high-throughput RNAi technology enabled NIH scientists to turn off nearly 22,000 genes one at a time. This process helped scientists identify dozens of genes that may regulate the clearance of damaged mitochondria. Researchers continue to study how these genes regulate the removal of damaged mitochondria from cells and the genes identified in this study may represent new therapeutic targets for PD.

One mechanism that helps regulate the health of mitochondria is autophagy, which allows for the breakdown and recycling of cellular components. Scientists have long observed that disruptions in the autophagy processes are associated with cell death in the substantia nigra and the accumulation of proteins in the brains of people with PD as well as other neurodegenerative diseases.

Ubiquitin-Proteasome System

Another area of PD research focuses on the ubiquitin-proteasome system (UPS), which helps cells stay healthy by getting rid of abnormal proteins. A chemical called ubiquitin acts as a "tag" that marks certain proteins in the cell for degradation by proteasomes, structures inside cells that launch chemical reactions that break peptide bonds. Researchers believe that if this disposal symptom fails to work correctly, toxins and other substances may accumulate to harmful levels, leading to cell death. Impairment of the UPS is believed to play a key role in several neurodegenerative disorders, including Alzheimer, Parkinson, and Huntington diseases.

The contribution of UPS to the development of PD appears to be multifactorial, meaning UPS influences the interactions of several genes. NINDS-funded researchers have found that UPS is critical for the degradation of misfolded alpha-synuclein in cells. Conversely, evidence suggests that abnormal or misfolded alpha-synuclein may also inhibit the proper functioning of UPS. A feedback loop may exist whereby abnormal alpha-synuclein inhibits the functions of UPS, causing more abnormal alpha-synuclein to accumulate and additional suppression of UPS activity. NINDS-funded researchers have also identified proteins that accumulate in the absence of parkin that contribute to the loss of dopaminergic neurons.

Several NINDS-funded investigators are exploring ways of enhancing UPS function as a potential therapeutic strategy.

Cell-to-Cell Transmission of Abnormally-Folded Proteins

Researchers have learned more about how PD-related damage spreads to various parts of the brain and nervous system. A characteristic pattern has emerged by which Lewy bodies are distributed in various regions of the brain. The earliest brain changes appear to involve Lewy bodies in the brain stem region (medulla oblongata and pontine tegmentum, as well as the olfactory bulb).

Braak staging is a six-tier classification method used to identify the degree of postmortem pathology resulting from PD. According to this classification, people in Braak stages 1 and 2 are generally thought to be presymptomatic. As the disease advances to Braak stages 3 and 4, Lewy bodies spread to the substantia nigra, areas of the midbrain, the basal forebrain, and the neocortex.

More recent evidence suggests that even before such brain changes have occurred, alpha-synuclein aggregates and Lewy bodies can be found in the nervous system of the gastrointestinal tract and in the salivary glands, a finding that supports the theory that PD many originate not in the brain but in the autonomic nervous system. Nonmotor symptoms such as constipation may in fact be a sign of the disease affecting nerves outside the brain before the disease moves into the brain where it later affects regions that control movement.

Researchers at the Udall Center at the Perelman School of Medicine of the University of Pennsylvania injected mice with a synthetic form of abnormal alpha-synuclein and found that misfolded alpha-synuclein appeared to spread throughout the brain. The researchers hypothesize that the injected abnormal alpha-synuclein may act like a seed that triggers the mouse's own alpha-synuclein to misfold, leading to a cell-to-cell transmission of PD-like brain changes, especially in regions of the brain important for motor function. The mice also exhibited PD-like motor symptoms.

Understanding more about how abnormal proteins spread through the nervous system may provide a potential window for a therapeutic strategy that interrupts the process of protein transmission and slows or halts disease progression. For example, NINDS-funded investigators are looking at immune therapy and antibodies or immunization against alpha-synuclein, to block PD transmission in the brains of mice.

Environmental Influences

Environmental circumstances are thought to impact the development of PD. Exposure to certain toxins may have a direct link to the development of PD. This was the case among people exposed to MPTP, a by-product accidentally produced in the manufacture of a synthetic opioid with effects similar to morphine. During the 1980s, street drugs contaminated with this substance caused a syndrome similar to PD. MPTP is also structurally similar to some pesticides. The brain converts MPTP into MPP+, which is toxic to substantia nigra neurons. MPP+ exposure produces severe, permanent parkinsonism and has been used to create animal models of PD.

In other cases, exposure to the metal manganese among those with working in the mining, welding, and steel industries has been associated with an increased risk of developing parkinsonism. Some evidence suggests that exposure to certain herbicides such as paraquat and maneb increase the risk of PD. Scientists believe that there are other yet-to-be identified environmental factors that play a role in PD among people who are already genetically susceptible to developing the disease.

The National Institute of Environmental Health Sciences (NIEHS) is the lead institute at the NIH investigating the association between PD and environmental influences such as pesticides and solvents as well as other factors like traumatic brain injury. For example, NIEHS is funding a project at the University of Washington aimed at developing and validating biomarkers to identify early-stage neurological disease processes associated with toxic agents such as chemicals, metals, and pesticides. Animal models are being developed to study the impact of pesticides on farmworkers and metals on professional welders.

The NIEHS also funds the Parkinson, Genes & Environment study. The study is designed to determine the role genes as well dietary, lifestyle, and environmental factors play on the risk for developing PD and their potential to cause the illness. The more than 500,000 study participants were originally recruited in 1995 as part of the National Institutes of Health-American Association of Retired Persons (NIH-AARP) Diet and Health Study. Researchers will continue to follow participants over time to address some of the most interesting theories about the causes of PD. Already they have found, for example, that people who consume low levels of healthy dietary fats, such as those from fish, or high levels of saturated fats are more vulnerable to developing PD after being exposed to neurotoxins such as pesticides. The findings need to be confirmed, however, they suggest the possibility that diets rich in healthy fats and low in saturated fats may reduce the risk of PD.

The development of PD is a complex interplay between environmental, genetic, and lifestyle factors. Scientists are increasingly aware that in any given individual, there may be multiple factors that cause the disease.

In some cases, environmental factors may also have a protective effect. Population-based studies have suggested, for example, that people with high levels of vitamin D in their blood have a much lower risk of developing PD compared with people with very low concentrations of vitamin D. Further research is need to determine if vitamin D deficiency puts people at higher risk for PD, but such findings suggest the possibility that vitamin D supplements may have a beneficial effect. However, there may be genetic factors that cause people with low vitamin D levels to have higher rates of PD in which case vitamin D supplements would not be helpful.

To answer to this question, researchers at the Udall Center at the University of Miami are examining the pharmacogenetics of vitamin D. The investigators are studying a large dataset to confirm the finding that low levels of vitamin D is a risk factor for PD. At the same time, they are trying to identify any potential genetic modifiers of vitamin D's effect on PD risk.

Certain drugs and chemicals available as a supplement or in a person's diet also have been shown to have a neuroprotective effect for PD and other disorders. For example, regular use of caffeine (coffee, tea) was found to reduce the loss of dopamine-producing neurons. Studies hope to define the optimal caffeine dose in treating movement disorders like PD while gaining a better understanding of the mechanisms involving caffeine's benefit. Uric acid, because of its antioxidative effect, may lower the risk for multiple neurodegenerative disorders, in particular, PD. A preliminary clinical trial funded by the Michael J. Fox Foundation examined the effectiveness of the drug inosine to safely raise uric acid levels and possibly slow the progression of Parkinson disease.

Neuroinflammation

Neuroinflammation is a protective biological response designed to eliminate damaged cells and other harmful agents in nervous system tissue. Mounting evidence suggests that neuroinflammation plays a role in PD. Several lines of research funded by the NINDS are investigating this connection.

Compared to people without PD, those with PD tend to have higher levels of pro-inflammatory substances known as cytokines in their cerebrospinal fluid. Immune cells in the brain called microglia also are more likely to be activated in the brains of individuals with PD. Epidemiological studies suggest that rates of PD among people who frequently use non steroidal anti-inflammatory drugs (NSAIDS) are lower than in those who do not use NSAIDS.

Evidence from animal studies also suggests that elevated levels of the protein alpha-synuclein may trigger microglia to become activated in the brains of people with PD.

Scientists are investigating whether inflammation itself is a cause of brain cell death or if it is a response to an already occurring process that contributes to the development of a disease. If researchers can interrupt the neuroinflammatory processes, they may be able to develop neuroprotective treatments for people with PD that prevent or slow the progression of the disease by halting, or at least reducing, the loss of neurons.

Section 10.2

VA Research on Parkinson Disease

This section includes text excerpted from "Parkinson's
Disease," U.S. Department of Veterans Affairs (VA),
October 14, 2016.

Published Research

In 2001, U.S. Department of Veterans Affairs (VA) created six specialized centers to provide Veterans with Parkinson disease (PD) with
state of the art clinical care, education, research, and national outreach
and advocacy.

Known as the Parkinson Disease Research, Education, and Clinical Centers (PADRECCs), these centers are located in Philadelphia; Richmond, Va.; Houston; Los Angeles; San Francisco; and
the Seattle/Portland area. The centers also provide comprehensive
diagnosis and treatment services for other movement disorders,
including essential tremor, restless leg syndrome (RLS), dystonia,
Lewy body disease (LBD), progressive supranuclear palsy (PSP),
multiple system atrophy (MSA), and corticobasal degeneration
(CBD).

Researchers at these sites are studying the biochemical pathways
involving dopamine, and testing a variety of treatment approaches,
including medication, surgery, and electrical stimulation.

Warning Signs of PD

In December 2011, a team of VA researchers led by investigators at
the Spark M. Matsunaga VA Medical Center in Honolulu presented a
paper to the World Congress on PD and Related Disorders that found
impaired sense of smell, constipation, slow reaction time, excessive
daytime sleepiness and faulty executive function (the ability to manage
life tasks of all types) may all be warning signs of PD. The researchers
stated that combinations of these signs could predict up to a tenfold
higher risk of the disease.

Studies of Deep Brain Stimulation (DBS)

DBS is a surgical procedure used to treat a variety of disabling neurological symptoms, especially those related to PD. DBS uses a surgically implanted, battery operated device called a neurostimulator. The neurostimulator delivers electrical stimulation to targeted areas in the brain that control movement, blocking abnormal nerve signals that cause tremors and other systems.

The first experimental DBS implants took place in 1987, and the U.S. Food and Drug Administration (FDA) approved the use of the procedure in 2002.

In early 2009, VA, along with the National Institutes of Health (NIH), completed the first large scale trial of the results of DBS. The six year cooperative study the Chartered Society of Physiotherapy ((CSP) #468), conducted at seven VA medical centers and six university hospitals, looked at 255 PD patients aged 37–83 and compared symptoms between those who had undergone the surgery and those who had used drug therapy alone.

The researchers found patients who underwent DBS had better control of their limbs and could walk better than those using medication. They found that older patients, who had previously been excluded from brain stimulation research and treatment, benefited from DBS as much as younger patients.

Researchers also found that potential side effects from DBS included a decrease in neurocognitive functioning and increases in the rate of infections, falls, depression, gait and balance problems, and pain—and that these side effects were more likely to occur than side effects from medication.

In addition, DBS did not help other symptoms of PD, including depression; decline in mental ability; and trouble with gastrointestinal, urinary or sexual functions. On the whole, the researchers concluded that while DBS appears to be riskier than drug therapy, it may hold significant benefits for those with PD who no longer respond well to medication alone.

DBS improves movement related functioning—Researchers with CSP #468 have continued to publish articles based on their findings on DBS. In one 2012 study, researchers found that DBS produced marked improvements in movement related functioning. Patients, on average, gained four to five hours a day free of troubling motor symptoms such as shaking, slowed movement or stiffness. The effects were greatest at six months, and leveled off slightly by three years.

Suicide no more likely with DBS than with medication—In another study, published in 2013, researchers looked at two types of DBS procedures, and at patients taking medication. They found that attempted suicide, or suicidal thinking, was no more common among patients who had undergone either form of the procedure than in those taking medication alone. Some previous international studies had raised the question of whether suicide was an important cause of mortality following DBS procedures.

DBS implantation location—Another study of the two forms of DBS procedures was published in 2015 by researchers from the Edward Hines, Jr. VA Hospital in Hines, Ill., the Jesse Brown VA Medical Center in Chicago, and three Chicago area schools of medicine.

Researchers found that, 6–12 months after DBS surgery, patients whose neurostimulator was implanted in their brain's subthalamic nucleus had a significantly greater increase in their use of medication for mental health issues than those whose neurostimulator was implanted in their brains' globus pallidus internus. The study found no significant differences in the two groups' use of outpatient or inpatient healthcare, however.

PD and Exercise

Research has demonstrated the great benefits of exercise for patients with PD. Not only have exercise programs been shown to improve motor function and reduce the risk of falls, but they also improve overall quality of life and possibly slow the course of the disease.

Walking improves PD symptoms—A 2014 study led by researchers with the Iowa City VA HealthCare System (HCS) and the University of Iowa found that patients who walked briskly for 45 minutes, three times a week, showed improvements in their Parkinson symptoms. They were also less depressed and less tired.

The study suggests that walking provides a safe and easily accessible way of improving the symptoms of PD. While previous studies had shown that moderately strenuous exercise is helpful, this research showed that even moderate walking can make a significant difference.

Low intensity workouts improve mobility—Researchers studying 67 patients with PD at the VA Maryland HealthCare System learned, in 2013, that low intensity workouts, stretching, and resistance exercise all improved the mobility of patients with Parkinson disease. Those who walked on a treadmill at a comfortable pace for nearly an hour showed the most consistent improvement in gait and mobility.

New exercise programs—Currently, a research team at the VA Boston Healthcare System is evaluating the effectiveness of a home-based approach to providing the benefits of a safe exercise program to people with PD. The program will be centered on remote, real-time instruction and supervision. Ideally, it will make the benefits of exercise available to PD patients who cannot travel to exercise locations.

Another current study, taking place at the VA Portland Health-Care System, is looking at whether people with PD can significantly improve their mobility and cognition functioning after participating in six weeks of group exercise and another six weeks of education on how to live better with a chronic disease. The study also hopes to determine if already-existing deficits in cognition functions can predict whether or not exercise programs help PD patients.

PD and Mental Symptoms

Antipsychotic drugs linked to mortality—According to a 2016 VA study, up to 60 percent of PD patients experience psychosis (a mental disorder characterized by symptoms that indicate impaired contact with reality) at some point during the course of their illness. Physicians commonly prescribe antipsychotic drugs to treat the condition.

The study, led by researchers at the Corporal Michael J. Crescenz VA Medical Center in Philadelphia, the VA Ann Arbor Healthcare System, and the University of Pennsylvania, looked at 15,000 VA PD patients. It found that those who began using antipsychotic drugs were more than twice as likely to die during the following six months, compared to a matched set of PD patients who did not use such drugs.

The relative risk of the drugs varied by the specific drug prescribed: mortality was 2.16 times higher for quetiapine compared with nontreatment; 2.46 for risperidone; 2.79 for olanzapine; and 5.08 for haloperidol. First-generation, or "typical," antipsychotics, which include haloperidol, were collectively associated with about 50 percent greater relative mortality risk compared with more recently developed "atypical" antipsychotics such as risperidone and quetiapine.

The research team did not find any clues that pointed to a specific cause or mechanism for the higher death rate. They are conducting a follow-up study that might shed more light on this issue. In the interim, the first author, Dr. Daniel Weintraub of the Corporal Michael

J. Crescenz VA Medical Center's PADRECC, suggested that antipsychotic drugs should not be prescribed to Parkinson patients without careful consideration.

PD's effect on cognitive impairment—In 2015, researchers from the Crescenz VA Medical Center and the University of Pennsylvania reported on a study in which they followed a cohort of patients with PD and baseline normal cognition skills (the activities of thinking, understanding, learning and remembering) for a minimum of two years and a maximum of six.

After one year, 8.5 percent of the patients had developed mild cognitive impairment, and by the end of six years that increased to 47.4 percent. All of the patients who had had mild cognitive impairment at the end of the first year developed dementia by the end of the study. The research team concluded that the transition from normal cognition in PD patients to cognitive impairment, including dementia, occurs frequently and quickly.

PD and Genomics

In 2010, researchers with several institutions, including the VA Puget Sound HealthCare System, found that a group of genes that help control the body's immune response may figure in the development of PD. The team examined the genetic makeup and health histories of nearly 4,000 people, half of whom had PD.

They found those with the disease were more likely to have certain variations in a group of immune genes known as the human leukocyte antigen system. The study provided important evidence of a role for the immune system in the development of PD.

In 2013, VA researchers and their colleagues published the results of a study that found that the E4 variant of the apolipoprotein-E (*APOE*) gene is more common in people with dementia who have either PD, Alzheimer disease, or Lewy body disease (a neurodegenerative disorder that causes dementia).

In genetic studies of donated brain tissue, *APOE* was found in 7 percent of people without dementia. It was found far more often in Alzheimer patients with and without Lewy body disease, people with only Lewy body disease, and patients with PD.

Because PD is characterized by a loss of dopamine-producing cells in the brain, scientists have been trying for decades to find a way to repair faulty dopamine neurons and put them back into patients, where they will start producing dopamine again.

PD and Gene Therapy

Creating new dopamine neurons—In 2015, researchers with the VA Western New York HealthCare System (WNYHS), the State University of New York at Buffalo, and Harvard University, along with collaborators in China, reported on a method to convert skin cells into neurons that produce dopamine.

Their research was based on the discovery that transcription factor protein p53 acts as a gatekeeper protein. (Transcription factors are proteins that control which genes are turned on or off in the human genome, by binding to deoxyribonucleic acid (DNA) and other proteins. Gatekeepers are proteins that directly control the cell cycle.)

By lowering the expression of p53 at the right time of the cell cycles, the team was able to turn patients' skin cells into dopamine neurons. These neurons, generated in a dish, can then be transplanted into the patients' brains to replace their faulty neurons. The neurons can also be used to efficiently screen new treatments for PD.

According to the paper's senior author, Dr. Jian Feng of China, the paper's findings are important for basic cell biology, not only for PD. The ability to lower the expression of p53 is a generic way to change cells from one type to another, thereby changing the way scientists work with all cells. It will also allow researchers to generate tissue similar to those in the body, even brain tissue.

Preventing PD with gene therapy—Researchers with the VA Pittsburgh Healthcare System (PHS) and the University of Pittsburgh School of Medicine (UPSOM) found, in 2015, that gene therapy to reduce the production of a brain protein can successfully prevent the development of PD in rats.

Aggregates or deposits of a protein called alpha synuclein within neurons are found in people with PD. PD is also linked to a dysfunction of mitochondria, the powerhouses of the cell that produce energy for the body.

According to the research team, their study was the first to show that mitochondria and α-synuclein can interact in a damaging way in vulnerable cells, and that targeting α-synuclein might be an effective way to treat the disease.

In their study, the team blocked the expression of alpha synuclein in rats' brains by injecting the rats with a harmless virus called Adeno-associated 2 (AAV2). They then exposed the rats to a naturally occurring pesticide called rotenone, which creates Parkinson like body chemistry changes in rats exposed to it.

They found that their gene therapy protected the rats from the effects of rotenone, and concluded that gene therapy aimed at reducing alpha synuclein production has a protective effect and successfully prevented the development of PD in a rat model.

The team is now working to identify the pathways by which alpha synuclein affects the mitochondrial function and will work to develop potential drug therapies that target this mechanism. They hope to be able to translate their approach into human clinical trials soon.

Section 10.3

Scientists Find a Role for Parkinson Gene in the Brain

This section includes text excerpted from "Scientists Find a Role for Parkinson's Gene in the Brain," National Institute of Neurological Disorders and Stroke (NINDS), October 25, 2017.

A new study published in the journal *Neuron* sheds light on the normal function of *LRRK2*, the most common genetic cause for late onset Parkinson disease. The study was supported by the National Institute of Neurological Disorders and Stroke (NINDS), part of the National Institutes of Health (NIH).

For more than 10 years, scientists have known that mutations in the *LRRK2* gene can lead to Parkinson disease, yet both its role in the disease and its normal function in the brain remain unclear. In a study in mice, researchers have now found that *LRRK* is necessary for the survival of dopamine containing neurons in the brain, the cells most affected by Parkinson. Importantly, this finding could alter the design of treatments against the disease.

"Since its discovery, researchers have been trying to define *LRRK2* function and how mutations may lead to Parkinson disease," said Beth Anne Sieber, Ph.D., program director at NINDS. "The findings in this chapter emphasize the importance of understanding the normal role for genes associated with neurodegenerative disorders."

81

LRRK2 is found along with a closely related protein, *LRRK1*, in the brain. A mutation in *LRRK2* alone can eventually produce Parkinson disease symptoms and brain pathology in humans as they age. In mice, however, *LRRK2* loss or mutation does not lead to the death of dopamine producing neurons, possibly because *LRRK1* plays a complementary or compensatory role during the relatively short, two year mouse lifespan.

"Parkinson linked mutations such as *LRRK2* have subtle effects that do not produce symptoms until late in life. Understanding the normal function of these types of genes will help us figure out what has gone wrong to cause disease," said Jie Shen, Ph.D., director of the NINDS Morris K. Udall Center of Excellence for Parkinson Disease at Brigham and Women's Hospital and senior author of this study.

To better understand the roles of these related proteins in brain function using animal models, Shen and her colleagues created mice lacking both *LRRK1* and *LRRK2*. They observed a loss of dopamine containing neurons in areas of the brain consistent with PD beginning around 15 months of age. When the researchers looked at the affected brain cells more closely, they saw the buildup of a protein called α-synuclein, a hallmark of Parkinson, and defects in pathways that clear cellular "garbage." At the same time, more dopamine containing neurons also began to show signs of apoptosis, the cells' "self-destruct" mechanism.

"Our findings show that *LRRK* is critical for the survival of the populations of neurons affected by Parkinson disease," said Dr. Shen.

While the deletion of both *LRRK1* and *LRRK2* did not affect overall brain size or cells in such areas of the brain as the cerebral cortex and cerebellum, the mice showed other significant effects such as a decrease in body weight and a lifespan of only 15–16 months. Thus, the scientists were unable to study other Parkinson related effects such as changes in behavior and movement nor were they able to conduct a long-term analysis of how *LRRK's* absence affects the brain.

Interestingly, the most common disease linked mutation in *LRRK2* is thought to make the protein more active. As a result, most efforts to develop a treatment against that mutation have focused on inhibiting *LRRK2* activity.

"The fact that the absence of *LRRK* leads to the death of dopamine containing neurons suggests that the use of inhibitory drugs as a treatment for Parkinson disease might not be the best approach," said Dr. Shen.

Dr. Shen and her colleagues are now developing mice that have *LRRK1* and 2 removed only in the dopamine containing neurons of the brain. This specific deletion will allow the researchers to study longer-term and behavioral changes while avoiding the other consequences that lead to a shortened lifespan.

Section 10.4

Stem Cells in PD Treatment

This section includes text excerpted from "Patient-Derived Stem Cells Could Improve Drug Research for Parkinson's," National Institutes of Health (NIH), July 4, 2012. Reviewed January 2018.

Researchers have taken a step toward personalized medicine for Parkinson disease, by investigating signs of the disease in patient derived cells and testing how the cells respond to drug treatments. The study was funded by the National Institutes of Health (NIH).

The researchers collected skin cells from patients with genetically inherited forms of Parkinson and reprogrammed those cells into neurons. They found that neurons derived from individuals with distinct types of Parkinson showed common signs of distress and vulnerability—in particular, abnormalities in the cellular energy factories known as mitochondria. At the same time, the cells' responses to different treatments depended on the type of Parkinson each patient had.

"These findings suggest new opportunities for clinical trials of Parkinson disease, in which cell reprogramming technology could be used to identify the patients most likely to respond to a particular intervention," said Margaret Sutherland, Ph.D., a program director at NIH's National Institute of Neurological Disorders and Stroke (NINDS).

A consortium of researchers conducted the study with primary funding from NINDS. The consortium is led by Ole Isacson, M.D., Ph.D., a professor of neurology at McLean Hospital and Harvard Medical School in Boston.

The NINDS consortium's first goal was to transform the patients' skin cells into induced pluripotent stem (iPS) cells, which are adult cells that have been reprogrammed to behave like embryonic stem cells. The consortium researchers then used a combination of growth conditions and growth stimulating molecules to coax these iPS cells into becoming neurons, including the type that die in Parkinson disease.

Parkinson disease affects a number of brain regions, including a motor control area of the brain called the substantia nigra. There, it destroys neurons that produce the chemical dopamine. Loss of these neurons leads to involuntary shaking, slowed movements, muscle stiffness and other symptoms. Medications can help manage the symptoms, but there is no treatment to slow or stop the disease.

Most cases of Parkinson are sporadic, meaning that the cause is unknown. However, genetics plays a strong role. There are 17 regions of the genome with common variations that affect the risk of developing Parkinson disease. Researchers have also identified nine genes that, when mutated, can cause the disease.

Dr. Isacson and his collaborators derived iPS cells from five people with genetic forms of Parkinson disease. By focusing on genetic cases, rather than sporadic cases, they hoped they would have a better chance of seeing patterns in the disease process and in treatment responses. Three of the individuals had mutations in a gene called *LRRK2*, and two others were siblings who had mutations in the gene *PINK1*. The researchers also derived iPS cells from two of the siblings' family members who did not have Parkinson or any known mutations linked to it.

Because prior studies have suggested that Parkinson disease involves a breakdown of mitochondrial function, the researchers looked for signs of impaired mitochondria in patient derived neurons. Mitochondria turn oxygen and glucose into cellular energy. The researchers found that oxygen consumption rates were lower in patient cells with *LRRK2* mutations, and higher in cells with the *PINK1* mutation. In *PINK1* mutant cells, the researchers also found increased vulnerability to oxidative stress, a damaging process that in theory can be counteracted with antioxidants.

Next, the researchers tested if neurons derived from patients and healthy volunteers were vulnerable to a variety of toxins, including some that target mitochondria. Compared to neurons from healthy individuals, patient derived neurons were more likely to become damaged or die after exposure to mitochondrial toxins. Patient derived neurons also suffered more damage from the toxins than did patient derived skin cells.

Next, the researchers attempted to rescue the toxin exposed cells with various drug treatments that have shown promise in animal models of Parkinson, including the antioxidant coenzyme Q10 and the immunosuppressant rapamycin. All patient derived neurons—whether they carried *LRRK2* or *PINK1* mutations—had beneficial responses to coenzyme Q10. However, the patient derived neurons differed in their response to rapamycin; the drug helped prevent damage to neurons with *LRRK2* mutations, but it did not protect the neurons with *PINK1* mutations.

These results hint that iPS cell technology could be used to help define subgroups of patients for clinical trials. To date, interventional trials for Parkinson disease have not focused on specific groups of patients or forms of the disease, because there have been few clues to point investigators toward individualized treatments. Although the current study focused on genetic forms of Parkinson, iPS cell technology could be used to define disease mechanisms and the most promising treatments for sporadic Parkinson as well.

The NINDS Parkinson Disease iPS Cell Research Consortium is one of three such consortia funded by NINDS. One of the consortia is focused on developing iPS cells for the study of Huntington disease (HD), and another focuses on amyotrophic lateral sclerosis (ALS) and frontotemporal dementia (FTD).

The Huntington disease consortium reported successful derivation of iPS cells and iPS generated neurons from patients. Cells from patients with both early and later onset disease showed severe defects in physiology, metabolism, and cell viability, compared to cells from healthy volunteers. These results were reported in the June 28th issue of Cell Stem Cell. The consortium is led by Leslie Thompson, PhD, a professor of psychiatry and human behavior at the University of California, Irvine.

Skin cell and iPS cell lines developed by the consortia are available to both academic and industry researchers through the NINDS human cell line repository at the Coriell Institute. To date the NINDS repository has distributed more than 200 cell lines worldwide.

Chapter 11

Deep Brain Stimulation for PD

Deep brain stimulation (DBS) is a surgical procedure used to treat several disabling neurological symptoms—most commonly the debilitating motor symptoms of Parkinson disease (PD), such as tremor, rigidity, stiffness, slowed movement, and walking problems. The procedure is also used to treat essential tremor and dystonia. The procedure is used only for individuals whose symptoms cannot be adequately controlled with medications. However, only individuals who improve to some degree after taking medication for Parkinson benefit from DBS. A variety of conditions may mimic PD but do not respond to medications or DBS. DBS uses a surgically implanted, battery operated medical device called an implantable pulse generator (IPG) similar to a heart pacemaker and approximately the size of a stopwatch to deliver electrical stimulation to specific areas in the brain that control movement, thus blocking the abnormal nerve signals that cause PD symptoms.

Before the procedure, a neurosurgeon uses magnetic resonance imaging (MRI) or computed tomography (CT) scanning to identify and locate the exact target within the brain for surgical intervention. Some surgeons may use microelectrode recording which involves a small wire that monitors the activity of nerve cells in the target area to

This chapter includes text excerpted from "Deep Brain Stimulation for Parkinson's Disease," National Institute of Neurological Disorders and Stroke (NINDS), May 15, 2014. Reviewed January 2018.

more specifically identify the precise brain area that will be stimulated. Generally, these areas are the thalamus, subthalamic nucleus, and globus pallidus. There is a low chance that placement of the stimulator may cause bleeding or infection in the brain.

The DBS system consists of three components: the lead, the extension, and the IPG. The lead (also called an electrode)—a thin, insulated wire—is inserted through a small opening in the skull and implanted in the brain. The tip of the electrode is positioned within the specific brain area.

The extension is an insulated wire that is passed under the skin of the head, neck, and shoulder, connecting the lead to the implantable pulse generator. The IPG (the "battery pack") is the third component and is usually implanted under the skin near the collarbone. In some cases it may be implanted lower in the chest or under the skin over the abdomen.

Once the system is in place, electrical impulses are sent from the IPG up along the extension wire and the lead and into the brain. These impulses block abnormal electrical signals and alleviate PD motor symptoms.

Treatment

Unlike previous surgeries for PD, DBS involves minimal permanent surgical changes to the brain. Instead, the procedure uses electrical stimulation to regulate electrical signals in neural circuits to and from identified areas in the brain to improve PD symptoms. Thus, if DBS causes unwanted side effects or newer, more promising treatments develop in the future, the implantable pulse generator can be removed, and the DBS procedure can be halted. Also, stimulation from the IPG is easily adjustable—without further surgery—if the person's condition changes. Some people describe the pulse generator adjustments as "programming."

Prognosis

Although most individuals still need to take medication after undergoing DBS, many people with Parkinson disease experience considerable reduction of their motor symptoms and are able to reduce their medications. The amount of reduction varies but can be considerably reduced in most individuals, and can lead to a significant improvement in side effects such as dyskinesias (involuntary movements caused by long-term use of levodopa). In some cases, the stimulation itself can suppress dyskinesias without a reduction in medication. DBS does not improve cognitive symptoms in PD and indeed may worsen them, so it is not generally used if there are signs of dementia. DBS changes the brain firing pattern but does not slow the progression of the neurodegeneration.

Chapter 12

Complementary and Alternative Medicine for PD

Parkinson Disease

Parkinson disease is a progressive neurodegenerative disease, the second most common disorder of this type after Alzheimer disease. It progresses slowly as small clusters of dopaminergic neurons in the midbrain die. The gradual loss of these neurons results in reduction of a critical neurotransmitter called dopamine, a chemical responsible for transmitting messages to parts of the brain that coordinate muscle movement.

Mind and Body Practices

Tai Chi

There is some evidence that tai chi, along with medication, may improve some symptoms of Parkinson disease, such as balance and functional mobility.

This chapter contains text excerpted from the following sources: Text under the heading "Parkinson Disease" is excerpted from "Parkinson Disease," National Institute of Environmental Health Sciences (NIEHS), September 15, 2017; Text beginning with the heading "Mind and Body Practices" is excerpted from "Parkinson Disease and Complementary Health Approaches: What the Science Says," National Center for Complementary and Integrative Health (NCCIH), December 2016.

Efficacy

- A 2015 systematic review and meta analysis of 15 randomized controlled trials involving 799 participants found positive
  evidence of tai chi plus medication for Parkinson disease for
  improvements in motor function, balance, and functional reach;
  however, no significant difference was found between tai chi plus
  medication and medication alone for gait or quality of life.

- A 2015 systematic review of 64 studies of nonpharmacologic
  approaches to improve balance in Parkinson disease found some
  evidence that tai chi may help improve balance and motor control abilities; however, a randomized controlled trial showed that
  16 weeks of tai chi training were ineffective in gait performance,
  gait initiation, or the reduction of disability related to Parkinson
  disease.

- A systematic review and meta-analysis of seven randomized controlled trials and one nonrandomized controlled trial involving
  a total of 470 participants found that tai chi showed beneficial
  effects in improving motor function, balance, and functional
  mobility in participants with Parkinson disease, but not in
  improving gait velocity, step length, or gait endurance. However,
  when compared to other active therapies, tai chi only showed
  better effects in improving balance.

- A systematic review and meta analysis of 10 randomized controlled trials involving a total of 409 participants with mild to
  moderate Parkinson disease concluded that tai chi, performed
  with medication, resulted in improvements in mobility and
  balance.

Safety

- Tai chi is generally considered safe for most people. A systematic review and meta analysis of 10 randomized controlled trials
  concluded that tai chi was safe and popular among participants
  with Parkinson disease who are at an early stage of disease.

Acupuncture

Clinical studies in China have shown a positive benefit of acupuncture in treating symptoms of Parkinson disease; however, large and
well controlled clinical trials are needed before a conclusion about the
efficacy of acupuncture for this condition can be drawn. The American

Academy of Neurology (AAN) practice parameter on neuroprotective strategies and alternative therapies for Parkinson disease concluded that there is insufficient evidence to support or refute the use of acupuncture in Parkinson disease.

Efficacy

- The American Academy of Neurology's practice parameter on neuroprotective strategies and alternative therapies for Parkinson disease concluded that there is insufficient evidence to support or refute the use of acupuncture in Parkinson disease.

- A 2015 systematic review and meta analysis of 27 studies involving 2,314 participants evaluating the effectiveness of traditional Chinese medicine as an adjunct therapy for Parkinson disease found that acupuncture (based on two studies of 98 participants) as adjunct therapy was markedly beneficial for improving some Parkinson related symptoms compared to routine treatment alone.

- A review of 11 studies concluded that the lack of randomized controlled trials and small sample size were not sufficient to demonstrate favorable effects of acupuncture on Parkinson disease.

Safety

- Acupuncture is generally safe and well tolerated in most people when it is performed by a licensed practitioner.

Massage Therapy

There is insufficient evidence to determine whether massage therapy has any beneficial effect on symptoms of Parkinson disease.

Efficacy

- The American Academy of Neurology's practice parameter on neuroprotective strategies and alternative therapies for Parkinson disease concluded that there is insufficient evidence to support or refute manual therapy, including massage therapy, biofeedback, or Alexander technique in the treatment of Parkinson disease.

- A randomized controlled pilot study of 45 participants with Parkinson disease found that salivary cortisol (a natural biomarker for stress) concentrations were significantly reduced immediately following the tactile massage intervention, but there were no significant differences in reduction compared to the control group and no long-term effect.

Safety

- Massage therapy is generally safe and well tolerated in most people when it is performed by a licensed practitioner.

Dance

There is some limited evidence that dance, such as the Argentine tango, can be a supportive approach for people with Parkinson disease and has the potential to improve specific symptoms of Parkinson, including motor severity and balance over the short-term.

Efficacy

- A 2015 systematic review and meta analysis of 13 studies evaluated research results on the effectiveness of Argentine tango for people with Parkinson disease and found significant overall effects in favor of tango for motor severity and balance. However, the studies were small and many were conducted by the same research groups.

- A clinical trial involving 31 participants examined the effects of adapted tango on spatial cognition and disease severity in Parkinson disease and found that the tango participants improved on disease severity and spatial cognition, compared with the control group. Improvements among the tango participants were also seen in balance and executive function.

- A randomized controlled trial of 52 participants with Parkinson disease found that those who participated in a community based Argentine tango class reported increased participation in complex daily activities, recovery of activities lost since the onset of Parkinson disease, and engagement in new activities.

- When comparing the differential effects of tango versus other types of dance for Parkinson disease, a 2015 study of 11 participants concluded that tango dance interventions may preferentially improve mobility and motor signs in people with Parkinson disease, compared to other dance interventions.

- A 2015 randomized controlled trial of 20 participants examined the effects of virtual reality dance exercise on people with Parkinson disease and found that virtual reality dance exercise had a positive effect on balance, activities of daily living, and depressive disorder status.

- A systematic review and meta analysis of five randomized controlled trials found that dance as an intervention for Parkinson disease significantly improved motor scores, balance, and gait speed when compared to no treatment. When compared with other exercise interventions, significant improvements in balance and quality of life were found.

Safety

- Dance interventions in people with Parkinson disease are generally considered safe when practiced in a controlled environment. Dancing with a partner may provide an added safety element in preventing falls by holding on to the partner.

Natural Products

Coenzyme Q10

The American Academy of Neurology's practice parameter on neuroprotective strategies and alternative therapies for Parkinson disease concluded that there is insufficient evidence to support or refute the use of coenzyme Q10 for neuroprotection.

Efficacy

- The American Academy of Neurology's practice parameter on neuroprotective strategies and alternative therapies for Parkinson disease concluded that there is insufficient evidence to support or refute the use of coenzyme Q10 for neuroprotection. The guidelines state, "Three single Class I studies using the unified Parkinson disease rating scale (UPDRS) as the outcome measure suggest there is no evidence of neuroprotection for riluzole, coenzyme Q, or pramipexole (as compared to levodopa). However, the studies of riluzole and coenzyme Q were underpowered to rule out a possible benefit, particularly if modest."

- A randomized clinical trial of 600 participants with Parkinson disease concluded that coenzyme Q10 was safe and well tolerated in this population, but showed no evidence of clinical benefit.

- A randomized controlled trial of 80 participants with early Parkinson disease found that less disability developed in subjects assigned to coenzyme Q10 than in those assigned to placebo; however, the results did not reach statistical significance.

Safety

- Studies have not reported serious side effects related to CoQ10 use. The most common side effects of CoQ10 include insomnia, increased liver enzymes, rashes, nausea, upper abdominal pain, dizziness, sensitivity to light, irritability, headaches, heartburn, and fatigue.
- CoQ10 may make warfarin less effective.

Creatine

There is insufficient evidence to determine whether creatine used alone or as an adjuvant treatment is efficacious for Parkinson disease.

Efficacy

- A Cochrane systematic review (CSR) of 2 randomized controlled trials involving 194 participants concluded that the evidence base on the effects of creatine in Parkinson disease is limited by risk of bias, small sample sizes, and short duration of clinical trials, and does not provide a reliable basis on which treatment decisions can be made.

Safety

- The Cochrane systematic review found that creatine appears to be safe and well tolerated; however, there was a higher rate of patients with gastrointestinal complaints in the creatine group compared to the placebo group at two years follow up.

Mucuna pruriens *(Velvet bean)*

There is insufficient evidence to support or refute the use of *Mucuna pruriens* for the treatment of Parkinson disease symptoms.

Efficacy

The American Academy of Neurology's practice parameter on neuroprotective strategies and alternative therapies for Parkinson disease concluded that there is insufficient evidence to support or refute the use of *Mucuna pruriens* for the treatment of motor symptoms of Parkinson disease.

A preliminary pilot study of eight participants with Parkinson disease with a short duration L-dopa response and disabling peak dose dyskinesias found that the seed powder formulation of *Mucuna pruriens* contains a considerable quantity of L-dopa and has a rapid onset of action with a slightly longer duration of therapeutic response compared with standard L-dopa. *Mucuna pruriens*'s long-term efficacy and safety has not yet been established.

Safety

- The safety of Mucuna pruriens has not yet been established.

Vitamin E

The American Academy of Neurology's practice parameter on neuroprotective strategies and alternative therapies for Parkinson disease concluded that Vitamin E is probably ineffective for the treatment of Parkinson disease.

Efficacy

- The American Academy of Neurology's practice parameter on neuroprotective strategies and alternative therapies for Parkinson disease concluded that vitamin E is probably ineffective for the treatment of Parkinson disease and recommended that for patients with Parkinson disease, vitamin E should not be considered for symptomatic treatment.

- A large clinical trial involving 800 participants with early stage Parkinson disease evaluated the effects of deprenyl (a monoamine oxidase inhibitor) and tocopherol (a component of vitamin E) on the progression of disability and found that tocopherol did not delay the onset of disability associated with Parkinson.

Safety

- High doses of alpha tocopherol supplements can cause hemorrhage and interrupt blood coagulation in animals, and *in vitro* data suggest that high doses inhibit platelet aggregation.

- Results from a large, the Selenium and Vitamin E Cancer Prevention Trial (SELECT) show that vitamin E supplements (400 international units (IU)/day) may harm adult men in the general population by increasing their risk of prostate cancer. Follow up studies are assessing whether the cancer risk was associated with baseline blood levels of vitamin E and selenium prior to supplementation as well as whether changes in one or more genes might increase a man's risk of developing prostate cancer while taking vitamin E.

Chapter 13

Nutrition and PD

Chapter Contents

Section 13.1

Eating Right If You Have PD

This section includes text excerpted from "Nutrition for Parkinson's Disease," U.S. Department of Veterans Affairs (VA), September 2009. Reviewed January 2018.

Leading a healthy lifestyle is important for managing Parkinson disease. Follow the tips given below and you will be on your way to good health.

- **Eat three meals a day.** Eating during the day will give you more energy and help you to feel better. Eating more often can also help prevent feelings of nausea and poor appetite.

- **Maintain a healthy body weight.** Most people with Parkinson experience unwanted weight loss. If you have unwanted weight loss, add snacks between each meal.

- **Eat slowly.** Many people with Parkinson experience chewing, swallowing, and coordination difficulties which requires more time to eat a meal. Plan your day around meal times giving yourself plenty of time.

- **Eat a variety of food groups.** Eating a variety of foods such as: whole grains, vegetables, fruit, milk/dairy, and meat/beans will help you get enough vitamins, minerals and calories.

- **Increase your intake of calcium and vitamin D.** People with Parkinson are at an increased risk for osteoporosis, a disease caused by low bone-mineral density. To prevent broken bones eat a diet rich in calcium and vitamin D. Diet alone may not provide enough calcium and vitamin D. Ask your provider if you need a supplement.

- **Good sources of calcium:**
  - Low fat dairy products (milk, yogurt, cottage cheese, etc.).
  - Deep green vegetables (broccoli, collard greens, spinach, kale, etc.).

- Calcium fortified breads and cereals.
- 100 percent fruit juice fortified with calcium.
- **Good sources of Vitamin D:**
  - 15–30 minutes in the sunshine.
  - Low fat dairy products fortified with Vitamin D.
  - Fatty fish (salmon, sardines, tuna, herring, trout).
  - 100 percent fruit juice fortified with Vitamin D.
- **Drink plenty of fluids.** Aim for drinking 6–8 cups of noncaffeinated fluids every day. Water and other fluids are needed to prevent constipation and to keep the body working well.
- **Tips for drinking more fluids:**
  - Have a bottle of water with you at all times.
  - Use a squirt bottle or straw if it makes it easier for you to drink.
  - Keep a bottle or pitcher of water in the fridge at all times for cool refreshing water at any hour.
  - Soups, ice cream, popsicles, and gelatin count as fluids.
- **Eat More Fiber.** Many people with Parkinson experience constipation. Eating more fiber will help. Remember to increase your fluids with an increase in fiber.
- **Good sources of Fiber:**
  - Whole grain breads and cereals
  - Bran cereal and muffins
  - Oatmeal
  - Beans (kidney, baked, navy, etc.)
  - Corn
  - Peas
  - Carrots
  - Bananas
  - Prunes

- **Be active.** Exercise improves mobility, flexibility, balance and mood. It can also help prevent constipation. Do as much activity as your stage of Parkinson allows you to do. Work with your physical therapist to find exercises that you enjoy and will help to keep you moving.

- **Possible exercises include:**
  - Walking
  - Swimming
  - Arm circles
  - Shoulder shrugs
  - Dancing
  - Biking
  - Leg lifts
  - Arm curls
  - Stretching

Section 13.2

Swallowing Problems Sometimes Associated with PD

This section includes text excerpted from "Dysphagia,"
National Institute on Deafness and Other Communication
Disorders (NIDCD), March 6, 2017.

What Is Dysphagia?

People with dysphagia have difficulty swallowing and may even experience pain while swallowing (odynophagia). Some people may be completely unable to swallow or may have trouble safely swallowing liquids, foods, or saliva. When that happens, eating becomes a challenge. Often, dysphagia makes it difficult to take in enough calories and fluids to nourish the body and can lead to additional serious medical problems.

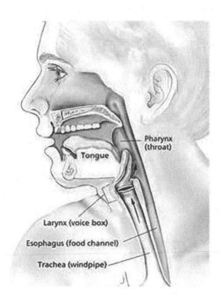

Figure 13.1. *Parts of the Mouth and Neck Involved in Swallowing*

How Do We Swallow?

Swallowing is a complex process. Some 50 pairs of muscles and many nerves work to receive food into the mouth, prepare it, and move it from the mouth to the stomach. This happens in three stages. During the first stage, called the oral phase, the tongue collects the food or liquid, making it ready for swallowing. The tongue and jaw move solid food around in the mouth so it can be chewed. Chewing makes solid food the right size and texture to swallow by mixing the food with saliva. Saliva softens and moistens the food to make swallowing easier. Normally, the only solid we swallow without chewing is in the form of a pill or caplet. Everything else that we swallow is in the form of a liquid, a puree, or a chewed solid.

The second stage begins when the tongue pushes the food or liquid to the back of the mouth. This triggers a swallowing response that passes the food through the pharynx, or throat. During this phase, called the pharyngeal phase, the larynx (voice box) closes tightly and breathing stops to prevent food or liquid from entering the airway and lungs.

The third stage begins when food or liquid enters the esophagus, the tube that carries food and liquid to the stomach. The passage through

103

the esophagus, called the esophageal phase, usually occurs in about three seconds, depending on the texture or consistency of the food, but can take slightly longer in some cases, such as when swallowing a pill.

How Does Dysphagia Occur?

Dysphagia occurs when there is a problem with the neural control or the structures involved in any part of the swallowing process. Weak tongue or cheek muscles may make it hard to move food around in the mouth for chewing. A stroke or other nervous system disorder may make it difficult to start the swallowing response, a stimulus that allows food and liquids to move safely through the throat. Another difficulty can occur when weak throat muscles, such as after cancer surgery, cannot move all of the food toward the stomach. Dysphagia may also result from disorders of the esophagus.

What Are Some Problems Caused by Dysphagia?

Dysphagia can be serious. Someone who cannot swallow safely may not be able to eat enough of the right foods to stay healthy or maintain an ideal weight.

Food pieces that are too large for swallowing may enter the throat and block the passage of air. In addition, when foods or liquids enter the airway of someone who has dysphagia, coughing or throat clearing sometimes cannot remove it. Food or liquid that stays in the airway may enter the lungs and allow harmful bacteria to grow, resulting in a lung infection called aspiration pneumonia.

Swallowing disorders may also include the development of a pocket outside the esophagus caused by weakness in the esophageal wall. This abnormal pocket traps some food being swallowed. While lying down or sleeping, someone with this problem may draw undigested food into the throat. The esophagus may also be too narrow, causing food to stick. This food may prevent other food or even liquids from entering the stomach.

What Causes Dysphagia?

Dysphagia has many possible causes and happens most frequently in older adults. Any condition that weakens or damages the muscles and nerves used for swallowing may cause dysphagia. For example, people with diseases of the nervous system, such as cerebral palsy or Parkinson disease, often have problems swallowing. Additionally, stroke or head injury may weaken or affect the coordination of the swallowing muscles or limit sensation in the mouth and throat.

People born with abnormalities of the swallowing mechanism may not be able to swallow normally. Infants who are born with an opening in the roof of the mouth (cleft palate (CP)) are unable to suck properly, which complicates nursing and drinking from a regular baby bottle.

In addition, cancer of the head, neck, or esophagus may cause swallowing problems. Sometimes the treatment for these types of cancers can cause dysphagia. Injuries of the head, neck, and chest may also create swallowing problems. An infection or irritation can cause narrowing of the esophagus. Finally, for people with dementia, memory loss, and cognitive decline may make it difficult to chew and swallow.

How Is Dysphagia Treated?

There are different treatments for various types of dysphagia. Medical doctors and speech language pathologists who evaluate and treat swallowing disorders use a variety of tests that allow them to look at the stages of the swallowing process. One test, the Flexible Endoscopic Evaluation of Swallowing with Sensory Testing (FEESST), uses a lighted fiber optic tube, or endoscope, to view the mouth and throat while examining how the swallowing mechanism responds to such stimuli as a puff of air, food, or liquids.

A videofluoroscopic swallow study (VFSS) is a test in which a clinician takes a videotaped X-ray of the entire swallowing process by having you consume several foods or liquids along with the mineral barium to improve visibility of the digestive tract. Such images help identify where in the swallowing process you are experiencing problems. Speech language pathologists use this method to explore what changes can be made to offer a safe strategy when swallowing. The changes may be in food texture, size, head and neck posture, or behavioral maneuvers, such as "chin tuck," a strategy in which you tuck your chin so that food and other substances do not enter the trachea when swallowing. If you are unable to swallow safely despite rehabilitation strategies, then medical or surgical intervention may be necessary for the short-term as you recover. In progressive conditions such as amyotrophic lateral sclerosis (ALS, or Lou Gehrig disease (LGD)), a feeding tube in the stomach may be necessary for the long term.

For some people, treatment may involve muscle exercises to strengthen weak facial muscles or to improve coordination. For others, treatment may involve learning to eat in a special way. For example, some people may have to eat with their head turned to one side or looking straight ahead. Preparing food in a certain way or avoiding certain foods may help in some situations. For instance, people who cannot swallow thin liquids may need to add special thickeners to their drinks. Other people may have to avoid hot or cold foods or drinks.

For some, however, consuming enough foods and liquids by mouth may no longer be possible. These individuals must use other methods to nourish their bodies. Usually this involves a feeding system, such as a feeding tube, that bypasses or supplements the part of the swallowing mechanism that is not working normally.

What Research Is Being Done on Dysphagia?

Scientists are conducting research that will improve the ability of physicians and speech language pathologists to evaluate and treat swallowing disorders. Every aspect of the swallowing process is being studied in people of all ages, including those who do not have dysphagia, to give researchers a better understanding of how normal and disordered processes compare.

Research has also led to new, safe ways to study tongue and throat movements during the swallowing process. These methods will help physicians and speech language pathologists safely evaluate a patient's progress during treatment.

Studies of treatment methods are helping scientists discover why some forms of treatment work with some people and not with others. This knowledge will help some people avoid serious lung infections and help others avoid tube feedings.

Chapter 14

Exercise and Physical Activity for Parkinson Disease

Parkinson Disease and Exercises[1]

Parkinson disease (PD) is a disabling neurodegenerative disease for which current treatments are suboptimal. As exercise is generally safe, inexpensive, and associated with secondary benefits, interest in exercise as a treatment for the motor symptoms of the disease is increasing. In this chapter, researchers offer compelling evidence that exercise can improve gait and fitness among individuals with PD. This research adds to the evidence regarding the value of interventions for PD beyond medications and surgery and offers an opportunity for patients to be active participants in their care.

This chapter includes text excerpted from documents published by two public domain sources. Text under headings marked 1 are excerpted from "The Benefits of Exercise in Parkinson Disease," U.S. Department of Health and Human Services (HHS), August 5, 2014. Reviewed January 2018; Text under headings marked 2 are excerpted from "Exercise and Physical Activity," U.S. Department of Veterans Affairs (VA), May 2017.

Types of Exercise[2]

- **Aerobic:** involves the cardiorespiratory system and should be done continuously for at least 10 minutes at a time.

  Examples: walking, jogging, bicycle riding (stationary or outside), swimming, water aerobics, dancing, tennis, golf (without a cart), raking leaves, pushing a lawn mower.

- **Flexibility or stretching:** helps with range of motion and posture, combats rigidity, releases muscle tension, improves circulation and balance.

  Examples: simple arm and leg stretches, head tilts and neck turns, trunk twists, tai chi, yoga.

- **Muscle strengthening and core:** involves external resistance against muscles.

  Examples: lifting weights with dumbbells or free weights, using resistance bands, Pilates, using weight machines.

- **Passive:** for people having a hard time moving by their self. Therapists or family members move arms and legs for them.

  Example: range of motion exercises.

Benefits of Exercise[1]

Researchers performed a comparative, prospective, randomized, single-blinded clinical trial of 3 types of exercise among patients with PD and gait impairment. 67 patients were randomized to either lower-intensity treadmill exercise, higher-intensity treadmill exercise, or a combination of stretching and resistance training. For their primary outcome of gait speed, all training types increased distance walked in 6 minutes at 4 months, but lower-intensity treadmill exercise led to the greatest increases. For their secondary outcome of cardiovascular fitness, both treadmill groups demonstrated improvement. In contrast, the stretching-resistance group improved muscle strength and motor scores on the Unified Parkinson Disease Rating Scale (UPDRS). They concluded that all 3 types of exercise have benefits, and patients may benefit most from a combination of lower-intensity training and stretching and resistance.

The investigation by the researchers adds to the growing body of literature demonstrating the value of exercise in PD. The Cochrane Collaboration examined randomized controlled trials that compared physiotherapy to placebo, and only 11 trials were eligible for their systematic review. At that time, researchers concluded that there was "insufficient evidence to support or refute the efficacy of physiotherapy in Parkinson disease." The evidence had increased, and Cochrane's updated review included 33 trials and discussed 6 additional ongoing studies. Using these new data, they concluded that while differences between physiotherapy and placebo groups in motor performance and other measures were small, they would be clinically meaningful to patients. While the investigation by the researchers certainly stands out in its rigorous method and large patient participation, each study demonstrates the importance of exercise in improving the health and well-being of individuals with PD.

Beyond its benefits on physical health, exercise gives patients a more active role in the management of their PD. Patients are thirsting for such a role, which is consistent with a patient-centered care model in which healthcare is "closely congruent with and responsive to patients' wants, needs, and preferences." The study by the researchers provides physicians and patients with evidence about what patients can do to improve and take charge of their health.

Exercise programs among those with neurological disorders increase the patients' sense of self-efficacy, their sense of involvement in their care and overall belief in their abilities to perform certain activities. In addition, patient involvement leads to higher satisfaction with care, and greater likelihood of following provider recommendations. In essence, exercise puts the patient—not a pill—at the center of care, which is exactly where patients want and ought to be.

Exercise May Help These Symptoms[2]

- slowness
- stiffness or rigidity
- gait
- balance problems
- tremor
- constipation
- depression

Ideas and Tips for Exercise[2]

- Popular Parkinson community suggestions include: walking, water exercises, bicycling, dancing, tai chi, yoga, boxing, Nintendo Wii or Microsoft Kinect Xbox games.
- Pick something fun. What activities did you enjoy as a youth?

- Try several things until you find something you like to do regularly.

- Pair with music to stay motivated and keep the intensity up.

- Go for a walk each day. Wear a pedometer and count your steps.

- Find out what is available in your community. Inquire at your hospital, clinic, support group, local gym, Young Men's Christian Association (YMCA), dance studio, or parks and recreation department.

- Ask for a referral to a rehabilitation doctor, physical therapist, occupational therapist, or kinesiotherapist.

Chapter 15

Driving and PD

You have been a safe driver for years. For you, driving means freedom and control. As you get older, changes in your physical and mental health can affect how safely you drive. Parkinson disease is a disorder of the central nervous system that weakens certain nerve cells in the brain over time. It changes the way your body moves. While it can occur at any age, it especially affects people 60 and older. If you have Parkinson, it can interfere with your daily activities, including driving safely. Early symptoms vary from person to person, but often include slow movement; stiffness of the arms, legs, or trunk; tremors or shaking while at rest; and problems with balance and falls.

How Can Parkinson Affect the Way I Drive?

Parkinson can cause your arms, hands, or legs to shake, even when you are relaxed. It can make it hard to keep your balance and to start moving when you have been still. It also may prevent you from:

- Reacting quickly to road hazards.

- Turning the steering wheel.

- Using the gas pedal or pushing down the brake when you need to react quickly.

- Driving safely at night because of changes in your vision.

This chapter includes text excerpted from "Driving When You Have Parkinson's Disease," National Highway Traffic Safety Administration (NHTSA), February 24, 2015.

What Should I Do If I Have Any of These Signs?

As soon as you notice any of these warning signs:

• Tell your family or someone close to you.

• Talk to your healthcare provider about ways to treat your condition. Some drugs may affect your ability to drive safely.

• Stay active. Exercise regularly to strengthen muscles you need to drive safely.

What Can I Do When Parkinson Affects My Driving Safety?

It is important to know how Parkinson is changing your driving safety. Your healthcare provider may suggest that you see a specialist to help you adjust to these changes.

Two types of specialists can help you:

1. **A driver rehabilitation specialist** can test how well you drive on and off the road. This specialist also can help you decide when you need to stop driving. To find a driver rehabilitation specialist, go to www.aota.org/olderdriver. Under "Driving & Community Mobility," click the button in the center of the page marked "Search for a Driver Rehabilitation Specialist." This will link you to a national database. There you can search for names and addresses of local driver rehabilitation specialists.

2. **An occupational therapist with special training in driving skills assessment and remediation.** To find an occupational therapist, contact local hospitals and rehabilitation centers.

What Can I Do If I Have to Limit or Stop Driving?

If you have Parkinson, you still may be able to drive safely during the early stages of the disease. Your healthcare provider will tell you what to do to manage your symptoms so you stay safe on the road.

Even if you have to limit or give up driving, you can stay active and do the things you like to do.

First, plan ahead. Talk with family and friends about how you can shift from driver to passenger. Below are some ways to get where you want to go and see the people you want to see:

- Rides with family and friends.

- Taxis. Shuttle buses or vans.

- Public buses, trains, and subways.

- Walking.

- Paratransit services (special transportation services for people with disabilities; some offer door-to-door service).

Take someone with you. You may want to have a family member or friend go with you when you use public transportation or when you walk. Having someone with you can help you get where you want to go without confusion.

Find out about transportation services in your area. Many community-based volunteer programs offer free or low-cost transportation.

Where Can I Get Help with Transportation?

To find transportation services in your area, visit www.eldercare. gov or call the national ElderCare Locator at 800-677-1116, and ask for your local Office on Aging.

If you have a disability, check out Easter Seals Project ACTION at www.projectaction.org or call 800-659-6428. This project works with the transportation industry and the disability community to give people with disabilities more ways to get around.

Chapter 16

Employment with PD

Is Parkinson Disease a Disability Under the Americans with Disabilities Act (ADA)?

The ADA does not contain a list of medical conditions that constitute disabilities. Instead, the ADA has a general definition of disability that each person must meet. Therefore, some people with Parkinson disease will have a disability under the ADA and some will not.

A person has a disability if he/she has a physical or mental impairment that substantially limits one or more major life activities, a record of such an impairment, or is regarded as having an impairment.

Accommodating Employees with Parkinson Disease (PD)

People with Parkinson disease may develop some limitations but seldom develop all of them. Also, the degree of limitation will vary among individuals. Be aware that not all people with Parkinson disease will need accommodations to perform their jobs and many others may only need a few accommodations. The following is only a sample of the possibilities available. Numerous other accommodation solutions may exist.

This chapter includes text excerpted from "Employees with Parkinson's Disease Accommodation and Compliance Series," Office of Disability Employment Policy (ODEP), U.S. Department of Labor (DOL), February 15, 2017.

Questions to Consider

1. What limitations is the employee with Parkinson disease experiencing?

2. How do these limitations affect the employee and the employee's job performance?

3. What specific job tasks are problematic as a result of these limitations?

4. What accommodations are available to reduce or eliminate these problems? Are all possible resources being used to determine possible accommodations?

5. Has the employee with Parkinson disease been consulted regarding possible accommodations?

6. Once accommodations are in place, would it be useful to meet with the employee with Parkinson disease to evaluate the effectiveness of the accommodations and to determine whether additional accommodations are needed?

7. Do supervisory personnel and employees need training regarding Parkinson disease?

Accommodation Ideas

Fine Motor:

- Implement ergonomic workstation design
- Provide arm supports
- Provide alternative computer access and a keyguard
- Provide alternative telephone access
- Provide writing and grip aids
- Provide a page turner and a book holder
- Provide a note taker

Gross Motor:

- Reduce walking or provide a scooter or other mobility aid
- Provide parking close to the work-site
- Provide an accessible entrance

- Install automatic door openers
- Provide an accessible route of travel to other work areas used by the employee
- Move workstation close to other work areas, office equipment, and break rooms

Fatigue/Weakness:

- Reduce or eliminate physical exertion and workplace stress
- Schedule periodic rest breaks away from the workstation
- Allow a flexible work schedule and flexible use of leave time
- Allow work from home
- Make sure materials and equipment are within reach range

Speech:

- Provide speech amplification, speech enhancement, or other communication device
- Use written communication, such as email or fax
- Transfer to a position that does not require a lot of communication
- Allow periodic rest breaks

Medical Treatment Allowances:

- Provide flexible schedules
- Provide flexible leave
- Allow a self-paced workload with flexible hours
- Allow employee to work from home
- Provide part-time work schedules

Depression and Anxiety:

- Reduce distractions in work environment
- Provide to-do lists and written instructions
- Remind employee of important deadlines and meetings
- Allow time off for counseling

- Provide clear expectations of responsibilities and consequences
- Provide sensitivity training to co-workers
- Allow breaks to use stress management techniques
- Develop strategies to deal with work problems before they arise
- Allow telephone calls during work hours to doctors and others for support
- Provide information on counseling and employee assistance programs

Cognitive Impairment:

- Provide written job instructions when possible with more structure
- Prioritize job assignments
- Allow flexible work hours
- Allow periodic rest breaks to reorient
- Provide memory aids, such as schedulers or organizers
- Minimize distractions
- Allow a self-paced workload
- Reduce job stress

Activities of Daily Living (ADL):

- Allow use of a personal attendant at work
- Allow use of a service animal at work
- Make sure the facility is accessible
- Move workstation closer to the restroom
- Allow longer breaks
- Refer to appropriate community services

Situations and Solutions

- A secretary with Parkinson disease and hand tremors was having difficulty using a keyboard, writing, manipulating manuals, and filing. She was accommodated with a keyguard, typing aid, page turner, and open files.

- A supervisor with Parkinson disease was having difficulty managing fatigue. The employer provided a private rest area with a cot so the individual could take breaks throughout the day.

- A file clerk with Parkinson disease was having difficulty meeting the physical demands of the job, including walking between work areas, standing at filing cabinets, and carrying files. The individual was accommodated with a power scooter with a basket and a stand/lean stool.

- A technician with Parkinson disease was having difficulty concentrating. The employee's supervisor provided written job instructions when possible and allowed the individual to have periodic rest breaks. In addition, she was moved to a corner cubicle where distractions were minimized with strategically placed baffles.

- A customer service representative with Parkinson disease was having difficulty manipulating his mouse, writing, standing to greet people, and communicating effectively. He was accommodated with a trackball, writing aid, stool with lift cushion, and speech amplification.

- A technical consultant was having difficulty using the computer in the afternoons due to fatigue. He was accommodated with speech recognition and an ergonomic workstation.

- An office assistant with tremors and fatigue caused by Parkinson disease was having difficulty typing the number of words per minute required by her employer. The individual rearranged her workstation to reduce distractions and her employer offered flexible scheduling. Her word processing software was programmed with macros to reduce keystrokes and she was given speech recognition software.

- A consultant with Parkinson disease was having difficulty getting to work on time. He was accommodated with flexible scheduling so he could use public transportation.

- A teacher with Parkinson disease was having difficulty standing in front of the classroom to write on the board. The individual was accommodated with a scooter and a laptop and PC projector. She was then able to remain seated while using the computer and projector to display information to the class.

- An engineer with Parkinson disease was having difficulty concentrating and communicating. The individual was accommodated with a quiet office free from distractions. In addition, her supervisor implemented a policy of scheduled interruptions with written reminders and assignments. The individual was also provided with a communication device.

Chapter 17

Caring for PD Patients

Physical and Mental Changes to Expect

Parkinson disease (PD) is a chronic and complex neurological disease, not an acute illness. Symptoms of PD vary widely and disease progression can vary considerably from one person to another. But for most people, PD presents as a slow, progressive illness and persons with PD often live an average lifespan. PD is typically thought of as a movement (motor) disorder with symptoms of slowness, stiffness, and tremor. However, a number of nonmotor symptoms commonly occur as well, and may appear before the motor impairments. Nonmotor symptoms can cause problems with thinking, depression and anxiety, loss of smell, vision changes, constipation and sleep disturbances. These nonmotor symptoms are important to quality of life and are often more bothersome than the motor symptoms. It is important to talk to the healthcare team about all symptoms so they can be addressed properly. Symptoms can be controlled by medication and other therapies. However, in the advanced stages of the disease, symptoms such as increased falls and impaired thought processes may become serious enough to warrant in-home support services or long-term care placement such as an assisted living facility or nursing home.

- **Physical changes may include:** Tremor; slowness of movement; stiffness of the arms, legs or trunk; balance problems;

This chapter includes text excerpted from "I'm Caring for a Veteran with Parkinson's Disease (PD)—What Do I Need to Know?" U.S. Department of Veterans Affairs (VA), July 1, 2013. Reviewed January 2018.

freezing of gait; small, cramped handwriting; reduced arm swing; loss of facial expression; softness of voice; tendency to fall backwards; walking with a series of quick, small steps; constipation; erectile dysfunction; bladder control problems; drooling; sleep problems; loss of sense of smell; vision changes; and restless leg syndrome.

- **Mental changes may include:** Difficulty with attention, focus, planning, multitasking; visual spatial functions (driving); apathy or lack of motivation; hallucinations (seeing things that aren't really there) and/or delusions (believing things that aren't true); impulsive behavior (gambling, shopping, eating, sexual behaviors); problems with memory.

- **Emotional changes may include:** Anxiety and depression.

Caregiving Tips

1. **Educate yourself and find a good doctor:** Keep up to date on your loved one's disease and do not be afraid to ask questions at doctor visits. Being educated helps you better understand what is happening to your loved one. Always bring an updated list of medications to all doctor appointments. Consider finding a neurologist who specializes in movement disorder.

2. **Hospitalization and PD:** Being hospitalized can be stressful for both the person with PD and his/her caregiver. Often, it becomes the caregiver's responsibility to educate hospital staff on the importance of the medication schedule and ensuring the patient is receiving his/her medications on time, as they may not be knowledgeable about PD management and treatment. Contact the patient's movement disorder specialist or treating neurologist to make them aware of the hospitalization and ask him/her to contact the hospital neurologist to discuss the treatment plan.

3. **Take care of yourself:** Address your own medical needs, eat well, exercise, sleep and take time for yourself. It is important to maintain your health so you can continue to provide the best care for the person with PD. Do not allow the disease to become you or the center of your life. Maintain a healthy social life and hobbies you had before you became a caregiver.

4. **Be realistic and access help:** Know what you can do and recognize when you have given all that you can. Access community resources such as home healthcare, respite, adult day healthcare, nursing home, etc. If family members or friends offer to help, let them, and be specific in ways they can help.

5. **Depression:** Be aware of the signs and symptoms of depression for both you and the patient and do not delay in seeking support or professional counseling. Keep contact information for a psychiatrist/therapist and other emergency phone numbers handy.

6. **Breathe/meditate:** Try yoga, tai chi, and/or deep breathing. These exercises will help slow your heart rate and calm your emotional state which, in turn, will help you think more clearly and feel refreshed.

7. **Emotional support:** Consider attending a support group where you can share your concerns and feelings and talk with other caregivers. This can help reduce any feelings of being alone. Support groups offer mutual support as well as valuable information on PD.

8. **Positive thinking and humor:** Think "I can do this!" Laughing is a great stress reliever.

9. **Long-term care planning:** It is important to explore future plans such as advance directives, living wills and care at home versus nursing home placement, etc. Be sure to discuss these issues and decisions with loved ones to ensure their wishes are followed.

What Does This Mean for Me?

It is possible to live well with PD despite the physical, and/or cognitive changes that come with the disease progression. PD is often considered a family disease because of the effect it may have on the person's family and friends. Being a caregiver is an important role and most often performed by the spouse, or an adult child. In the early and middle stages of the disease, the role is often described as a partnership. The care partner and the person with PD have a dynamic relationship as both adjust to sharing duties and working together. In the later stages of the disease, caring for someone with PD may become physically and emotionally draining. It is important for caregivers to remember that it is okay to ask for help, and to acknowledge that one person cannot do it alone. Caregivers often feel empowered and supported by staying engaged in social activities, building a strong backup team, and attending support groups.

Part Three

Other Hypokinetic Movement Disorders: Slowed or Absent Movements

Chapter 18

Amyotrophic Lateral Sclerosis (ALS)

What Is Amyotrophic Lateral Sclerosis (ALS)?

Amyotrophic lateral sclerosis (ALS) is a rare group of neurological diseases that mainly involve the nerve cells (neurons) responsible for controlling voluntary muscle movement. Voluntary muscles produce movements like chewing, walking, breathing, and talking. The disease is progressive, meaning the symptoms get worse over time. Currently, there is no cure for ALS and no effective treatment to halt, or reverse, the progression of the disease.

ALS belongs to a wider group of disorders known as motor neuron diseases, which are caused by gradual deterioration (degeneration) and death of motor neurons. Motor neurons are nerve cells that extend from the brain to the spinal cord and to muscles throughout the body. These motor neurons initiate and provide vital communication links between the brain and the voluntary muscles.

Messages from motor neurons in the brain (called upper motor neurons) are transmitted to motor neurons in the spinal cord and to motor nuclei of brain (called lower motor neurons) and from the spinal cord and motor nuclei of brain to a particular muscle or muscles.

This chapter includes text excerpted from "Amyotrophic Lateral Sclerosis (ALS) Fact Sheet," National Institute of Neurological Disorders and Stroke (NINDS), June 2013. Reviewed January 2018.

In ALS, both the upper motor neurons and the lower motor neurons degenerate or die, and stop sending messages to the muscles. Unable to function, the muscles gradually weaken, start to twitch (called fasciculations), and waste away (atrophy). Eventually, the brain loses its ability to initiate and control voluntary movements.

Early symptoms of ALS usually include muscle weakness or stiffness. Gradually all muscles under voluntary control are affected, and individuals lose their strength and the ability to speak, eat, move, and even breathe.

Most people with ALS die from respiratory failure, usually within 3–5 years from when the symptoms first appear. However, about 10 percent of people with ALS survive for 10 or more years.

Who Gets ALS?

Centers for Disease Control and Prevention (CDC) estimated that between 14,000–15,000 Americans have ALS. ALS is a common neuromuscular disease worldwide. It affects people of all races and ethnic backgrounds.

There are several potential risk factors for ALS including:

- **Age.** Although the disease can strike at any age, symptoms most commonly develop between the ages of 55 and 75.

- **Gender.** Men are slightly more likely than women to develop ALS. However, as age the difference between men and women disappears.

- **Race and ethnicity.** Most likely to develop the disease are Caucasians and non-Hispanics.

Some studies suggest that military veterans are about 1.5–2 times more likely to develop ALS. Although the reason for this is unclear, possible risk factors for veterans include exposure to lead, pesticides, and other environmental toxins. ALS is recognized as a service-connected disease by the U.S. Department of Veterans Affairs (VA).

Sporadic ALS

The majority of ALS cases (90 percent or more) are considered sporadic. This means the disease seems to occur at random with no clearly associated risk factors and no family history of the disease. Although family members of people with sporadic ALS are at an increased risk for the disease, the overall risk is very low and most will not develop ALS.

Familial (Genetic) ALS

About 5–10 percent of all ALS cases are familial, which means that an individual inherits the disease from his or her parents. The familial form of ALS usually only requires one parent to carry the gene responsible for the disease. Mutations in more than a dozen genes have been found to cause familial ALS. About 25–40 percent of all familial cases (and a small percentage of sporadic cases) are caused by a defect in a gene known as "chromosome 9 open reading frame 72," or *C9ORF72*. Interestingly, the same mutation can be associated with atrophy of frontal-temporal lobes of the brain causing frontal-temporal lobe dementia. Some individuals carrying this mutation may show signs of both motor neuron and dementia symptoms (ALS-FTD). Another 12–20 percent of familial cases result from mutations in the gene that provides instructions for the production of the enzyme copper-zinc superoxide dismutase 1 (*SOD1*).

What Are the Symptoms?

The onset of ALS can be so subtle that the symptoms are overlooked but gradually these symptoms develop into more obvious weakness or atrophy that may cause a physician to suspect ALS. Some of the early symptoms include:

- fasciculations (muscle twitches) in the arm, leg, shoulder, or tongue
- muscle cramps
- tight and stiff muscles (spasticity)
- muscle weakness affecting an arm, a leg, neck, or diaphragm.
- slurred and nasal speech
- difficulty chewing or swallowing

For many individuals the first sign of ALS may appear in the hand or arm as they experience difficulty with simple tasks such as buttoning a shirt, writing, or turning a key in a lock. In other cases, symptoms initially affect one of the legs, and people experience awkwardness when walking or running or they notice that they are tripping or stumbling more often.

When symptoms begin in the arms or legs, it is referred to as "limb onset" ALS. Other individuals first notice speech or swallowing problems, termed "bulbar onset" ALS.

Regardless of where the symptoms first appear, muscle weakness and atrophy spread to other parts of the body as the disease progresses. Individuals may develop problems with moving, swallowing (dysphagia), speaking or forming words (dysarthria), and breathing (dyspnea).

Although the sequence of emerging symptoms and the rate of disease progression vary from person to person, eventually individuals will not be able to stand or walk, get in or out of bed on their own, or use their hands and arms.

Individuals with ALS usually have difficulty swallowing and chewing food, which makes it hard to eat normally and increases the risk of choking. They also burn calories at a faster rate than most people without ALS. Due to these factors, people with ALS tend to lose weight rapidly and can become malnourished.

Because people with ALS usually retain their ability to perform higher mental processes such as reasoning, remembering, understanding, and problem solving, they are aware of their progressive loss of function and may become anxious and depressed.

A small percentage of individuals may experience problems with language or decision-making, and there is growing evidence that some may even develop a form of dementia over time.

Individuals with ALS will have difficulty breathing as the muscles of the respiratory system weaken. They eventually lose the ability to breathe on their own and must depend on a ventilator. Affected individuals also face an increased risk of pneumonia during later stages of the disease. Besides muscle cramps that may cause discomfort, some individuals with ALS may develop painful neuropathy (nerve disease or damage).

How Is ALS Diagnosed?

No one test can provide a definitive diagnosis of ALS. ALS is primarily diagnosed based on detailed history of the symptoms and signs observed by a physician during physical examination along with a series of tests to rule out other mimicking diseases. However, the presence of upper and lower motor neuron symptoms strongly suggests the presence of the disease.

Physicians will review an individual's full medical history and conduct a neurologic examination at regular intervals to assess whether symptoms such as muscle weakness, atrophy of muscles, and spasticity are getting progressively worse.

ALS symptoms in the early stages of the disease can be similar to those of a wide variety of other, more treatable diseases or disorders. Appropriate tests can exclude the possibility of other conditions.

Muscle and Imaging Tests

Electromyography (EMG), a special recording technique that detects electrical activity of muscle fibers, can help diagnose ALS. Another common test is a nerve conduction study (NCS), which measures electrical activity of the nerves and muscles by assessing the nerve's ability to send a signal along the nerve or to the muscle. Specific abnormalities in the NCS and EMG may suggest, for example, that the individual has a form of peripheral neuropathy (damage to peripheral nerves outside of the brain and spinal cord) or myopathy (muscle disease) rather than ALS.

A physician may also order a magnetic resonance imaging (MRI) test, a noninvasive procedure that uses a magnetic field and radio waves to produce detailed images of the brain and spinal cord. Standard MRI scans are generally normal in people with ALS. However, they can reveal other problems that may be causing the symptoms, such as a spinal cord tumor, a herniated disk in the neck that compresses the spinal cord, syringomyelia (a cyst in the spinal cord), or cervical spondylosis (abnormal wear affecting the spine in the neck).

Laboratory Tests

Based on the person's symptoms, test results, and findings from the examination, a physician may order tests on blood and urine samples to eliminate the possibility of other diseases.

Tests for Other Diseases and Disorders

Infectious diseases such as human immunodeficiency virus (HIV), human T-cell leukemia virus (HTLV), polio, and West Nile virus can, in some cases, cause ALS-like symptoms. Neurological disorders such as multiple sclerosis, postpolio syndrome, multifocal motor neuropathy, and spinal and bulbar muscular atrophy (Kennedy disease) also can mimic certain features of the disease and should be considered by physicians attempting to make a diagnosis. Fasciculations and muscle cramps also occur in benign conditions.

Because of the prognosis carried by this diagnosis and the variety of diseases or disorders that can resemble ALS in the early stages of the disease, individuals may wish to obtain a second neurological opinion.

What Causes ALS?

The cause of ALS is not known, and scientists do not yet know why ALS strikes some people and not others. However, evidence from scientific studies suggests that both genetics and environment play a role in the development of ALS.

Genetics

An important step toward determining ALS risk factors was made in 1993 when scientists supported by the National Institute of Neurological Disorders and Stroke (NINDS) discovered that mutations in the *SOD1* gene were associated with some cases of familial ALS. Although it is still not clear how mutations in the *SOD1* gene lead to motor neuron degeneration, there is increasing evidence that the gene playing a role in producing mutant SOD1 protein can become toxic.

Since then, more than a dozen additional genetic mutations have been identified and each of these gene discoveries is providing new insights into possible mechanisms of ALS. The discovery of certain genetic mutations involved in ALS suggests that changes in the processing of ribonucleic acid (RNA) molecules may lead to ALS-related motor neuron degeneration. RNA molecules are one of the major macromolecules in the cell involved in directing the synthesis of specific proteins as well as gene regulation and activity.

Other gene mutations indicate defects in the natural process in which malfunctioning proteins are broken down and used to build new ones, known as protein recycling. Still others point to possible defects in the structure and shape of motor neurons, as well as increased susceptibility to environmental toxins. Overall, it is becoming increasingly clear that a number of cellular defects can lead to motor neuron degeneration in ALS.

Another important discovery was made when scientists found that a defect in the *C9ORF72* gene is not only present in a significant subset of individuals with ALS but also in some people with a type of frontotemporal dementia (FTD). This observation provides evidence for genetic ties between these two neurodegenerative disorders. Most researchers now believe ALS and some forms of FTD are related disorders.

Environmental Factors

In searching for the cause of ALS, researchers are also studying the impact of environmental factors. Researchers are investigating a number of possible causes such as exposure to toxic or infectious agents, viruses, physical trauma, diet, and behavioral and occupational factors. For example, researchers have suggested that exposure to toxins during warfare, or strenuous physical activity, are possible reasons for why some veterans and athletes may be at increased risk of developing ALS.

Although there has been no consistent association between any environmental factor and the risk of developing ALS, future research may show that some factors are involved in the development or progression of the disease.

How Is ALS Treated?

No cure has yet been found for ALS. However, there are treatments available that can help control symptoms, prevent unnecessary complications, and make living with the disease easier.

Supportive care is best provided by multidisciplinary teams of healthcare professionals such as physicians; pharmacists; physical, occupational, and speech therapists; nutritionists; social workers; respiratory therapists and clinical psychologists; and home care and hospice nurses. These teams can design an individualized treatment plan and provide special equipment aimed at keeping people as mobile, comfortable, and independent as possible.

Medication

The U.S. Food and Drug Administration (FDA) has approved the drugs riluzole (Rilutek) and edaravone (Radicava) to treat ALS. Riluzole is believed to reduce damage to motor neurons by decreasing levels of glutamate, which transports messages between nerve cells and motor neurons. Clinical trials in people with ALS showed that riluzole prolongs survival by a few months, particularly in the bulbar form of the disease, but does not reverse the damage already done to motor neurons. Edaravone has been shown to slow the decline in clinical assessment of daily functioning in persons with ALS.

Physicians can also prescribe medications to help manage symptoms of ALS, including muscle cramps, stiffness, excess saliva, and phlegm, and the pseudobulbar affect (involuntary or uncontrollable episodes of crying and/or laughing, or other emotional displays). Drugs also are available to help individuals with pain, depression, sleep disturbances, and constipation. Pharmacists can give advice on the proper use of medications and monitor a person's prescriptions to avoid risks of drug interactions.

Physical Therapy

Physical therapy and special equipment can enhance an individual's independence and safety throughout the course of ALS. Gentle, low-impact aerobic exercise such as walking, swimming, and stationary bicycling can strengthen unaffected muscles, improve cardiovascular health, and help people fight fatigue and depression. Range of motion and stretching exercises can help prevent painful spasticity and shortening (contracture) of muscles.

Physical therapists can recommend exercises that provide these benefits without overworking muscles. Occupational therapists can suggest devices such as ramps, braces, walkers, and wheelchairs that help individuals conserve energy and remain mobile.

Speech Therapy

People with ALS who have difficulty speaking may benefit from working with a speech therapist, who can teach adaptive strategies to speak louder and more clearly. As ALS progresses, speech therapists can help people maintain the ability to communicate. They can recommend aids such as computer-based speech synthesizers that use eye-tracking technology and can help people develop ways for responding to yes-or-no questions with their eyes or by other nonverbal means.

Some people with ALS may choose to use voice banking while they are still able to speak as a process of storing their own voice for future use in computer-based speech synthesizers. These methods and devices help people communicate when they can no longer speak or produce vocal sounds.

Nutritional Support

Nutritional support is an important part of the care of people with ALS. It has been shown that individuals with ALS will get weaker if they lose weight. Nutritionists can teach individuals and caregivers how to plan and prepare small meals throughout the day that provide enough calories, fiber, and fluid and how to avoid foods that are difficult to swallow. People may begin using suction devices to remove excess fluids or saliva and prevent choking. When individuals can no longer get enough nourishment from eating, doctors may advise inserting a feeding tube into the stomach. The use of a feeding tube also reduces the risk of choking and pneumonia that can result from inhaling liquids into the lungs.

Breathing Support

As the muscles responsible for breathing start to weaken, people may experience shortness of breath during physical activity and difficulty breathing at night or when lying down. Doctors may test an individual's breathing to determine when to recommend a treatment called noninvasive ventilation (NIV). NIV refers to breathing support that is usually delivered through a mask over the nose and/or mouth. Initially, NIV may only be necessary at night. When muscles are no longer able to maintain normal oxygen and carbon dioxide levels, NIV may be used full-time. NIV improves the quality of life and prolongs survival for many people with ALS. Because the muscles that control breathing become weak, individuals with ALS may also have trouble generating a strong cough. There are several techniques to help people increase forceful coughing, including mechanical cough assist devices and breath stacking. In breath stacking, a person takes a series of small breaths without exhaling until the lungs are full, briefly holds the breath, and then expels the air with a cough.

As the disease progresses and muscles weaken further, individuals may consider forms of mechanical ventilation (respirators) in which a machine inflates and deflates the lungs. Doctors may place a breathing tube through the mouth or may surgically create a hole at the front of the neck and insert a tube leading to the windpipe (tracheostomy). The tube is connected to a respirator.

Individuals with ALS and their families often consider several factors when deciding whether and when to use ventilation support. These devices differ in their effect on a person's quality of life and in cost. Although ventilation support can ease problems with breathing and prolong survival, it does not affect the progression of ALS. People may choose to be fully informed about these considerations and the long-term effects of life without movement before they make decisions about ventilation support.

What Research Is Being Done?

Cellular Defects

Scientists are seeking to understand the mechanisms that selectively trigger motor neurons to degenerate in ALS, and to find effective approaches to halt the processes leading to cell death. Using both animal models and cell culture systems, scientists are trying to determine how and why ALS-causing gene mutations lead to the destruction of neurons. These animal models include fruit flies, zebrafish, and rodents.

Initially, genetically modified animal models focused on mutations in the *SOD1* gene but more recently, models have been developed for defects in the *C9ORF72*, *TARDP*, *FUS*, *PFN1*, *TUBA4A*, and *UBQLN2* genes. Research in these models suggests that, depending on the gene mutation, motor neuron death is caused by a variety of cellular defects, including in the processing of RNA molecules and recycling of proteins, and structural impairments of motor neurons. Increasing evidence also suggests that various types of glial support cells and inflammation cells of the nervous system may play an important role in the disease.

Stem Cells

In addition to animal models, scientists are also using innovative stem cells models to study ALS. Scientists have developed ways to take skin or blood cells from individuals with ALS and turn them into stem cells, which are capable of becoming any cell type in the body, including motor neurons and other cell types that may be involved in the disease. NINDS is supporting research on the development of stem cell lines for a number of neurodegenerative diseases, including ALS.

Familial versus Sporadic ALS

Overall, the work in familial ALS is already leading to a greater understanding of the more common sporadic form of the disease. Because familial ALS and sporadic ALS show many of the same signs and symptoms, some researchers believe that some familial ALS, genes may also be involved in sporadic ALS.

Clinical research studies supported by NINDS are looking into how ALS symptoms change over time in people with *C9ORF72* mutations. Other NINDS-supported research studies are working to identify additional genes that may cause or put a person at risk for either familial or sporadic ALS.

Additionally, researchers are looking at the potential role of epigenetics in the development of ALS. Epigenetic changes can switch genes on and off, and thus can profoundly affect the human condition in both health and disease. These changes can occur in response to multiple factors, including external or environmental conditions and events. Although this research is still at a very exploratory stage, scientists hope that understanding epigenetics can offer new information about how ALS develops.

Biomarkers

Biomarkers are biological measures that help to identify the presence or rate of progression of a disease or the effectiveness of a therapeutic intervention. Since ALS is difficult to diagnose, biomarkers could potentially help clinicians diagnose ALS earlier and faster.

Additionally, biomarkers are needed to help predict and accurately measure disease progression and enhance clinical studies aimed at developing more effective treatments. Biomarkers can be molecules derived from a bodily fluid (such as those in the blood and cerebrospinal fluid), an image of the brain or spinal cord, or a measure of the ability of a nerve or muscle to process electrical signals. The NINDS is supporting research on the development biomarkers for ALS.

New Treatment Options

Potential therapies for ALS are being investigated in a range of disease models. This work involves tests of drug-like compounds, gene therapy approaches, antibodies, and cell-based therapies. For example, NINDS-supported scientists are investigating whether lowering levels of the SOD1 enzyme in the brain and spinal cord of individuals with *SOD1* gene mutations would slow the rate of disease progression.

Other NINDS scientists are studying the use of glial-restricted progenitor cells (which have the ability to develop into other support cells) to slow disease progression and improve respiratory function. Additionally, a number of exploratory treatments are being tested in people with ALS. Investigators are optimistic that these and other basic, translational, and clinical research studies will eventually lead to new and more effective treatments for ALS.

Chapter 19

Cerebellar or Spinocerebellar Degeneration

Chapter Contents

Section 19.1

Ataxia-Telangiectasia (AT)

This section contains text excerpted from the following sources:
Text beginning with the heading "What Is Ataxia Telangiectasia
(AT)?" is excerpted from "Ataxia Telangiectasia," Genetic and Rare
Diseases Information Center (GARD), National Center for Advancing
Translational Sciences (NCATS), April 15, 2016; Text beginning
with the heading "What Is the Prognosis for AT?" is excerpted from
"Ataxia Telangiectasia Information Page," National Institute of
Neurological Disorders and Stroke (NINDS), September 18, 2011.
Reviewed January 2018.

What Is Ataxia Telangiectasia (AT)?

Ataxia telangiectasia (AT) is rare condition that affects the nervous
system, the immune system, and many other parts of the body. Signs
and symptoms of the condition usually begin in early childhood, often
before age 5. The condition is typically characterized by cerebellar
ataxia (uncoordinated muscle movements), oculomotor apraxia, telan-
giectasias, choreoathetosis (uncontrollable movements of the limbs), a
weakened immune system with frequent infections, and an increased
risk of cancers such as leukemia and lymphoma. AT is caused by
changes (mutations) in the *ATM* gene and is inherited in an autosomal
recessive manner. Treatment is supportive and based on the signs and
symptoms present in each person.

What Are the Signs and Symptoms of AT?

Ataxia-telangiectasia affects the nervous system, immune system,
and other body systems. This disorder is characterized by progressive
difficulty with coordinating movements (ataxia) beginning in early
childhood, usually before age 5. Affected children typically develop
difficulty walking, problems with balance and hand coordination, involuntary jerking movements (chorea), muscle twitches (myoclonus), and
disturbances in nerve function (neuropathy). The movement problems
typically cause people to require wheelchair assistance by adolescence.
People with this disorder also have slurred speech and trouble moving

their eyes to look side-to-side (oculomotor apraxia). Small clusters of enlarged blood vessels called telangiectases, which occur in the eyes and on the surface of the skin, are also characteristic of this condition.

Affected individuals tend to have high amounts of a protein called alpha-fetoprotein (AFP) in their blood. The level of this protein is usually increased in the bloodstream of pregnant women. The effect of abnormally high levels of AFP in people with ataxia-telangiectasia is unknown.

People with ataxia-telangiectasia often have a weakened immune system, and many develop chronic lung infections. They are also at an increased risk of developing cancer, particularly leukemia and lymphoma. Affected individuals are very sensitive to the effects of radiation exposure, including medical X-rays. Although people with ataxia-telangiectasia usually live into adulthood, their life expectancy is reduced.

What Is the Prognosis for AT?

Average lifespan has been improving for years, for unknown reasons, and varies with the severity of the underlying mutations, ATM (ataxia-telangiectasia mutated) protein levels, and residual ATM kinase activity. Some individuals with later onset of disease and slower progression survive into their 50s.

What Treatment Options Are Available for AT?

There is no cure for AT and, currently, no way to slow the progression of the disease. Treatment is symptomatic and supportive. Physical and occupational therapy help to maintain flexibility. Speech therapy is important, teaching children to control air flow to the vocal cords. Gamma-globulin injections may be useful if immunoglobulin levels are sufficiently reduced to weaken the immune system. High-dose vitamin regimens and antioxidants such as alpha lipoic acid also may also be used.

Section 19.2

Friedreich Ataxia

This section includes text excerpted from "Friedreich Ataxia,"
Genetic and Rare Diseases Information Center (GARD), National
Center for Advancing Translational Sciences (NCATS), May 22, 2015.

What Is Friedreich Ataxia?

Friedreich ataxia is an inherited condition that affects the nervous system and causes movement problems. People with this condition develop impaired muscle coordination (ataxia) that worsens over time. Other features include the gradual loss of strength and sensation in the arms and legs, muscle stiffness (spasticity), and impaired speech. Many individuals have a form of heart disease called hypertrophic cardiomyopathy. Some develop diabetes, impaired vision, hearing loss, or an abnormal curvature of the spine (scoliosis). Most people with Friedreich ataxia begin to experience the signs and symptoms around puberty. This condition is caused by mutations in the *FXN* gene and is inherited in an autosomal recessive pattern.

What Are the Signs and Symptoms of Friedreich Ataxia?

Symptoms usually begin between the ages of 5 and 15 but can, on occasion, appear in adulthood or even as late as age 75. The first symptom is usually difficulty walking (gait ataxia). The ataxia gradually worsens and slowly spreads to the arms and then the trunk. Over time, muscles begin to weaken and waste away, especially in the feet, lower legs, and hands. Other symptoms include loss of tendon reflexes, especially in the knees and ankles. There is often a gradual loss of sensation in the extremities, which may spread to other parts of the body. Slurred speech (dysarthria), fatigue, and involuntary eye movements (nystagmus) are also common. Most people with Friedreich ataxia develop scoliosis (a curving of the spine to one side), which, if severe, may impair breathing.

Other symptoms that may occur include chest pain, shortness of breath, and heart palpitations. These symptoms are the result of various forms of heart disease that often accompany Friedreich ataxia, such as cardiomyopathy (enlargement of the heart), myocardial fibrosis (formation of fiber-like material in the muscles of the heart), and cardiac failure. Heart rhythm abnormalities such as tachycardia (fast heart rate) and heart block (impaired conduction of cardiac impulses within the heart) are also common. About 20 percent of people with Friedreich ataxia develop carbohydrate intolerance and 10 percent develop diabetes mellitus. Some people lose hearing or eyesight.

The rate of progression varies from person to person. Generally, within 10–20 years after the first symptoms appear, people with Friedreich ataxia need to consistently use a wheelchair. Life expectancy may be affected, and many people with Friedreich ataxia die in adulthood from the associated heart disease. However, some people with less severe symptoms of Friedreich ataxia live much longer, sometimes into their sixties or seventies.

What Causes Friedreich Ataxia?

Friedreich ataxia is caused by mutations in the *FXN* gene. This gene provides instructions for making a protein called frataxin. One region of the *FXN* gene contains a segment of deoxyribonucleic acid (DNA) known as a GAA trinucleotide repeat. This segment is made up of a series of three DNA building blocks (one guanine and two adenines) that appear multiple times in a row. Normally, this segment is repeated 5–33 times within the *FXN* gene. In people with Friedreich ataxia, the GAA segment is repeated 66 to more than 1,000 times. The length of the GAA trinucleotide repeat appears to be related to the age at which the symptoms of Friedreich ataxia appear.

The abnormally long GAA trinucleotide repeat disrupts the production of frataxin, which severely reduces the amount of this protein in cells. Certain nerve and muscle cells cannot function properly with a shortage of frataxin, leading to the characteristic signs and symptoms of Friedreich ataxia.

Is Friedreich Ataxia Inherited?

Friedreich ataxia is inherited in an autosomal recessive manner. This means that to be affected, a person must have a mutation in both copies of the responsible gene in each cell. The parents of an affected person usually each carry one mutated copy of the gene and are referred to as carriers. Carriers typically do not show signs or symptoms of the condition. When two carriers of an autosomal recessive condition have children, each child has a 25 percent (1 in 4) risk to have the condition, a 50 percent (1 in 2) risk to be a carrier like each of the parents, and a 25 percent chance to not have the condition and not be a carrier.

What Is the Diagnosis for Friedreich Ataxia?

Making a diagnosis for a genetic or rare disease can often be challenging. Healthcare professionals typically look at a person's medical history, symptoms, physical exam, and laboratory test results in order to make a diagnosis. The following resources provide information relating to diagnosis and testing for this condition. If you have questions about getting a diagnosis, you should contact a healthcare professional.

Section 19.3

Machado-Joseph Disease

This section includes text excerpted from "Machado-Joseph Disease Fact Sheet," National Institute of Neurological Disorders and Stroke (NINDS), February 2010. Reviewed January 2018.

What Is Machado-Joseph Disease?

Machado-Joseph disease (MJD)—also called spinocerebellar ataxia Type 3 (SCA3)—is one of approximately 30 recognized, dominantly inherited forms of ataxia. Ataxia is a general term meaning lack of muscle control or coordination. MJD is characterized by slowly progressive clumsiness in the arms and legs, a staggering lurching gait that can be mistaken for drunkenness, difficulty with speech and swallowing, impaired eye movements sometimes accompanied by double vision or bulging eyes, and lower limb spasticity. Some individuals develop dystonia (sustained muscle contractions that cause twisting of the body and limbs, repetitive movements, and abnormal postures) or symptoms similar to those of Parkinson disease. Others may develop fasciculations (twitching) of the face or tongue, neuropathy, or problems with urination and the autonomic nervous system.

The clinical manifestations of MJD can be highly variable, even among affected persons in the same family. This wide range in symptoms reflects the particular type of mutation that causes MJD: a repeat expansion in the deoxyribonucleic acid (DNA) code that varies in size among affected persons. The longer the expansion, typically the more severe the disease. In other words, longer repeat expansions tend to cause disease that begins earlier in life and shows a broader range of neurological symptoms. In most individuals with MJD, symptoms typically begin in the third to fifth decade of life but can start as early as young childhood or as late as 70 years of age.

MJD is a progressive disease, meaning that symptoms worsen with time. Life expectancy ranges from the mid-30s for those with the most severe forms of early onset MJD to a nearly normal life expectancy for those with mild, late onset forms. The cause of death for those who die early from the disease is often aspiration pneumonia.

The name "Machado-Joseph" comes from two families of Portuguese/Azorean descent who were among the first families described with the unique symptoms of the disease in the 1970s. The prevalence of the disease is highest among people of Portuguese/Azorean descent. For example, among immigrants of Portuguese ancestry in New England, the prevalence is around one in 4,000, and the highest prevalence in the world, about 1 in 140, occurs on the small Azorean island of Flores. Soon after the gene defect was discovered, a hereditary ataxia in European families known as SCA3 was found to be caused by the exact same mutation. Thus, SCA3 and MJD are the same disorder.

What Are the Different Types of MJD?

All persons with MJD have the same disease gene mutation: a DNA repeat expansion in the *ATXN3* gene. The wide range in symptoms among affected individuals led researchers to separate the disease into distinct types that are broadly distinguished by age of onset and range of symptoms. Type I MJD is characterized by onset between about 10 and 30 years of age, with faster progression and more dystonia and rigidity than ataxia. Type II, the most common type of MJD, generally begins between the ages of about 20 and 50 years, has an intermediate rate of progression, and causes various symptoms, including prominent ataxia, spastic gait, and enhanced reflex responses. Individuals affected by type III MJD have the latest onset of disease (beginning between approximately 40 and 70 years of age) which progresses relatively slowly and is characterized as much by peripheral neuromuscular involvement (muscle twitching, weakness, atrophy, and abnormal sensations such as numbness, tingling, cramps, and pain in the hands and feet) as by ataxia. Most individuals with MJD, but especially those with types I and II, experience one or more problems with vision, including double vision or blurred vision, loss of ability to distinguish color and/or contrast, and inability to control eye movements. Some individuals also experience prominent Parkinson disease-like symptoms, such as slowness of movement, rigidity or stiffness of the limbs and trunk, and tremor or trembling in the hands.

What Causes MJD?

MJD is classified as one of many dominantly inherited ataxias, specifically the spinocerebellar ataxias or SCAs. In the SCAs, of which nearly 30 separate genetic causes have been identified, degeneration of cells in the hindbrain leads to impaired coordination of movement. The hindbrain includes the cerebellum (a large bundle of brain tissue resembling a bun located at the back of the head), the brainstem, and the upper part of the spinal cord. MJD is inherited in an autosomal dominant pattern, meaning that an affected person has a single disease-causing MJD allele (an allele is half of a pair of genes located at the same position on a person's chromosomes) and a normal MJD allele, and can pass on either allele to the next generation. Any child of an affected parent has a 50 percent chance of inheriting the disease allele. If the child inherits the disease-causing gene, he or she will eventually develop symptoms of the disease. A child who does not inherit the disease allele will not develop the disease and cannot pass it on to the next generation.

MJD belongs to a class of genetic disorders called expanded repeat diseases. Mutations in expanded repeat diseases are abnormally long repeats of a normal repetition of three letters of the DNA genetic code. In the case of MJD, the code sequence "CAG" is repeated in the *ATXN3* gene, which produces the disease protein called ataxin-3. This protein, when mutated, is prone to fold abnormally and accumulate in affected brain cells. The accumulated ataxin-3 protein forms abnormal clumps known as inclusion bodies, which are located in the nucleus of the cell. While the clumps themselves may not be toxic to brain cells, they do reflect a problem in protein folding that likely affects normal properties of the ataxin-3 protein.

One unusual feature of MJD and many other expanded repeat diseases is a phenomenon called anticipation. Anticipation is the remarkable fact that children of affected parents tend to develop symptoms of the disease earlier in life and may experience more severe symptoms.

This is due to the tendency for the expanded repeat mutation to further expand when being passed to the next generation, especially when passed from the father. Because longer expansions tend to cause earlier and more severe disease, this molecular growth from one generation to the next likewise causes, on average, an earlier age of onset in subsequent generations. Though longer repeats tend to cause earlier onset disease, it is impossible to predict precisely the time and course of the disease for an individual based solely on the repeat length.

On a worldwide basis, MJD or SCA3 appears to be the most prevalent autosomal dominant inherited form of ataxia.

How Is MJD Diagnosed?

Physicians diagnose MJD by recognizing the symptoms of the disease and by taking a family history. They ask detailed questions about family members who show (or showed) symptoms of the disease, the kinds of symptoms seen in these relatives, the age(s) of disease onset, and the progression and severity of symptoms. A definitive diagnosis of MJD can be made only with a genetic test. The genetic test for MJD (SCA3) is highly accurate. Those individuals who are at risk for MJD (i.e., have an affected parent) but do not have any symptoms can undergo presymptomatic testing to determine whether they carry the disease allele (and thus will later develop the disease). Obtaining presymptomatic testing is a highly personal decision that at-risk individuals should make only after fully considering the potential pros and cons. Many at-risk persons choose not to undergo this test out of concern for job discrimination and difficulty in obtaining or maintaining insurance, among other reasons.

How Is MJD Treated?

MJD is incurable, but some symptoms of the disease can be treated. Levodopa therapy (used in treating individuals with Parkinson disease) can ease parkinsonian features (stiffness and slowness of movements, often accompanied by a tremor) for many years. Antispasmodic drugs, such as baclofen, can help reduce spasticity. Botulinum toxin can treat severe spasticity and some symptoms of dystonia, but it should be used as a last resort due to possible side effects, such as swallowing problems (dysphagia). Speech problems (dysarthria) and dysphagia can be treated with medication and speech therapy. Wearing prism glasses can reduce blurred or double vision, but eye surgery has only short-term benefits due to the progressive degeneration of eye muscles. Physiotherapy can help individuals cope with disability associated with gait problems, and physical aids, such as walkers and wheelchairs, can assist people with everyday activities. Daytime sleepiness, a common complaint in MJD (as is sleep disturbance in general), can be treated with modafanil and should prompt a formal sleep evaluation. Other problems, such as cramps and urinary dysfunction, can be treated with medications and medical care.

Chapter 20

Cerebral Palsy

Cerebral palsy (CP) is a group of disorders that affect a person's ability to move and maintain balance and posture. CP is the most common motor disability in childhood. Cerebral means having to do with the brain. Palsy means weakness or problems with using the muscles. CP is caused by abnormal brain development or damage to the developing brain that affects a person's ability to control his or her muscles.

The symptoms of CP vary from person to person. A person with severe CP might need to use special equipment to be able to walk, or might not be able to walk at all and might need lifelong care. A person with mild CP, on the other hand, might walk a little awkwardly, but might not need any special help. CP does not get worse over time, though the exact symptoms can change over a person's lifetime.

Causes and Risk Factors

CP is caused by abnormal development of the brain or damage to the developing brain that affects a child's ability to control his or her muscles. There are several possible causes of the abnormal development or damage. People used to think that CP was mainly caused by lack of oxygen during the birth process. Now, scientists think that this causes only a small number of CP cases.

This chapter includes text excerpted from "Cerebral Palsy (CP)," Centers for Disease Control and Prevention (CDC), February 3, 2017.

The brain damage that leads to CP can happen before birth, during birth, within a month after birth, or during the first years of a child's life, while the brain is still developing. CP related to brain damage that occurred before or during birth is called congenital CP. The majority of CP (85–90 percent) is congenital. In many cases, the specific cause is not known. A small percentage of CP is caused by brain damage that occurs more than 28 days after birth. This is called acquired CP, and usually is associated with an infection (such as meningitis) or head injury.

Types of CP

Doctors classify CP according to the main type of movement disorder involved. Depending on which areas of the brain are affected, one or more of the following movement disorders can occur:

- Stiff muscles (spasticity)
- Uncontrollable movements (dyskinesia)
- Poor balance and coordination (ataxia)

There are four main types of CP:

Spastic CP

The most common type of CP is spastic CP. Spastic CP affects about 80 percent of people with CP.

People with spastic CP have increased muscle tone. This means their muscles are stiff and, as a result, their movements can be awkward. Spastic CP usually is described by what parts of the body are affected:

- **Spastic diplegia/diparesis.** In this type of CP, muscle stiffness is mainly in the legs, with the arms less affected or not affected at all. People with spastic diplegia might have difficulty walking because tight hip and leg muscles cause their legs to pull together, turn inward, and cross at the knees (also known as scissoring).

- **Spastic hemiplegia/hemiparesis.** This type of CP affects only one side of a person's body; usually the arm is more affected than the leg.

- **Spastic quadriplegia/quadriparesis.** Spastic quadriplegia is the most severe form of spastic CP and affects all four limbs, the trunk, and the face. People with spastic quadriparesis usually cannot walk and often have other developmental disabilities

150

such as intellectual disability; seizures; or problems with vision, hearing, or speech.

Dyskinetic CP (Also Includes Athetoid, Choreoathetoid, and Dystonic Cerebral Palsies)

People with dyskinetic CP have problems controlling the movement of their hands, arms, feet, and legs, making it difficult to sit and walk. The movements are uncontrollable and can be slow and writhing or rapid and jerky. Sometimes the face and tongue are affected and the person has a hard time sucking, swallowing, and talking. A person with dyskinetic CP has muscle tone that can change (varying from too tight to too loose) not only from day to day, but even during a single day.

Ataxic CP

People with ataxic CP have problems with balance and coordination. They might be unsteady when they walk. They might have a hard time with quick movements or movements that need a lot of control, like writing. They might have a hard time controlling their hands or arms when they reach for something.

Mixed CP

Some people have symptoms of more than one type of CP. The most common type of mixed CP is spastic dyskinetic CP.

Early Signs

The signs of CP vary greatly because there are many different types and levels of disability. The main sign that a child might have CP is a delay reaching motor or movement milestones (such as rolling over, sitting, standing, or walking). Following are some other signs of possible CP. It is important to note that some children without CP also might have some of these signs.

In a Baby Younger than 6 Months of Age

- His head lags when you pick him up while he's lying on his back
- He feels stiff
- He feels floppy

- When held cradled in your arms, he seems to overextend his back and neck, constantly acting as if he is pushing away from you

- When you pick him up, his legs get stiff and they cross or scissor

In a Baby Older than 6 Months of Age

- She doesn't roll over in either direction

- She cannot bring her hands together

- She has difficulty bringing her hands to her mouth

- She reaches out with only one hand while keeping the other fisted

In a Baby Older than 10 Months of Age

- He crawls in a lopsided manner, pushing off with one hand and leg while dragging the opposite hand and leg

- He scoots around on his buttocks or hops on his knees, but does not crawl on all fours

Screening and Diagnosis

Diagnosing CP at an early age is important to the well being of children and their families. Diagnosing CP can take several steps:

Developmental Monitoring

Developmental monitoring (also called surveillance) means tracking a child's growth and development over time. If any concerns about the child's development are raised during monitoring, then a developmental screening test should be given as soon as possible.

Developmental Screening

During developmental screening a short test is given to see if the child has specific developmental delays, such as motor or movement delays. If the results of the screening test are cause for concern, then the doctor will make referrals for developmental and medical evaluations.

Developmental and Medical Evaluations

The goal of a developmental evaluation is to diagnose the specific type of disorder that affects a child.

Treatments and Intervention Services

There is no cure for CP, but treatment can improve the lives of those who have the condition. It is important to begin a treatment program as early as possible.

After a CP diagnosis is made, a team of health professionals works with the child and family to develop a plan to help the child reach his or her full potential. Common treatments include medicines; surgery; braces; and physical, occupational, and speech therapy. No single treatment is the best one for all children with CP. Before deciding on a treatment plan, it is important to talk with the child's doctor to understand all the risks and benefits.

Intervention Services

Both early intervention and school aged services are available through the Individuals with Disabilities Education Act (IDEA). Part C of IDEA deals with early intervention services (birth through 36 months of age), while Part B applies to services for school aged children (3 through 21 years of age). Even if your child has not been diagnosed with CP, he or she may be eligible for IDEA services.

Chapter 21

Charcot-Marie-Tooth Disease

What Is Charcot-Marie-Tooth Disease (CMT)?

Charcot-Marie-Tooth disease (CMT) is one of the most common inherited neurological disorders, affecting approximately 1 in 2,500 people in the United States. The disease is named for the three physicians who first identified it in 1886—Jean-Martin Charcot and Pierre Marie in Paris, France, and Howard Henry Tooth in Cambridge, England. CMT, also known as hereditary motor and sensory neuropathy (HMSN) or peroneal muscular atrophy, comprises a group of disorders that affect peripheral nerves. The peripheral nerves lie outside the brain and spinal cord and supply the muscles and sensory organs in the limbs. Disorders that affect the peripheral nerves are called peripheral neuropathies.

What Are the Symptoms of CMT?

The neuropathy of CMT affects both motor and sensory nerves. (Motor nerves cause muscles to contract and control voluntary muscle activity such as speaking, walking, breathing, and swallowing.) A typical feature includes weakness of the foot and lower leg muscles, which may result in foot drop and a high-stepped gait with frequent tripping or falls. Foot deformities, such as high arches and hammertoes

---

This chapter includes text excerpted from "Charcot-Marie-Tooth Disease Fact Sheet," National Institute of Neurological Disorders and Stroke (NINDS), April 2007. Reviewed January 2018.

(a condition in which the middle joint of a toe bends upwards) are also characteristic due to weakness of the small muscles in the feet. In addition, the lower legs may take on an "inverted champagne bottle" appearance due to the loss of muscle bulk. Later in the disease, weakness and muscle atrophy may occur in the hands, resulting in difficulty with carrying out fine motor skills (the coordination of small movements usually in the fingers, hands, wrists, feet, and tongue).

Onset of symptoms is most often in adolescence or early adulthood, but some individuals develop symptoms in mid-adulthood. The severity of symptoms varies greatly among individuals and even among family members with the disease. Progression of symptoms is gradual. Pain can range from mild to severe, and some people may need to rely on foot or leg braces or other orthopedic devices to maintain mobility. Although in rare cases, individuals may have respiratory muscle weakness, CMT is not considered a fatal disease and people with most forms of CMT have a normal life expectancy.

What Causes CMT?

A nerve cell communicates information to distant targets by sending electrical signals down a long, thin part of the cell called the axon. In order to increase the speed at which these electrical signals travel, the axon is insulated by myelin, which is produced by another type of cell called the Schwann cell. Myelin twists around the axon like a jelly-roll cake and prevents the loss of electrical signals. Without an intact axon and myelin sheath, peripheral nerve cells are unable to activate target muscles or relay sensory information from the limbs back to the brain.

CMT is caused by mutations in genes that produce proteins involved in the structure and function of either the peripheral nerve axon or the myelin sheath. Although different proteins are abnormal in different forms of CMT disease, all of the mutations affect the normal function of the peripheral nerves. Consequently, these nerves slowly degenerate and lose the ability to communicate with their distant targets. The degeneration of motor nerves results in muscle weakness and atrophy in the extremities (arms, legs, hands, or feet), and in some cases the degeneration of sensory nerves results in a reduced ability to feel heat, cold, and pain.

The gene mutations in CMT disease are usually inherited. Each of us normally possesses two copies of every gene, one inherited from each parent. Some forms of CMT are inherited in an autosomal dominant fashion, which means that only one copy of the abnormal gene is needed to cause the disease. Other forms of CMT are inherited in an autosomal recessive fashion, which means that both copies of the abnormal gene must be present to cause the disease. Still other forms of CMT are inherited in an X-linked fashion, which means that the abnormal gene is located on the X chromosome. The X and Y chromosomes determine an individual's sex. Individuals with two X chromosomes are female and individuals with one X and one Y chromosome are male.

In rare cases the gene mutation causing CMT disease is a new mutation which occurs spontaneously in the individual's genetic material and has not been passed down through the family.

How Is CMT Diagnosed?

Diagnosis of CMT begins with a standard medical history, family history, and neurological examination. Individuals will be asked about the nature and duration of their symptoms and whether other family members have the disease. During the neurological examination a physician will look for evidence of muscle weakness in the individual's arms, legs, hands, and feet, decreased muscle bulk, reduced tendon reflexes, and sensory loss. Doctors look for evidence of foot deformities, such as high arches, hammer toes, inverted heel, or flat feet. Other orthopedic problems, such as mild scoliosis or hip dysplasia, may also be present. A specific sign that may be found in people with CMT1 is nerve enlargement that may be felt or even seen through the skin. These enlarged nerves, called hypertrophic nerves, are caused by abnormally thickened myelin sheaths.

If CMT is suspected, the physician may order electrodiagnostic tests. This testing consists of two parts: nerve conduction studies and electromyography (EMG). During nerve conduction studies, electrodes are placed on the skin over a peripheral motor or sensory nerve. These electrodes produce a small electric shock that may cause mild discomfort. This electrical impulse stimulates sensory and motor nerves and provides quantifiable information that the doctor can use to arrive at a diagnosis. EMG involves inserting a needle electrode through the skin to measure the bioelectrical activity of muscles. Specific abnormalities in the readings signify axon degeneration. EMG may be useful in further characterizing the distribution and severity of peripheral nerve involvement.

Genetic testing is available for some types of CMT and results are usually enough to confirm a diagnosis. In addition, genetic counseling is available to assist individuals in understanding their condition and plan for the future.

If all the diagnostic work-up in inconclusive or genetic testing comes back negative, a neurologist may perform a nerve biopsy to confirm the diagnosis. A nerve biopsy involves removing a small piece of peripheral nerve through an incision in the skin. This is most often done by removing a piece of the nerve that runs down the calf of the leg. The nerve is then examined under a microscope. Individuals with CMT1 typically show signs of abnormal myelination. Specifically, "onion bulb" formations may be seen which represent axons surrounded by layers of demyelinating and remyelinating Schwann cells. Individuals with CMT1 usually show signs of axon degeneration. Recently, skin biopsy has been used to study unmyelinated and myelinated nerve fibers in a minimally invasive way, but their clinical use in CMT has not yet been established.

How Is CMT Treated?

There is no cure for CMT, but physical therapy, occupational therapy, braces and other orthopedic devices, and even orthopedic surgery can help individuals cope with the disabling symptoms of the disease. In addition, pain-killing drugs can be prescribed for individuals who have severe pain.

Physical and occupational therapy, the preferred treatment for CMT, involves muscle strength training, muscle and ligament stretching, stamina training, and moderate aerobic exercise. Most therapists recommend a specialized treatment program designed with the approval of the person's physician to fit individual abilities and needs. Therapists also suggest entering into a treatment program early; muscle strengthening may delay or reduce muscle atrophy, so strength training is most useful if it begins before nerve degeneration and muscle weakness progress to the point of disability.

Stretching may prevent or reduce joint deformities that result from uneven muscle pull on bones. Exercises to help build stamina or increase endurance will help prevent the fatigue that results from performing everyday activities that require strength and mobility. Moderate aerobic activity can help to maintain cardiovascular fitness and overall health. Most therapists recommend low-impact or no-impact exercises, such as biking or swimming, rather than activities such as walking or jogging, which may put stress on fragile muscles and joints.

Many CMT patients require ankle braces and other orthopedic devices to maintain everyday mobility and prevent injury. Ankle braces can help prevent ankle sprains by providing support and stability during activities such as walking or climbing stairs. High-top shoes or boots can also provide support for weak ankles. Thumb splints can help with hand weakness and loss of fine motor skills. Assistive devices should be used before disability sets in because the devices may prevent muscle strain and reduce muscle weakening. Some individuals with CMT may decide to have orthopedic surgery to reverse foot and joint deformities.

Chapter 22

Muscular Dystrophy

What Is Muscular Dystrophy?

Muscular dystrophy (MD) refers to a group of more than 30 inherited diseases that cause muscle weakness and muscle loss. Some forms of MD appear in infancy or childhood, while others may not appear until middle age or even later. In addition, the types of MD differ in the areas of the body they affect and in the severity of the symptoms. All forms of MD grow worse as the person's muscles get weaker. Most people with MD eventually lose their ability to walk.

What Causes Muscular Dystrophy?

MD is generally an inherited disease caused by gene mutations (changes in the DNA sequence) that affect proteins in muscles. In some cases, the mutation was not inherited from a person's parents but instead happened spontaneously. Such a mutation can then be inherited by the affected person's offspring.

Hundreds of genes are involved in making the proteins that affect muscles. Each type of MD is caused by a genetic mutation that is specific to that type. Some of the forms, like limb-girdle and distal, are caused by defects in the same gene.

MD is not contagious and cannot be caused by injury or activity.

This chapter includes text excerpted from "Muscular Dystrophy: Condition Information," *Eunice Kennedy Shriver* National Institute of Child Health and Human Development (NICHD), December 1, 2016.

161

What Are the Types of Muscular Dystrophy?

There are more than 30 forms of muscular dystrophy (MD), with information on the primary types included in the table below.

Table 22.1. Types of Muscular Dystrophy

Type of Muscular Dystrophy	What It Is	Common Symptoms	How It Develops
Duchenne	The most common and severe form of MD among children, DMD accounts for more than 50 percent of all cases. DMD is caused by a deficiency of dystrophin, a protein that helps strengthen muscle fibers and protect them from injury.	Weakness begins in the upper legs and pelvis. People with DMD may also: • Fall down a lot • Have trouble rising from a lying or sitting position • Waddle when walking • Have difficulty running and jumping • Have calf muscles that appear large because of fat accumulation	DMD appears typically in boys between ages 3 and 5 and progresses rapidly. Most people with DMD are unable to walk by age 12 and may later need a respirator to breathe. They usually die in their late teens or early 20s from heart trouble, respiratory complications, or infection.
Becker	Also caused by a deficiency of dystrophin, and with symptoms similar to those of DMD, Becker can progress slowly or quickly.	Patients with Becker MD may: • Walk on their tiptoes • Fall down a lot • Have difficulty rising from the floor • Have cramping in their muscles	Becker MD appears primarily in males between ages 11 and 25. Some people may never need to use a wheelchair, while others lose the ability to walk during their teens, mid-30s, or later.

Table 22.1. Continued

Type of Muscular Dystrophy	What It Is	Common Symptoms	How It Develops
Myotonic	The most common adult form of MD, myotonic MD appears in two forms, type 1 and type 2. Type 1 is more common and is caused by an abnormally large number of repeats of a three-letter "word" (CTG) in genetic code. While most people have up to 37 repeats of CTG, people with myotonic can have up to 4,000. The number of repeats may reflect the severity of symptoms.	Myotonic MD causes an inability to relax muscles following a sudden contraction. Other symptoms include: • Long, thin face and neck • Swallowing difficulties • Drooping eyelids, cataracts, and other vision problems • Baldness at the front of the scalp • Weight loss • Increased sweating Drowsiness • Heart problems that may lead to death during the 30s or 40s • Irregular menstrual periods • Infertility • Impotence	Myotonic MD affects both men and women between ages 20 and 30.
Emery-Dreifuss	Affecting boys primarily, the two forms of Emery-Dreifuss MD are caused by defects in the proteins that surround the nucleus in cells.	Weakness begins in the upper arm and lower leg muscles. People with this form may also: • Develop chronic shortening of muscles around joints (preventing them from moving freely), in the spine, ankles, knees, elbows, and back of the neck • Have elbows locked in a flexed position • Develop shoulder deterioration • Have a rigid spine • Walk on their toes • Experience mild weakness in their facial muscles	Symptoms usually begin by age 10 but can appear in patients up to their mid-20s. People with this form often develop heart problems by age 30, and they may die in mid-adulthood from progressive pulmonary or cardiac failure.

Table 22.1. Continued

Type of Muscular Dystrophy	What It Is	Common Symptoms	How It Develops
Facioscapulohumeral	FSHD refers to the areas affected: the face (facio), the shoulders (scapulo), and the upper arms (humeral). Researchers don't know what gene causes FSHD. They do know where the defect occurs and that it affects specific muscle groups.	FSHD MD often appears first in the eyes (difficulty in opening and shutting) and mouth (inability to smile or pucker). Other symptoms may include: • Muscle wasting that causes shoulders to appear slanted and shoulder blades to appear "winged" • Impaired reflexes only at the biceps and triceps • Trouble swallowing, chewing, or speaking • Hearing problems • Swayback curve in the spine, called lordosis	FSHD affects teen boys and girls typically but may occur as late as age 40. Most individuals have a normal life span, but symptoms can vary from mild to severely disabling.
Limb-girdle	Affecting both males and females, different types of limb-girdle are caused by different gene mutations. Patients with limb-girdle inherit a defective gene from either parent, or, in the more severe form, the same defective gene from both parents.	Patients with limb-girdle MD may: • First develop weakness around the hips, which then spreads to the shoulders, legs, and neck • Fall down a lot • Have trouble rising from chairs, climbing stairs, or carrying things • Waddle when they walk • Have a rigid spine	This form of MD can appear in childhood but most often appears in adolescence or young adulthood. Limb-girdle can progress quickly or slowly, but most patients become severely disabled (with muscle damage and inability to walk) within 20 years of developing the disease.

Table 22.1. Continued

Type of Muscular Dystrophy	What It Is	Common Symptoms	How It Develops
Distal	Distal MDs refer to a group of diseases that affect the muscles of the forearms, hands, lower legs, and feet. They are caused by defects in the protein dysferlin and can occur in both men and women.	Distal MD may cause: • Inability to perform hand movements • Difficulty extending fingers • Trouble walking and climbing stairs • Inability to hop or stand on the heels	This form typically appears between ages 40 and 60. Distal MD is less severe and progresses more slowly than other forms of MD, but it can spread to other muscles. Patients may eventually need a ventilator.
Oculopharyngeal	This form occurs in both men and women, and it can be mild or severe. It is caused by a defect in a protein that binds to molecules that help make other proteins. It is common among Americans of French-Canadian descent, Jewish Ashkenazi, and Hispanics from the Southwest region.	Oculopharyngeal MD may cause: • Drooping eyelids and other vision problems • Swallowing problems • Muscle wasting and weakness in the neck, shoulders, and sometimes limbs • Heart problems	This form of MD typically appears in a person's 40s or 50s. Some people will eventually lose their ability to walk.

How Many People Are Affected by or Are at Risk of Muscular Dystrophy?

The incidence of MD in the United States varies, because different kinds of MD are rarer than others. The most common forms in children, Duchenne and Becker, affect approximately 1 in every 5,600–7,700 males ages 5–24. The most common adult form, type 1 myotonic MD, affects 1 in 8,000 worldwide.

What Are Common Symptoms of Muscular Dystrophy?

Muscle weakness that worsens over time is a common symptom of all forms of MD. Each form of MD varies in the order in which symptoms occur and in the parts of the body that are affected.

How Is Muscular Dystrophy Diagnosed?

The first step in diagnosing MD is a visit with a healthcare provider for a physical exam. The healthcare provider will ask a series of questions about the patient's family history and medical history, including any problems affecting the muscles that the patient may be experiencing.

The healthcare provider may order tests to determine whether the problems are a result of MD and, if so, what form of this disorder. The tests may also rule out other problems that could cause muscle weakness, such as surgery, toxic exposure, medications, or other muscle diseases. These tests may include:

- Blood tests
- Muscle biopsies
- Genetic testing
- Neurological tests
- Heart testing such as an electrocardiogram (ECG)
- Exercise assessments
- Imaging tests such as magnetic resonance imaging (MRI) and ultrasound imaging

What Are the Treatments for Muscular Dystrophy?

No treatment is currently available to stop or reverse any form of MD. Instead, certain therapies and medications aim to treat the various problems that result from MD and improve the quality of life for patients. These include the following:

Physical Therapy

Beginning physical therapy early can help keep muscles flexible and strong. A combination of physical activity and stretching exercises may be recommended.

Respiratory Therapy

Many people with MD do not realize they have little respiratory strength until they have difficulty coughing or an infection leads to pneumonia. Regular visits to a specialist early in the diagnosis of MD can help guide treatment before a respiratory problem occurs. Eventually, many MD patients require assisted ventilation.

Speech Therapy

MD patients who experience weakness in the facial and throat muscles may benefit from learning to slow the pace of their speech by pausing more between breaths and by using special communication equipment.

Occupational Therapy

As physical abilities change, occupational therapy can help patients with MD relearn these movements and abilities. Occupational therapy also teaches patients to use assistive devices such as wheelchairs and utensils.

Corrective Surgery

At various times and depending on the form of MD, many patients require surgery to treat the conditions that result from MD. People with myotonic MD may need a pacemaker to treat heart problems or surgery to remove cataracts, a clouding of the lens of the eye that blocks light from entering the eye.

Drug Therapy

Certain medications can help slow or control the symptoms of MD. These include the following:

- **Glucocorticoids**, such as prednisone. Studies show that daily treatment with prednisone can increase muscle strength, ability, and respiratory function and slow the progression of weakness. Side effects may include weight gain. Long-term use may result in brittle bones, cataracts, and high blood pressure. The National Institutes of Health (NIH)'s Therapeutics for Rare and Neglected Diseases (TRND) Program is collaborating on a new glucocorticoid treatment called VBP15. Early clinical trial results show that the treatment may have the same positive results as prednisone, but without the side effects.

- **Anticonvulsants**. Typically taken for epilepsy, these drugs may help control seizures and some muscle spasms.

- **Immunosuppressants**. Commonly given to treat autoimmune diseases such as lupus and eczema, immunosuppressant drugs may help delay some damage to dying muscle cells.

- **Antibiotics** to treat respiratory infections.

Chapter 23

Multiple Sclerosis

What Is Multiple Sclerosis (MS)?

Multiple sclerosis (MS) is a neuroinflammatory disease that affects myelin, a substance that makes up the membrane (called the myelin sheath) that wraps around nerve fibers (axons). Myelinated axons are commonly called white matter. Researchers have learned that MS also damages the nerve cell bodies, which are found in the brain's gray matter, as well as the axons themselves in the brain, spinal cord, and optic nerve (the nerve that transmits visual information from the eye to the brain). As the disease progresses, the brain's cortex shrinks (cortical atrophy).

The term multiple sclerosis refers to the distinctive areas of scar tissue (sclerosis or plaques) that are visible in the white matter of people who have MS. Plaques can be as small as a pinhead or as large as the size of a golf ball. Doctors can see these areas by examining the brain and spinal cord using a type of brain scan called magnetic resonance imaging (MRI).

While MS sometimes causes severe disability, it is only rarely fatal and most people with MS have a normal life expectancy.

This chapter includes text excerpted from "Multiple Sclerosis: Hope through Research," National Institute of Neurological Disorders and Stroke (NINDS), June 2012. Reviewed January 2018.

What Are Plaques Made of and Why Do They Develop?

Plaques, or lesions, are the result of an inflammatory process in the brain that causes immune system cells to attack myelin. The myelin sheath helps to speed nerve impulses traveling within the nervous system. Axons are also damaged in MS, although not as extensively, or as early in the disease, as myelin.

Under normal circumstances, cells of the immune system travel in and out of the brain patrolling for infectious agents (viruses, for example) or unhealthy cells. This is called the "surveillance" function of the immune system.

Surveillance cells usually won't spring into action unless they recognize an infectious agent or unhealthy cells. When they do, they produce substances to stop the infectious agent. If they encounter unhealthy cells, they either kill them directly or clean out the dying area and produce substances that promote healing and repair among the cells that are left.

Researchers have observed that immune cells behave differently in the brains of people with MS. They become active and attack what appears to be healthy myelin. It is unclear what triggers this attack. MS is one of many autoimmune disorders, such as rheumatoid arthritis, and lupus, in which the immune system mistakenly attacks a person's healthy tissue as opposed to performing its normal role of attacking foreign invaders like viruses and bacteria. Whatever the reason, during these periods of immune system activity, most of the myelin within the affected area is damaged or destroyed. The axons also may be damaged. The symptoms of MS depend on the severity of the immune reaction as well as the location and extent of the plaques, which primarily appear in the brain stem, cerebellum, spinal cord, optic nerves, and the white matter of the brain around the brain ventricles (fluid filled spaces inside of the brain).

What Are the Signs and Symptoms of MS?

The symptoms of MS usually begin over one to several days, but in some forms, they may develop more slowly. They may be mild or severe and may go away quickly or last for months. Sometimes the initial symptoms of MS are overlooked because they disappear in a day or so and normal function returns. Because symptoms come and go in the majority of people with MS, the presence of symptoms is called an attack, or in medical terms, an exacerbation. Recovery from symptoms is referred to as remission, while a return of symptoms is called a relapse. This form of MS is therefore called relapsing-remitting MS, in contrast to a more slowly developing form called primary progressive MS. Progressive MS can also be a second stage of the illness that follows years of relapsing-remitting symptoms.

A diagnosis of MS is often delayed because MS shares symptoms with other neurological conditions and diseases.

The first symptoms of MS often include:

- vision problems such as blurred or double vision or optic neuritis, which causes pain in the eye and a rapid loss of vision

- weak, stiff muscles, often with painful muscle spasms

- tingling or numbness in the arms, legs, trunk of the body, or face

- clumsiness, particularly difficulty staying balanced when walking

- bladder control problems, either inability to control the bladder or urgency

- dizziness that doesn't go away

  MS may also cause later symptoms such as:

- mental or physical fatigue which accompanies the above symptoms during an attack

- mood changes such as depression or euphoria

- changes in the ability to concentrate or to multitask effectively

- difficulty making decisions, planning, or prioritizing at work or in private life

Some people with MS develop transverse myelitis, a condition caused by inflammation in the spinal cord. Transverse myelitis causes loss of spinal cord function over a period of time lasting from several hours to several weeks. It usually begins as a sudden onset of lower back pain, muscle weakness, or abnormal sensations in the toes, and feet, and can rapidly progress to more severe symptoms, including paralysis. In most cases of transverse myelitis, people recover at least some function within the first 12 weeks after an attack begins. Transverse myelitis can also result from viral infections, arteriovenous malformations, or neuroinflammatory problems unrelated to MS. In such instances, there are no plaques in the brain that suggest previous MS attacks.

Neuromyelitis optica is a disorder associated with transverse myelitis as well as optic nerve inflammation. Patients with this disorder usually have antibodies against a particular protein in their spinal cord, called the aquaporin channel. These patients respond differently to treatment than most people with MS.

Most individuals with MS have muscle weakness, often in their hands and legs. Muscle stiffness and spasms can also be a problem. These symptoms may be severe enough to affect walking or standing. In some cases, MS leads to partial or complete paralysis. Many people with MS find that weakness and fatigue are worse when they have a fever or when they are exposed to heat. MS exacerbations may occur following common infections.

Tingling and burning sensations are common, as well as the opposite, numbness and loss of sensation. Moving the neck from side to side or flexing it back and forth may cause "Lhermitte sign," a characteristic sensation of MS that feels like a sharp spike of electricity coursing down the spine.

While it is rare for pain to be the first sign of MS, pain often occurs with optic neuritis and trigeminal neuralgia, a neurological disorder that affects one of the nerves that runs across the jaw, cheek, and face. Painful spasms of the limbs and sharp pain shooting down the legs or around the abdomen can also be symptoms of MS.

Most individuals with MS experience difficulties with coordination and balance at some time during the course of the disease. Some may have a continuous trembling of the head, limbs, and body, especially during movement, although such trembling is more common with other disorders such as Parkinson disease.

Fatigue is common, especially during exacerbations of MS. A person with MS may be tired all the time or may be easily fatigued from mental or physical exertion.

Urinary symptoms, including loss of bladder control and sudden attacks of urgency, are common as MS progresses. People with MS sometimes also develop constipation or sexual problems.

Depression is a common feature of MS. A small number of individuals with MS may develop more severe psychiatric disorders such as bipolar disorder, and paranoia, or experience inappropriate episodes of high spirits, known as euphoria.

People with MS, especially those who have had the disease for a long time, can experience difficulty with thinking, learning, memory, and judgment. The first signs of what doctors call cognitive dysfunction (CD) may be subtle. The person may have problems finding the right word to say, or trouble remembering how to do routine tasks on the job or at home. Day to day decisions that once came easily may now be made more slowly and show poor judgment. Changes may be so small or happen so slowly that it takes a family member or friend to point them out.

How Many People Have MS?

No one knows exactly how many people have MS. Experts think there are currently 250,000–350,000 people in the United States diagnosed with MS. This estimate suggests that approximately 200 new cases are diagnosed every week. Studies of the prevalence (the proportion of individuals in a population having a particular disease) of MS indicate that the rate of the disease increased steadily during the 20th century.

As with most autoimmune disorders, twice as many women are affected by MS as men. MS is more common in colder climates. People of Northern European descent appear to be at the highest risk for the disease, regardless of where they live. Native Americans of North and South America, as well as Asian American populations, have relatively low rates of MS.

What Causes MS?

The ultimate cause of MS is damage to myelin, nerve fibers, and neurons in the brain and spinal cord, which together make up the central nervous system (CNS). But how that happens, and why, are questions that challenge researchers. Evidence appears to show that MS is a disease caused by genetic vulnerabilities combined with environmental factors.

Although there is little doubt that the immune system contributes to the brain and spinal cord tissue destruction of MS, the exact target of the immune system attacks and which immune system cells cause the destruction isn't fully understood.

Researchers have several possible explanations for what might be going on. The immune system could be:

- fighting some kind of infectious agent (for example, a virus) that has components which mimic components of the brain (molecular mimickry)

- destroying brain cells because they are unhealthy

- mistakenly identifying normal brain cells as foreign

173

The last possibility has been the favored explanation for many years. Research now suggests that the first two activities might also play a role in the development of MS. There is a special barrier, called the blood-brain barrier, which separates the brain and spinal cord from the immune system. If there is a break in the barrier, it exposes the brain to the immune system for the first time. When this happens, the immune system may misinterpret the brain as "foreign."

Genetic Susceptibility

Susceptibility to MS may be inherited. Studies of families indicate that relatives of an individual with MS have an increased risk for developing the disease. Experts estimate that about 15 percent of individuals with MS have one or more family members or relatives who also have MS. But even identical twins, whose deoxyribonucleic acid (DNA) is exactly the same, have only a 1 in 3 chance of both having the disease. This suggests that MS is not entirely controlled by genes. Other factors must come into play.

Current research suggests that dozens of genes and possibly hundreds of variations in the genetic code (called gene variants) combine to create vulnerability to MS. Some of these genes have been identified. Most of the genes identified so far are associated with functions of the immune system. Additionally, many of the known genes are similar to those that have been identified in people with other autoimmune diseases as type 1 diabetes, rheumatoid arthritis, or lupus. Researchers continue to look for additional genes and to study how they interact with each other to make an individual vulnerable to developing MS.

Sunlight and Vitamin D

A number of studies have suggested that people who spend more time in the sun and those with relatively high levels of vitamin D are less likely to develop MS. Bright sunlight helps human skin produce vitamin D. Researchers believe that vitamin D may help regulate the immune system in ways that reduce the risk of MS. People from regions near the equator, where there is a great deal of bright sunlight, generally have a much lower risk of MS than people from temperate areas such as the United States and Canada. Other studies suggest that people with higher levels of vitamin D generally have less severe MS and fewer relapses.

Smoking

A number of studies have found that people who smoke are more likely to develop MS. People who smoke also tend to have more brain lesions and brain shrinkage than nonsmokers. The reasons for this are currently unclear.

Infectious Factors and Viruses

A number of viruses have been found in people with MS, but the virus most consistently linked to the development of MS is *Epstein Barr* virus (EBV), the virus that causes mononucleosis.

Only about 5 percent of the population has not been infected by EBV. These individuals are at a lower risk for developing MS than those who have been infected. People who were infected with EBV in adolescence or adulthood and who therefore develop an exaggerated immune response to EBV are at a significantly higher risk for developing MS than those who were infected in early childhood. This suggests that it may be the type of immune response to EBV that predisposes to MS, rather than EBV infection itself. However, there is still no proof that EBV causes MS.

Autoimmune and Inflammatory Processes

Tissue inflammation and antibodies in the blood that fight normal components of the body and tissue in people with MS are similar to those found in other autoimmune diseases. Along with overlapping evidence from genetic studies, these findings suggest that MS results from some kind of disturbed regulation of the immune system.

How Is MS Diagnosed?

There is no single test used to diagnose MS. Doctors use a number of tests to rule out or confirm the diagnosis. There are many other disorders that can mimic MS. Some of these other disorders can be cured, while others require different treatments than those used for MS. Therefore it is very important to perform a thorough investigation before making a diagnosis.

In addition to a complete medical history, physical examination, and a detailed neurological examination, a doctor will order an MRI scan of the head and spine to look for the characteristic lesions of

MS. MRI is used to generate images of the brain and/or spinal cord. Then a special dye or contrast agent is injected into a vein and the MRI is repeated. In regions with active inflammation in MS, there is disruption of the blood-brain barrier and the dye will leak into the active MS lesion.

Doctors may also order evoked potential tests, which use electrodes on the skin and painless electric signals to measure how quickly and accurately the nervous system responds to stimulation. In addition, they may request a lumbar puncture (sometimes called a "spinal tap") to obtain a sample of cerebrospinal fluid. This allows them to look for proteins and inflammatory cells associated with the disease and to rule out other diseases that may look similar to MS, including some infections and other illnesses. MS is confirmed when positive signs of the disease are found in different parts of the nervous system at more than one time interval and there is no alternative diagnosis.

What Is the Course of MS?

The course of MS is different for each individual, which makes it difficult to predict. For most people, it starts with a first attack, usually (but not always) followed by a full to almost full recovery. Weeks, months, or even years may pass before another attack occurs, followed again by a period of relief from symptoms. This characteristic pattern is called relapsing-remitting MS.

Primary-progressive MS is characterized by a gradual physical decline with no noticeable remissions, although there may be temporary or minor relief from symptoms. This type of MS has a later onset, usually after age 40, and is just as common in men as in women.

Secondary progressive MS begins with a relapsing-remitting course, followed by a later primary progressive course. The majority of individuals with severe relapsing-remitting MS will develop secondary progressive MS if they are untreated.

Finally, there are some rare and unusual variants of MS. One of these is Marburg variant MS (also called malignant MS), which causes a swift and relentless decline resulting in significant disability or even death shortly after disease onset. Balo Concentric Sclerosis (BCS), which causes concentric rings of demyelination that can be seen on an MRI, is another variant type of MS that can progress rapidly.

Determining the particular type of MS is important because the current disease modifying drugs have been proven beneficial only for the relapsing-remitting types of MS.

What Is an Exacerbation or Attack of MS?

An exacerbation — which is also called a relapse, flare up, or attack — is a sudden worsening of MS symptoms, or the appearance of new symptoms that lasts for at least 24 hours. MS relapses are thought to be associated with the development of new areas of damage in the brain. Exacerbations are characteristic of relapsing-remitting MS, in which attacks are followed by periods of complete or partial recovery with no apparent worsening of symptoms.

An attack may be mild or its symptoms may be severe enough to significantly interfere with life's daily activities. Most exacerbations last from several days to several weeks, although some have been known to last for months.

When the symptoms of the attack subside, an individual with MS is said to be in remission. However, MRI data have shown that this is somewhat misleading because MS lesions continue to appear during these remission periods. Patients do not experience symptoms during remission because the inflammation may not be severe or it may occur in areas of the brain that do not produce obvious symptoms. Research suggests that only about 1 out of every 10 MS lesions is perceived by a person with MS. Therefore, MRI examination plays a very important role in establishing an MS diagnosis, deciding when the disease should be treated, and determining whether treatments work effectively or not. It also has been a valuable tool to test whether an experimental new therapy is effective at reducing exacerbations.

Are There Treatments Available for MS?

There is still no cure for MS, but there are treatments for initial attacks, medications and therapies to improve symptoms, and recently developed drugs to slow the worsening of the disease. These new drugs have been shown to reduce the number and severity of relapses and to delay the long-term progression of MS.

Table 23.1. Disease Modifying Drugs

Trade Name	Generic Name
Avonex	interferon beta-1a
Betaseron	Interferon beta-1b
Rebif	interferon beta-1a
Copaxone	glatiramer acetate

Table 23.1. Continued

Trade Name	Generic Name
Tysabri	natalizumab
Novantrone	mitoxantrone
Gilenya	fingolimod

How Do Doctors Treat the Symptoms of MS?

MS causes a variety of symptoms that can interfere with daily activities but which can usually be treated or managed to reduce their impact. Many of these issues are best treated by neurologists who have advanced training in the treatment of MS and who can prescribe specific medications to treat the problems.

Vision Problems

Eye and vision problems are common in people with MS but rarely result in permanent blindness. Inflammation of the optic nerve or damage to the myelin that covers the optic nerve and other nerve fibers can cause a number of symptoms, including blurring, or graying of vision, blindness in one eye, loss of normal color vision, depth perception, or a dark spot in the center of the visual field (scotoma).

Uncontrolled horizontal or vertical eye movements (nystagmus) and "jumping vision" (opsoclonus) are common to MS, and can be either mild or severe enough to impair vision.

Double vision (diplopia) occurs when the two eyes are not perfectly aligned. This occurs commonly in MS when a pair of muscles that control a specific eye movement aren't coordinated due to weakness in one or both muscles. Double vision may increase with fatigue or as the result of spending too much time reading or on the computer. Periodically resting the eyes may be helpful.

Weak Muscles, Stiff Muscles, Painful Muscle Spasms, and Weak Reflexes

Muscle weakness is common in MS, along with muscle spasticity. Spasticity refers to muscles that are stiff or that go into spasms without any warning. Spasticity in MS can be as mild as a feeling of tightness in the muscles or so severe that it causes painful, uncontrolled spasms. It can also cause pain or tightness in and around the joints. It also frequently affects walking, reducing the normal flexibility, or "bounce" involved in taking steps.

Tremor

People with MS sometimes develop tremor, or uncontrollable shaking, often triggered by movement. Tremor can be very disabling. Assistive devices and weights attached to limbs are sometimes helpful for people with tremor. Deep brain stimulation and drugs such as clonazepam also may be useful.

Problems with Walking and Balance

Many people with MS experience difficulty walking. In fact, studies indicate that half of those with relapsing-remitting MS will need some kind of help walking within 15 years of their diagnosis if they remain untreated. The most common walking problem in people with MS experience is ataxia—unsteady, uncoordinated movements—due to damage with the areas of the brain that coordinate movement of muscles. People with severe ataxia generally benefit from the use of a cane, walker, or other assistive device. Physical therapy can also reduce walking problems in many cases.

In 2010, the FDA approved the drug dalfampridine to improve walking in patients with MS. It is the first drug approved for this use. Clinical trials showed that patients treated with dalfampridine had faster walking speeds than those treated with a placebo pill.

Fatigue

Fatigue is a common symptom of MS and may be both physical (for example, tiredness in the legs) and psychological (due to depression). Probably the most important measures people with MS can take to counter physical fatigue are to avoid excessive activity and to stay out of the heat, which often aggravates MS symptoms. On the other hand, daily physical activity programs of mild to moderate intensity can significantly reduce fatigue. An antidepressant such as fluoxetine may be prescribed if the fatigue is caused by depression. Other drugs that may reduce fatigue in some individuals include amantadine and modafinil.

Fatigue may be reduced if the person receives occupational therapy to simplify tasks and/or physical therapy to learn how to walk in a way that saves physical energy or that takes advantage of an assistive device. Some people benefit from stress management programs, relaxation training, membership in an MS support group, or individual psychotherapy. Treating sleep problems and MS symptoms that interfere with sleep (such as spastic muscles) may also help.

Pain

People with MS may experience several types of pain during the course of the disease.

Trigeminal neuralgia is a sharp, stabbing, facial pain caused by MS affecting the trigeminal nerve as it exits the brainstem on its way to the jaw and cheek. It can be treated with anticonvulsant or antispasmodic drugs, alcohol injections, or surgery.

People with MS occasionally develop central pain, a syndrome caused by damage to the brain and/or spinal cord. Drugs such as gabapentin and nortryptiline sometimes help to reduce central pain.

Burning, tingling, and prickling (commonly called "pins and needles") are sensations that happen in the absence of any stimulation. The medical term for them is "dysesthesias" They are often chronic and hard to treat.

Chronic back or other musculoskeletal pain may be caused by walking problems or by using assistive aids incorrectly. Treatments may include heat, massage, ultrasound treatments, and physical therapy to correct faulty posture and strengthen and stretch muscles.

Problems with Bladder Control and Constipation

The most common bladder control problems encountered by people with MS are urinary frequency, urgency, or the loss of bladder control. The same spasticity that causes spasms in legs can also affect the bladder. A small number of individuals will have the opposite problem—retaining large amounts of urine. Urologists can help with treatment of bladder related problems. A number of medical treatments are available. Constipation is also common and can be treated with a high fiber diet, laxatives, and other measures.

Sexual Issues

People with MS sometimes experience sexual problems. Sexual arousal begins in the central nervous system, as the brain sends messages to the sex organs along nerves running through the spinal cord. If MS damages these nerve pathways, sexual response—including arousal and orgasm—can be directly affected. Sexual problems may also stem from MS symptoms such as fatigue, cramped or spastic muscles, and psychological factors related to lowered selfesteem or depression. Some of these problems can be corrected with medications. Psychological counseling also may be helpful.

Depression

Studies indicate that clinical depression is more frequent among people with MS than it is in the general population or in persons with many other chronic, disabling conditions. MS may cause depression as part of the disease process, since it damages myelin and nerve fibers inside the brain. If the plaques are in parts of the brain that are involved in emotional expression and control, a variety of behavioral changes can result, including depression. Depression can intensify symptoms of fatigue, pain, and sexual dysfunction. It is most often treated with selective scrotonin reuptake inhibitor (SSRI) antidepressant medications, which are less likely than other antidepressant medications to cause fatigue.

Inappropriate Laughing or Crying

MS is sometimes associated with a condition called pseudobulbar affect that causes inappropriate and involuntary expressions of laughter, crying, or anger. These expressions are often unrelated to mood; for example, the person may cry when they are actually very happy, or laugh when they are not especially happy. In 2010 the FDA approved the first treatment specifically for pseudobulbar affect, a combination of the drugs dextromethorphan and quinidine. The condition can also be treated with other drugs such as amitriptyline or citalopram.

Cognitive Changes

Half to three quarters of people with MS experience cognitive impairment, which is a phrase doctors use to describe a decline in the ability to think quickly and clearly and to remember easily. These cognitive changes may appear at the same time as the physical symptoms or they may develop gradually over time. Some individuals with MS may feel as if they are thinking more slowly, are easily distracted, have trouble remembering, or are losing their way with words. The right word may often seem to be on the tip of their tongue.

Some experts believe that it is more likely to be cognitive decline, rather than physical impairment, that causes people with MS to eventually withdraw from the workforce. A number of neuropsychological tests have been developed to evaluate the cognitive status of individuals with MS. Based on the outcomes of these tests, a neuropsychologist can determine the extent of strengths and weaknesses in different cognitive areas. Drugs such as donepezil, which is usually used for Alzheimer disease, may be helpful in some cases.

Complementary and Alternative Therapies

Many people with MS use some form of complementary or alternative medicine. These therapies come from many disciplines, cultures, and traditions and encompass techniques as different as acupuncture, aromatherapy, ayurvedic medicine, touch and energy therapies, physical movement disciplines such as yoga, and tai chi, herbal supplements, and biofeedback.

Because of the risk of interactions between alternative and more conventional therapies, people with MS should discuss all the therapies they are using with their doctor, especially herbal supplements. Although herbal supplements are considered "natural," they have biologically active ingredients that could have harmful effects on their own or interact harmfully with other medications.

Chapter 24

Myasthenia

Chapter Contents

Section 24.1

Myasthenia Gravis

This section includes text excerpted from "Myasthenia
Gravis Fact Sheet," National Institute of Neurological
Disorders and Stroke (NINDS), May 2017.

What Is Myasthenia Gravis?

Myasthenia gravis is a chronic autoimmune neuromuscular disease
that causes weakness in the skeletal muscles, which are responsible
for breathing and moving parts of the body, including the arms and
legs. The name myasthenia gravis, which is Latin and Greek in origin,
means "grave, or serious, muscle weakness."

The hallmark of myasthenia gravis is muscle weakness that worsens after periods of activity and improves after periods of rest. Certain
muscles such as those that control eye and eyelid movement, facial
expression, chewing, talking, and swallowing are often (but not always)
involved in the disorder. The muscles that control breathing and neck
and limb movements may also be affected.

There is no known cure but with current therapies most cases of
myasthenia gravis are not as "grave" as the name implies. Available
treatments can control symptoms and often allow people to have a
relatively high quality of life. Most individuals with the condition have
a normal life expectancy.

What Causes Myasthenia Gravis?

Myasthenia gravis is caused by an error in the transmission of
nerve impulses to muscles. It occurs when normal communication
between the nerve and muscle is interrupted at the neuromuscular
junction—the place where nerve cells connect with the muscles they
control.

Neurotransmitters are chemicals that neurons, or brain cells,
use to communicate information. Normally when electrical signals
or impulses travel down a motor nerve, the nerve endings release a
neurotransmitter called acetylcholine. Acetylcholine travels from the

nerve ending and binds to acetylcholine receptors on the muscle. The binding of acetylcholine to its receptor activates the muscle and causes a muscle contraction.

In myasthenia gravis, antibodies (immune proteins) block, alter, or destroy the receptors for acetylcholine at the neuromuscular junction, which prevents the muscle from contracting. In most individuals with myasthenia gravis, this is caused by antibodies to the acetylcholine receptor itself. However, antibodies to other proteins, such as muscle-specific kinase (MuSK) protein, can also lead to impaired transmission at the neuromuscular junction.

These antibodies are produced by the body's own immune system. Myasthenia gravis is an autoimmune disease because the immune system—which normally protects the body from foreign organisms—mistakenly attacks itself.

The thymus is a gland that controls immune function and maybe associated with myasthenia gravis. Located in the chest behind the breastbone, the gland is largest in children. It grows gradually until puberty, and then gets smaller and is replaced by fat. Throughout childhood, the thymus plays an important role in the development of the immune system because it is responsible for producing T-lymphocytes or T cells, a specific type of white blood cell that protects the body from viruses and infections.

In many adults with myasthenia gravis, the thymus gland remains large. People with the disease typically have clusters of immune cells in their thymus gland similar to lymphoid hyperplasia—a condition that usually only happens in the spleen and lymph nodes during an active immune response. Some individuals with myasthenia gravis develop thymomas (tumors of the thymus gland). Thymomas are most often harmless, but they can become cancerous.

The thymus gland plays a role in myasthenia gravis, but its function is not fully understood. Scientists believe that the thymus gland may give incorrect instructions to developing immune cells, ultimately causing the immune system to attack its own cells and tissues and produce acetylcholine receptor antibodies—setting the stage for the attack on neuromuscular transmission.

What Are the Symptoms of Myasthenia Gravis?

Although myasthenia gravis may affect any skeletal muscle, muscles that control eye and eyelid movement, facial expression, and swallowing are most frequently affected. The onset of the disorder may be sudden and symptoms often are not immediately recognized as myasthenia gravis.

In most cases, the first noticeable symptom is weakness of the eye muscles. In others, difficulty swallowing and slurred speech may be the first signs. The degree of muscle weakness involved in myasthenia gravis varies greatly among individuals, ranging from a localized form limited to eye muscles (ocular myasthenia), to a severe or generalized form in which many muscles—sometimes including those that control breathing—are affected.

Symptoms may include:

- drooping of one or both eyelids (ptosis)
- blurred or double vision (diplopia) due to weakness of the muscles that control eye movements
- a change in facial expression
- difficulty swallowing
- shortness of breath
- impaired speech (dysarthria)
- weakness
- in the arms, hands, fingers, legs, and neck

Who Gets Myasthenia Gravis?

Myasthenia gravis affects both men and women and occurs across all racial and ethnic groups. It most commonly impacts young adult women (under 40) and older men (over 60), but it can occur at any age, including childhood. Myasthenia gravis is not inherited nor is it contagious. Occasionally, the disease may occur in more than one member of the same family.

Although myasthenia gravis is rarely seen in infants, the fetus may acquire antibodies from a mother affected with myasthenia gravis—a condition called neonatal myasthenia. Generally, neonatal myasthenia gravis is temporary and the child's symptoms usually disappear within two to three months after birth. Rarely, children of a healthy mother may develop congenital myasthenia. This is not an autoimmune disorder (it is caused by defective genes that produce abnormal proteins in the neuromuscular junction) and can cause similar symptoms to myasthenia gravis.

How Is Myasthenia Gravis Diagnosed?

A doctor may perform or order several tests to confirm the diagnosis, including:

- **A physical and neurological examination.** A physician will first review an individual's medical history and conduct a physical examination. In a neurological examination, the physician will check muscle strength and tone, coordination, sense of touch, and look for impairment of eye movements.

- **An edrophonium test.** This test uses injections of edrophonium chloride to briefly relieve weakness in people with myasthenia gravis. The drug blocks the breakdown of acetylcholine and temporarily increases the levels of acetylcholine at the neuromuscular junction. It is usually used to test ocular muscle weakness.

- **A blood test.** Most individuals with myasthenia gravis have abnormally elevated levels of acetylcholine receptor antibodies. A second antibody—called the antibody—has been found in about half of individuals with myasthenia gravis who do not anti-MuSK have acetylcholine receptor antibodies. A blood test can also detect this antibody. However, in some individuals with myasthenia gravis, neither of these antibodies is present. These individuals are said to have seronegative (negative antibody) myasthenia.

- **Electrodiagnostics.** Diagnostic tests include repetitive nerve stimulation, which repeatedly stimulates a person's nerves with small pulses of electricity to tire specific muscles. Muscle fibers in myasthenia gravis, as well as other neuromuscular disorders, do not respond as well to repeated electrical stimulation compared to muscles from normal individuals. Single fiber electromyography (EMG), considered the most sensitive test for myasthenia gravis, detects impaired nerve to muscle transmission. EMG can be very helpful in diagnosing mild cases of myasthenia gravis when other tests fail to demonstrate abnormalities.

- **Diagnostic imaging.** Diagnostic imaging of the chest using computed tomography (CT) or magnetic resonance imaging (MRI) may identify the presence of a thymoma.

- **Pulmonary function testing.** Measuring breathing strength can help predict if respiration may fail and lead to a myasthenic crisis.

Because weakness is a common symptom of many other disorders, the diagnosis of myasthenia gravis is often missed or delayed (sometimes up to two years) in people who experience mild weakness or in those individuals whose weakness is restricted to only a few muscles.

What Is a Myasthenic Crisis?

A myasthenic crisis is a medical emergency that occurs when the muscles that control breathing weaken to the point where individuals require a ventilator to help them breathe.

Approximately 15–20 percent of people with myasthenia gravis experience at least one myasthenic crisis. This condition usually requires immediate medical attention and may be triggered by infection, stress, surgery, or an adverse reaction to medication. However, up to one-half of people may have no obvious cause for their myasthenic crisis. Certain medications have been shown to cause myasthenia gravis. However, sometimes these medications may still be used if it is more important to treat an underlying condition.

How Is Myasthenia Gravis Treated?

Today, myasthenia gravis can generally be controlled. There are several therapies available to help reduce and improve muscle weakness.

- **Thymectomy.** This operation to remove the thymus gland (which often is abnormal in individuals with myasthenia gravis) can reduce symptoms and may cure some people, possibly by rebalancing the immune system. The National Institute of Neurological Disorders and Stroke (NINDS)-funded study found that thymectomy is beneficial both for people with thymoma and those with no evidence of the tumors. The clinical trial followed 126 people with myasthenia gravis and no visible thymoma and found that the surgery reduced muscle weakness and the need for immunosuppressive drugs.

- **Anticholinesterase medications.** Medications to treat the disorder include anticholinesterase agents such as mestinon or pyridostigmine, which slow the breakdown of acetylcholine at the neuromuscular junction and thereby improve neuromuscular transmission and increase muscle strength.

- **Immunosuppressive drugs.** These drugs improve muscle strength by suppressing the production of abnormal antibodies.

They include prednisone, azathioprine, mycophenolate mofetil, tacrolimus, and rituximab. The drugs can cause significant side effects and must be carefully monitored by a physician.

- **Plasmapheresis and intravenous immunoglobulin.** These therapies may be options in severe cases of myasthenia gravis. Individuals can have antibodies in their plasma (a liquid component in blood) that attack the neuromuscular junction. These treatments remove the destructive antibodies, although their effectiveness usually only lasts for a few weeks to months.

- **Plasmapheresis** is a procedure using a machine to remove harmful antibodies in plasma and replace them with good plasma or a plasma substitute.

- **Intravenous immunoglobulin** is a highly concentrated injection of antibodies pooled from many healthy donors that temporarily changes the way the immune system operates. It works by binding to the antibodies that cause myasthenia gravis and removing them from circulation.

What Is the Prognosis?

With treatment, most individuals with myasthenia can significantly improve their muscle weakness and lead normal or nearly normal lives. Sometimes the severe weakness of myasthenia gravis may cause respiratory failure, which requires immediate emergency medical care.

Some cases of myasthenia gravis may go into remission—either temporarily or permanently—and muscle weakness may disappear completely so that medications can be discontinued. Stable, long-lasting complete remissions are the goal of thymectomy and may occur in about 50 percent of individuals who undergo this procedure.

What Research Is Being Done?

Although there is no cure for myasthenia gravis, management of the disorder has improved over the past 30 years. There is a greater understanding about the structure and function of the neuromuscular junction, the fundamental aspects of the thymus gland and of autoimmunity, and the disorder itself. Technological advances have led to more timely and accurate diagnosis of myasthenia gravis and enhanced therapies have improved treatment options. Researchers are working to develop better medications, identify ways to diagnose and treat individuals, and improve treatment options.

Medication

Some people with myasthenia gravis do not respond favorably to available treatment options, which usually include long-term suppression of the immune system. Drugs are being tested, either alone or in combination with existing drug therapies, to see if they are effective in treating the disease.

Studies are investigating the use of therapy targeting the B cells that make antibodies (rituximab) or the process by which acetylcholine antibodies injure the neuromuscular junction (eculizumab). The drugs have shown promise in initial clinical trials.

Diagnostics and Biomarkers

In addition to developing new medications, researchers are trying to find better ways to diagnose and treat this disorder. For example, NINDS-funded researchers are exploring the assembly and function of connections between nerves and muscle fibers to understand the fundamental processes in neuromuscular development. This research could reveal new therapies for neuromuscular diseases like myasthenia gravis.

Researchers are also exploring better ways to treat myasthenia gravis by developing new tools to diagnose people with undetectable antibodies and identify potential biomarkers (signs that can help diagnose or measure the progression of a disease) to predict an individual's response to immunosuppressive drugs.

Treatment Options

Findings from a NINDS-supported study yielded conclusive evidence about the benefits of surgery for individuals without thymoma, a subject that had been debated for decades. Researchers hope that this trial will become a model for rigorously testing other treatment options, and that other studies will continue to examine different therapies to see if they are superior to standard care options.

Section 24.2

Congenital Myasthenia Syndrome (CMS)

This section includes text excerpted from "Congenital Myasthenic Syndrome," Genetics Home Reference (GHR), National Institutes of Health (NIH), January 16, 2018.

What Is Congenital Myasthenic Syndrome (CMS)?

CMS is a group of conditions characterized by muscle weakness (myasthenia) that worsens with physical exertion. The muscle weakness typically begins in early childhood but can also appear in adolescence or adulthood. Facial muscles, including muscles that control the eyelids, muscles that move the eyes, and muscles used for chewing, and swallowing, are most commonly affected. However, any of the muscles used for movement (skeletal muscles) can be affected in this condition. Due to muscle weakness, affected infants may have feeding difficulties. Development of motor skills such as crawling or walking may be delayed. The severity of the myasthenia varies greatly, with some people experiencing minor weakness and others having such severe weakness that they are unable to walk.

Some individuals have episodes of breathing problems that may be triggered by fevers or infection. Severely affected individuals may also experience short pauses in breathing (apnea) that can lead to a bluish appearance of the skin or lips (cyanosis).

How Prevalent Is CMS?

The prevalence of congenital myasthenic syndrome is unknown. At least 600 families with affected individuals have been described in the scientific literature.

Does CMS Cause due to Genetic Changes?

Mutations in many genes can cause congenital myasthenic syndrome. Mutations in the *CHRNE* gene are responsible for more than half of all cases. A large number of cases are also caused by mutations in the *RAPSN, CHAT, COLQ*, and *DOK7* genes. All of these genes provide instructions for producing proteins that are involved in the normal function of the neuromuscular junction. The neuromuscular junction is the area between the ends of nerve cells and muscle cells where signals are relayed to trigger muscle movement.

Gene mutations lead to changes in proteins that play a role in the function of the neuromuscular junction and disrupt signaling between the ends of nerve cells and muscle cells. Disrupted signaling between these cells results in an impaired ability to move skeletal muscles, muscle weakness, and delayed development of motor skills. The respiratory problems in congenital myasthenic syndrome result from impaired movement of the muscles of the chest wall and the muscle that separates the abdomen from the chest cavity (the diaphragm).

Mutations in other genes that provide instructions for proteins involved in neuromuscular signaling have been found to cause some cases of congenital myasthenic syndrome, although these mutations account for only a small number of cases. Some people with congenital myasthenic syndrome do not have an identified mutation in any of the genes known to be associated with this condition.

Inheritance Pattern

This condition is most commonly inherited in an autosomal recessive pattern, which means both copies of the gene in each cell have mutations. The parents of an individual with an autosomal recessive condition each carry one copy of the mutated gene, but they typically do not show signs and symptoms of the condition.

Rarely, this condition is inherited in an autosomal dominant pattern, which means one copy of the altered gene in each cell is sufficient to cause the disorder. In some cases, an affected person inherits the mutation from one affected parent. Other cases result from new mutations in the gene and occur in people with no history of the disorder in their family.

Chapter 25

Myoclonus

What Is Myoclonus?

Myoclonus describes a symptom and not a diagnosis of a disease. It refers to sudden, involuntary jerking of a muscle or group of muscles. Myoclonic twitches or jerks usually are caused by sudden muscle contractions, called positive myoclonus, or by muscle relaxation, called negative myoclonus. Myoclonic jerks may occur alone or in sequence, in a pattern or without pattern. They may occur infrequently or many times each minute. Myoclonus sometimes occurs in response to an external event or when a person attempts to make a movement. The twitching cannot be controlled by the person experiencing it.

In its simplest form, myoclonus consists of a muscle twitch followed by relaxation. A hiccup is an example of this type of myoclonus. Other familiar examples of myoclonus are the jerks or "sleep starts" that some people experience while drifting off to sleep. These simple forms of myoclonus occur in normal, healthy persons and cause no difficulties. When more widespread, myoclonus may involve persistent, shock-like contractions in a group of muscles. In some cases, myoclonus begins in one region of the body and spreads to muscles in other areas. More severe cases of myoclonus can distort movement and severely limit a person's ability to eat, talk, or walk. These types of myoclonus may indicate an underlying disorder in the brain or nerves.

This chapter includes text excerpted from "Myoclonus Fact Sheet," National Institute of Neurological Disorders and Stroke (NINDS), July 2012. Reviewed January 2018.

What Are the Causes of Myoclonus?

Myoclonus may develop in response to infection, head or spinal cord injury, stroke, brain tumors, kidney or liver failure, lipid storage disease, chemical or drug poisoning, or other disorders. Prolonged oxygen deprivation to the brain, called hypoxia, may result in posthypoxic myoclonus. Myoclonus can occur by itself, but most often it is one of several symptoms associated with a wide variety of nervous system disorders. For example, myoclonic jerking may develop in patients with multiple sclerosis, Parkinson disease (PD), Alzheimer disease (AD), or Creutzfeldt-Jakob disease (CJD). Myoclonic jerks commonly occur in persons with epilepsy, a disorder in which the electrical activity in the brain becomes disordered leading to seizures.

What Are the Types of Myoclonus?

Classifying the many different forms of myoclonus is difficult because the causes, effects, and responses to therapy vary widely. Listed below are the types most commonly described.

- **Action myoclonus** is characterized by muscular jerking triggered or intensified by voluntary movement or even the intention to move. It may be made worse by attempts at precise, coordinated movements. Action myoclonus is the most disabling form of myoclonus and can affect the arms, legs, face, and even the voice. This type of myoclonus often is caused by brain damage that results from a lack of oxygen and blood flow to the brain when breathing or heartbeat is temporarily stopped.

- **Cortical reflex myoclonus** is thought to be a type of epilepsy that originates in the cerebral cortex—the outer layer, or "gray matter," of the brain, responsible for much of the information processing that takes place in the brain. In this type of myoclonus, jerks usually involve only a few muscles in one part of the body, but jerks involving many muscles also may occur. Cortical reflex myoclonus can be intensified when individuals attempt to move in a certain way (action myoclonus) or perceive a particular sensation.

- **Essential myoclonus** occurs in the absence of epilepsy or other apparent abnormalities in the brain or nerves. It can occur randomly in people with no family history, but it also can appear among members of the same family, indicating that it sometimes may be an inherited disorder. Essential myoclonus tends to be stable without increasing in severity over time. In some families, there is an association of essential myoclonus, essential tremor, and even myoclonus dystonia (a form of dystonia). Another form of essential myoclonus may be a type of epilepsy with no known cause.

- **Palatal myoclonus** is a regular, rhythmic contraction of one or both sides of the rear of the roof of the mouth, called the soft palate. These contractions may be accompanied by myoclonus in other muscles, including those in the face, tongue, throat, and diaphragm. The contractions are very rapid, occurring as often as 150 times a minute, and may persist during sleep. The condition usually appears in adults and can last indefinitely. Some people with palatal myoclonus regard it as a minor problem, although some occasionally complain of a "clicking" sound in the ear, a noise made as the muscles in the soft palate contract. The disorder can cause discomfort and severe pain in some individuals.

- **Progressive myoclonus epilepsy (PME)** is a group of diseases characterized by myoclonus, epileptic seizures, and other serious symptoms such as trouble walking or speaking. These rare disorders often get worse over time and sometimes are fatal. Studies have identified many forms of PME. Lafora body disease is inherited as an autosomal recessive disorder, meaning that the disease occurs only when a child inherits two copies of a defective gene, one from each parent. Lafora body disease is characterized by myoclonus, epileptic seizures, and dementia (progressive loss of memory and other intellectual functions). A second group of PME diseases belonging to the class of cerebral storage diseases usually involves myoclonus, visual problems, dementia, and dystonia (sustained muscle contractions that cause twisting movements or abnormal postures). Another group of PME disorders in the class of system degenerations often is accompanied by action myoclonus, seizures, and problems with balance and walking. Many of these PME diseases begin in childhood or adolescence.

- **Reticular reflex myoclonus** is thought to be a type of generalized epilepsy that originates in the brain stem, the part of the brain that connects to the spinal cord and controls vital functions such as breathing and heartbeat. Myoclonic jerks usually affect the whole body, with muscles on both sides of the body

195

affected simultaneously. In some people, myoclonic jerks occur in only a part of the body, such as the legs, with all the muscles in that part being involved in each jerk. Reticular reflex myoclonus can be triggered by either a voluntary movement or an external stimulus.

- **Stimulus-sensitive myoclonus** is triggered by a variety of external events, including noise, movement, and light. Surprise may increase the sensitivity of the individual.

- **Sleep myoclonus** occurs during the initial phases of sleep, especially at the moment of dropping off to sleep. Some forms appear to be stimulus-sensitive. Some persons with sleep myoclonus are rarely troubled by, or need treatment for, the condition. However, myoclonus may be a symptom in more complex and disturbing sleep disorders, such as restless legs syndrome (RLS), and may require treatment by a doctor.

How Is Myoclonus Treated?

Treatment of myoclonus focuses on medications that may help reduce symptoms. The drug of first choice to treat myoclonus, especially certain types of action myoclonus, is clonazepam, a type of tranquilizer. Dosages of clonazepam usually are increased gradually until the individual improves or side effects become harmful. Drowsiness and loss of coordination are common side effects. The beneficial effects of clonazepam may diminish over time if the individual develops a tolerance for the drug.

Many of the drugs used for myoclonus, such as barbiturates, levetiracetam, phenytoin, and primidone, are also used to treat epilepsy. Barbiturates slow down the central nervous system and cause tranquilizing or antiseizure effects. Phenytoin, levetiracetam, and primidone are effective antiepileptic drugs, although phenytoin can cause liver failure or have other harmful long-term effects in individuals with PME. Sodium valproate is an alternative therapy for myoclonus and can be used either alone or in combination with clonazepam. Although clonazepam and/or sodium valproate are effective in the majority of people with myoclonus, some people have adverse reactions to these drugs.

Some studies have shown that doses of 5-hydroxytryptophan (5-HTP), a building block of serotonin, leads to improvement in people with some types of action myoclonus and PME. However, other studies indicate that 5-HTP therapy is not effective in all people with myoclonus, and, in fact, may worsen the condition in some individuals. These differences in the effect of 5-HTP on individuals with myoclonus have not yet been explained, but they may offer important clues to underlying abnormalities in serotonin receptors.

The complex origins of myoclonus may require the use of multiple drugs for effective treatment. Although some drugs have a limited effect when used individually, they may have a greater effect when used with drugs that act on different pathways or mechanisms in the brain. By combining several of these drugs, scientists hope to achieve greater control of myoclonic symptoms. Some drugs currently being studied in different combinations include clonazepam, sodium valproate, levetiracetam, and primidone. Hormonal therapy also may improve responses to antimyoclonic drugs in some people.

What Do Scientists Know about Myoclonus?

Although rare cases of myoclonus are caused by an injury to the peripheral nerves (defined as the nerves outside the brain and spinal cord, or the central nervous system (CNS)), most myoclonus is caused by a disturbance of the central nervous system. Studies suggest that several locations in the brain are involved in myoclonus. One such location, for example, is in the brain stem close to structures that are responsible for the startle response, an automatic reaction to an unexpected stimulus involving rapid muscle contraction.

The specific mechanisms underlying myoclonus are not yet fully understood. Scientists believe that some types of stimulus-sensitive myoclonus may involve overexcitability of the parts of the brain that control movement. These parts are interconnected in a series of feedback loops called motor pathways. These pathways facilitate and modulate communication between the brain and muscles. Key elements of this communication are chemicals known as neurotransmitters, which carry messages from one nerve cell, or neuron, to another. Neurotransmitters are released by neurons and attach themselves to receptors on parts of neighboring cells. Some neurotransmitters may make the receiving cell more sensitive, while others tend to make the receiving cell less sensitive. Laboratory studies suggest that an imbalance between these chemicals may underlie myoclonus.

Some researchers speculate that abnormalities or deficiencies in the receptors for certain neurotransmitters may contribute to some forms of myoclonus. Receptors that appear to be related to myoclonus include those for two important inhibitory neurotransmitters: serotonin and gamma-aminobutyric acid (GABA). Other receptors with links to myoclonus include those for opiates and glycine, the latter an inhibitory neurotransmitter that is important for the control of motor and sensory functions in the spinal cord. More research is needed to determine how these receptor abnormalities cause or contribute to myoclonus.

Chapter 26

Progressive Supranuclear Palsy (PSP)

What Is Progressive Supranuclear Palsy (PSP)?

PSP is an uncommon brain disorder that affects movement, control of walking (gait) and balance, speech, swallowing, vision, mood and behavior, and thinking. The disease results from damage to nerve cells in the brain. Its long name indicates that the disease worsens (progressive) and causes weakness (palsy) by damaging certain parts of the brain above nerve cell clusters called nuclei (supranuclear). These nuclei particularly control eye movements. One of the classic signs of the disease is an inability to aim and move the eyes properly, which individuals may experience as blurring of vision.

Estimates vary, but only about 3–6 in every 100,000 people world-wide, or approximately 20,000 Americans, have PSP—making it much less common than Parkinson disease (PD) (another movement disorder in which an estimated 50,000 Americans are diagnosed each year). Symptoms of PSP begin on average after age 60, but may occur earlier. Men are affected more often than women.

PSP was first described as a distinct disorder in 1964, when three scientists published a paper that distinguished the condition from PD.

This chapter includes text excerpted from "Progressive Supranuclear Palsy Fact Sheet," National Institute of Neurological Disorders and Stroke (NINDS), September 2015.

It was sometimes referred to as Steele-Richardson-Olszewski syndrome, reflecting the combined names of the scientists who defined the disorder.

Currently there is no effective treatment for PSP, but some symptoms can be managed with medication or other interventions.

What Are the Symptoms?

The pattern of signs and symptoms can be quite different from person to person. The most frequent first symptom of PSP is a loss of balance while walking. Individuals may have unexplained falls or a stiffness and awkwardness in gait.

As the disease progresses, most people will begin to develop a blurring of vision and problems controlling eye movement. In fact, eye problems, in particular slowness of eye movements, usually offer the first definitive clue that PSP is the proper diagnosis. Individuals affected by PSP especially have trouble voluntarily shifting their gaze vertically (i.e., downward and/or upward) and also can have trouble controlling their eyelids. This can lead to a need to move the head to look in different directions, involuntary closing of the eyes, prolonged or infrequent blinking, or difficulty in opening the eyes. Another common visual problem is an inability to maintain eye contact during a conversation. This can give the mistaken impression that the person is hostile or uninterested.

People with PSP often show alterations of mood and behavior, including depression and apathy. Some show changes in judgment, insight, and problem solving, and may have difficulty finding words. They may lose interest in ordinary pleasurable activities or show increased irritability and forgetfulness. Individuals may suddenly laugh or cry for no apparent reason, they may be apathetic, or they may have occasional angry outbursts, also for no apparent reason. Speech usually becomes slower and slurred and swallowing solid foods or liquids can be difficult. Other symptoms include slowed movement, monotone speech, and a mask-like facial expression. Since many symptoms of PSP are also seen in individuals with PD, particularly early in the disorder, PSP is often misdiagnosed as PD.

How Is PSP Different from PD?

Both PSP and PD cause stiffness, movement difficulties, and clumsiness, but PSP is more rapidly progressive as compared to PD. People with PSP usually stand exceptionally straight or occasionally even tilt their heads backward (and tend to fall backward). This is termed "axial rigidity." Those with PD usually bend forward. Problems with speech and swallowing are much more common and severe in PSP than in PD, and tend to show up earlier in the course of the disease. Eye movements are abnormal in PSP but close to normal in PD. Both diseases share other features: onset in late middle age, bradykinesia (slow movement), and rigidity of muscles. Tremor, very common in individuals with PD, is rare in PSP. Although individuals with PD markedly benefit from the drug levodopa, people with PSP respond minimally and only briefly to this drug. Also, people with PSP show accumulation of the protein tau in affected brain cells, while people with PD show accumulation of a different protein, called alpha-synuclein.

What Causes PSP?

The exact cause of PSP is unknown. The symptoms of PSP are caused by a gradual deterioration of brain cells in a few specific areas in the brain, mainly in the region called the brain stem. One of these areas, the substantia nigra, is also affected in PD, and damage to this region of the brain accounts in part for the motor symptoms that PSP and PD have in common.

The hallmark of the disease is the accumulation of abnormal deposits of the protein tau in nerve cells in the brain, so that the cells do not work properly and die. The protein tau is associated with microtubules—structures that support a nerve cell's long processes, or axons, that transmit information to other nerve cells. The accumulation of tau puts PSP in the group of disorders called the tauopathies, which also includes other disorders such as Alzheimer disease (AD), corticobasal degeneration, and some forms of frontotemporal degeneration. Scientists are looking at ways to prevent the harmful clumping of tau in treating each of these disorders.

PSP is usually sporadic, meaning that occurs infrequently and without known cause; in very few cases the disease results from mutations in the *MAPT* gene, which then provides faulty instructions for making tau to the nerve cell. Genetic factors have not been implicated in most individuals.

There are several theories about PSP's cause. A central hypothesis in many neurodegenerative diseases is that once the abnormal aggregates of proteins like tau form in a cell, they can affect a connected cell to also form the protein clumps. In this way the toxic protein aggregates spreads through the nervous system. How this process is triggered remains unknown. One possibility is that an unconventional infectious agent takes years or decades to start producing visible effects (as is seen in disorders like Creutzfeldt-Jakob Disease (CJD)). Another possibility is that random genetic mutations, of the kind that occur in all of us all the time, happen to occur in particular cells or certain genes, in just the right combination to injure these cells. A third possibility is that there is exposure to some unknown chemical in the food, air, or water which slowly damages certain vulnerable areas of the brain. This theory stems from a clue found on the Pacific island of Guam, where a common neurological disease occurring only there and on a few neighboring islands shares some of the characteristics of PSP, AD, PD, and amyotrophic lateral sclerosis (ALS). Its cause is thought to be a dietary factor or toxic substance found only in that area.

Another possible cause of PSP is cellular damage caused by free radicals, which are reactive molecules produced continuously by all cells during normal metabolism. Although the body has built-in mechanisms for clearing free radicals from the system, scientists suspect that, under certain circumstances, free radicals can react with and damage other molecules. A great deal of research is directed at understanding the role of free radical damage in human diseases.

How Is PSP Diagnosed?

No specific laboratory tests or imaging approaches currently exist to definitively diagnose PSP. The disease is often difficult to diagnose because its symptoms can be very much like those of other movement disorders, and because some of the most characteristic symptoms may develop late or not at all. Initial complaints in PSP are typically vague and fall into these categories:

- Symptoms of disequilibrium, such as unsteady walking or abrupt and unexplained falls without loss of consciousness;

- Visual complaints, including blurred vision, difficulties in looking up or down, double vision, light sensitivity, burning eyes, or other eye trouble;

- Slurred speech; and

- Various mental complaints such as slowness of thought, impaired memory, personality changes, and changes in mood.

An initial diagnosis is based on the person's medical history and a physical and neurological exam. Diagnostic scans such as magnetic resonance imaging (MRI) may show shrinkage at the top of the brain stem. Other imaging tests can look at brain activity in known areas of degeneration.

PSP is often misdiagnosed because it is relatively rare and some of its symptoms are very much like those of PD. Memory problems and personality changes may also lead a physician to mistake PSP for depression, or even attribute symptoms to some form of dementia. The key to diagnosing PSP is identifying early gait instability and difficulty moving the eyes, speech and swallow abnormalities, as well as ruling out other similar disorders, some of which are treatable.

Is There Any Treatment?

There is currently no effective treatment for PSP, although scientists are searching for better ways to manage the disease. PSP symptoms usually do not respond to medications. Drugs prescribed to treat PD, such as ropinirole, rarely provide additional benefit. In some individuals the slowness, stiffness, and balance problems of PSP may respond to some degree to antiparkinsonian agents such as levodopa, but the effect is usually minimal and short-lasting. Excessive eye closing can be treated with botulinum injections. Some antidepressant drugs may provide benefit beyond treating depression, such as pain relief and decreasing drooling.

Recent approaches to therapeutic development for PSP have focused primarily on the clearance of abnormally accumulated tau in the brain. One ongoing clinical trial will determine the safety and tolerability of a compound that prevents accumulation of tau in preclinical models. Other studies are exploring improved tau imaging agents that will be used to assess disease progression and improvement in response to treatment.

Nondrug treatment for PSP can take many forms. Individuals frequently use weighted walking aids because of their tendency to fall backward. Bifocals or special glasses called prisms are sometimes prescribed for people with PSP to remedy the difficulty of looking down. Formal physical therapy is of no proven benefit in PSP, but certain exercises can be done to keep the joints limber.

A gastrostomy (a minimally invasive surgical procedure that involves the placement of a tube through the skin of the abdomen into the stomach for feeding purposes) may be necessary when there are swallowing disturbances or the definite risk of severe choking. Deep brain stimulation (DBS) (which uses a surgically implanted electrode and pulse generator to stimulate the brain in a way that helps to block signals that cause many of the motor symptoms) and other surgical procedures used in individuals with PD have not been proven effective in PSP.

What Is the Prognosis?

The disease gets progressively worse, with people becoming severely disabled within three to five years of onset. Affected individuals are predisposed to serious complications such as pneumonia, choking, head injury, and fractures. The most common cause of death is pneumonia. With good attention to medical and nutritional needs, it is possible for individuals with PSP to live a decade or more after the first symptoms of the disease.

Chapter 27

Rett Syndrome

What Is Rett Syndrome?

Rett syndrome was first reported by Dr. Andreas Rett in 1966. Rett syndrome is a complex neurological and developmental disorder in which early growth and development appear normal at first, but then the infant stops developing and affected children even lose skills and abilities. Rett syndrome occurs mostly in females.

Over time, the effects of Rett syndrome can lead to cognitive, sensory, emotional, motor, cardiac, and such autonomic nervous system problems as difficulties with digestion or breathing.

What Are the Types and Phases of Rett Syndrome?

There are two main types of Rett syndrome: classic and atypical. The two types may differ by their symptoms or by the specific gene mutation.

The majority of Rett syndrome patients have the classic form, which typically develops in four phases. Healthcare providers and researchers, relying on consensus criteria, view the progression of classic Rett syndrome as the following phases:

- **Early onset phase.** In this phase, development stalls or stops completely. Sometimes, the syndrome takes hold at such a

This chapter includes text excerpted from "Rett Syndrome—Condition Information," *Eunice Kennedy Shriver* National Institute of Child Health and Human Development (NICHD), December 1, 2016.

subtle pace that parents and healthcare providers do not notice it at first. Researchers once thought that this phase began around 6 months of age. However, after analyzing videotapes of Rett individuals taken from birth, they now know that some infants with Rett syndrome only seem to develop normally. In fact, these infants show problems with very early development. In one study, all of the infants with Rett syndrome showed problems with body movements from birth through age 6 months. Another 42 percent showed stereotyped hand movements during this time period.

- **Rapid destructive phase.** The child loses skills (regresses) quickly. Purposeful hand movements and speech are usually the first skills lost. Breathing problems and stereotypic hand movements such as wringing (clasping or squeezing), washing (a movement that resembles washing the hands), and clapping or tapping also tend to start during this stage.

- **Plateau phase.** The child's regression slows and other problems may seem to lessen, or there may even be improvement in some areas. Seizures and movement problems are common at this stage. Many people with Rett syndrome spend most of their lives in this stage.

- **Late motor deterioration phase.** Individuals in this stage may become stiff or lose muscle tone; some become immobile. Scoliosis (an abnormal curvature of the spine) may be present and even become severe enough to require bracing or surgery. Stereotypic hand movements and breathing problems seem to become less common.

What Are the Symptoms of Rett Syndrome?

The first symptom of Rett syndrome is usually the loss of muscle tone, called hypotonia. With hypotonia, an infant's arms and legs will appear "floppy."

Although hypotonia and other symptoms of Rett syndrome often present themselves in stages, some typical symptoms can occur at any stage. Symptoms may vary among patients and range from mild to severe.

Typical symptoms (may occur at any stage) can include:

- Loss of ability to grasp and intentionally touch things

- Loss of ability to speak. (Initially, a child may stop saying words or phrases that he or she once said; later, the child may make sounds, but not say any purposeful words.)

- Severe problems with balance or coordination, leading to loss of the ability to walk. (These problems may start out as clumsiness and trouble walking. About 60 percent of those with Rett syndrome are still able to walk later in life; others may become unable to sit up or walk or may become immobile.)

- Mechanical, repetitive hand movements, such as hand wringing, hand washing, or grasping

- Complications with breathing, including hyperventilation and breath holding when awake

- Anxiety and social behavioral problems

- Intellectual disability

In addition, a person with Rett syndrome may experience one or more of the following associated problems:

- Scoliosis, or curvature of the spine from side to side. (Approximately 80 percent of girls with Rett syndrome have scoliosis. In some cases, the curving of the spine can become so severe that the girls require surgery. For some, bracing relieves the problem, prevents it from getting worse, or delays or eliminates the need for surgery.)

- Seizures. (These may involve the whole body, or they may be staring spells with no movement.)

- Constipation and gastroesophageal reflux (GERD)

- Discomfort in the abdomen or gallbladder problems such as gallstones

- Cardiac or heart problems, usually problems with heart rhythm. (Some persons with Rett syndrome may have abnormally long pauses between heartbeats, as measured by an electrocardiogram, or they may experience other types of arrhythmia.)

- Trouble feeding oneself, swallowing, and chewing food. (In some cases, too, in spite of healthy appetites, girls with Rett syndrome do not gain weight or have trouble maintaining a healthy weight. As a result, some girls with Rett syndrome rely on feeding tubes.)

- Disrupted sleep patterns at night (during childhood) and increased sleep (after age 5). (Some researchers suggest that problems with sleep are among the earliest symptoms of Rett syndrome and can appear between 1–2 months of age. Such problems can lead to sudden death during sleep.)

- Excessive saliva and drooling

- Poor circulation in hands and legs

- Walking on toes or the balls of feet

- Walking with a wide gait (ataxia)

- Grinding the teeth (bruxism)

How Many People Are Affected by or at Risk of Rett Syndrome?

Current estimates suggest that Rett syndrome occurs in 1 out of every 10,000–15,000 girls born and affects 1 in 10,000–22,000 females in the United States.

What Causes Rett Syndrome?

Most cases of Rett syndrome are caused by a change (also called a mutation) in a single gene. In 1999, *Eunice Kennedy Shriver* National Institute of Child Health and Human Development (NICHD)-supported scientists discovered that most classic Rett syndrome cases are caused by a mutation within the Methylcytosine-binding protein 2 (*MECP2*) gene. The *MECP2* gene is located on the X chromosome. Between 90–95 percent of girls with Rett syndrome have a mutation in the *MECP2* gene. Among families with a child affected by Rett syndrome the chance of having a second child with the syndrome is less than 1 percent.

Eight mutations in the *MECP2* gene represent the most prevalent causes of Rett syndrome. The development and severity of Rett syndrome symptoms depend on the location and type of the mutation on the *MECP2* gene.

The *MECP2* gene makes a protein that is necessary for the development of the nervous system, especially the brain. The mutation causes the gene to either make insufficient amounts of this protein or to make a damaged protein that the body cannot use. In either case, if there is not enough of the working protein for the brain to develop normally, Rett syndrome develops.

Researchers are still trying to understand exactly how the brain uses this protein, called MeCP2, and how problems with this protein cause the typical features of Rett syndrome.

Mutations on two other genes can cause some of the atypical variants of Rett syndrome: Congenital Rett syndrome (Rolando variant) is associated with mutations of the *FOXG1* gene, and *CDKL5* mutations are linked with the early-onset, or Hanefeld, variant. Males affected by these types of mutations can survive infancy. Males can also have a duplication of a normal *MECP2* gene and survive, but are severely affected. Too much MeCP2 protein is as bad for development as too little.

Is Rett Syndrome Passed from One Generation to the Next?

In 99.9 percent of cases, the genetic change that causes Rett syndrome is spontaneous, meaning it happens randomly. Such random mutations are usually not inherited or passed from one generation to the next. However, in a very small percentage of families—about 1 percent—Rett mutations are inherited and passed on by female carriers.

Why Do Mostly Females and So Few Boys Have Rett Syndrome?

Two types of chromosomes determine the sex of an embryo: the X and the Y chromosomes. Girls have two X chromosomes, and boys have one X and one Y chromosome.

Because the mutated gene that causes Rett syndrome is located on the X chromosome, females have twice the opportunity to develop a mutation in one of their X chromosomes. Females with Rett syndrome usually have one mutated X chromosome and one normal X chromosome. Only one X chromosome in a given cell remains active throughout life and cells randomly determine which X chromosome will remain active. If the cells have an active mutated gene more often than the normal gene, the symptoms of Rett syndrome will be more severe. This random process allows most females with Rett syndrome to survive infancy.

Because most boys have only one X chromosome, when this gene is mutated to cause Rett syndrome the detrimental effects are not softened by the presence of a second, normal X chromosome. As a result, many males with Rett syndrome are stillborn or do not live past infancy.

Some boys with Rett syndrome, however, do live past infancy, likely for one of three reasons:

- Mosaicism, a condition in which individual cells within the same person have a different genetic makeup. This means that some of the X chromosome genes in a boy's body have the Rett mutation, and some genes do not have the mutation. When a lower percentage of genes have the Rett syndrome mutation, the symptoms are not as severe.

- A boy may have two X chromosomes and one Y chromosome (Klinefelter syndrome (KS)). Only one X chromosome will be active in each cell, so if one X carries a mutation in *MECP2*, the severity of symptoms will depend on how many cells have that the mutant X active in the body.

- The genetic mutation is less severe than that of other forms of Rett syndrome mutations.

Duplication of the *MECP2* gene can occur in boys and affects intellectual and physical function.

How Do Healthcare Providers Diagnose Rett Syndrome?

Blood Test

Genetic evaluation of a blood sample can identify whether a child has one of the known mutations that cause Rett syndrome. Even if a child has a mutation of the Methylcytosine-binding protein 2 (*MECP2*) gene (which also occurs in other conditions), the symptoms of Rett syndrome may not always be present, so healthcare providers also need to evaluate the child's symptoms to confirm a diagnosis.

Clinical Symptoms

A child must meet the following five necessary criteria to be diagnosed with classic Rett syndrome:

Main Diagnostic Criteria

- A pattern of development, regression, then recovery or stabilization

- Partial or complete loss of purposeful hand skills such as grasping with fingers, reaching for things, or touching things on purpose

- Partial or complete loss of spoken language

- Repetitive hand movements, such as wringing the hands, washing, squeezing, clapping, or rubbing

- Gait abnormalities, including walking on toes or with an unsteady, wide-based, stiff-legged gait

A slowing of head growth between 3 months and 4 years of age, leading to acquired microcephaly, is also characteristic of Rett syndrome and calls for a diagnosis to be considered.

Healthcare providers will also consider whether any of the following conditions are present. The presence of any of the symptoms below would rule out a Rett syndrome diagnosis.

Atypical Rett Syndrome

Genetic mutations causing some atypical variants of Rett syndrome have been identified. After a blood test to confirm a child's genetic makeup, a healthcare provider may diagnose the child with atypical Rett syndrome if the child demonstrates development, followed by regression and then recovery or stabilization. In addition, the healthcare provider will confirm at least two of the other four main criteria, and five of the 11 supportive criteria before making a diagnosis.

Other Possible Diagnoses

Sometimes Rett syndrome is misdiagnosed as regressive autism, cerebral palsy, or nonspecific developmental delays.

For some males, the features of Rett syndrome occur with another genetic condition called Klinefelter syndrome, in which a boy has two X chromosomes and one Y chromosome. This means that the boy may have one mutated *MECP2* gene and one normal *MECP2* gene, reducing the effects of the mutated gene.

What Are the Treatments for Rett Syndrome?

Most people with Rett syndrome benefit from well-designed interventions no matter what their age, but the earlier that treatment begins, the better. With therapy and assistance, people with Rett syndrome can participate in school and community activities.

These treatments, forms of assistance, and options for medication generally aim to slow the loss of abilities, improve or preserve movement, and encourage communication and social contact. A list of treatment options is presented below; the need for these treatments depends on the severity of different symptoms.

Physical Therapy / Hydrotherapy

- Improves or maintains mobility and balance

- Reduces misshapen back and limbs

- Provides weight-bearing training for patients with scoliosis (an abnormal curvature of the spine)

Occupational Therapy

- Improves or maintains use of hands

- Reduces stereotypic hand movements such as wringing, washing (a movement that resembles washing the hands), clapping, rubbing, or tapping

- Teaches self-directed activities like dressing and feeding

Speech-Language Therapy

- Teaches nonverbal communication

- Improves social interaction

Feeding Assistance

- Supplements calcium and minerals to strengthen bones and slow scoliosis

- High-calorie, high-fat diet to increase height and weight

- Insertion of a feeding tube if patients accidentally swallow their food into their lungs (aspiration)

Physical Assistance

- Braces or surgery to correct scoliosis

- Splints to adjust hand movements

Medication

- To reduce breathing problems

- To eliminate problems with abnormal heart rhythm
- To relieve indigestion and constipation
- To control seizures

Chapter 28

Spina Bifida

Spina bifida is a condition that affects the spine and is usually apparent at birth. It is a type of neural tube defect (NTD).

Spina bifida can happen anywhere along the spine if the neural tube does not close all the way. When the neural tube doesn't close all the way, the backbone that protects the spinal cord doesn't form and close as it should. This often results in damage to the spinal cord and nerves.

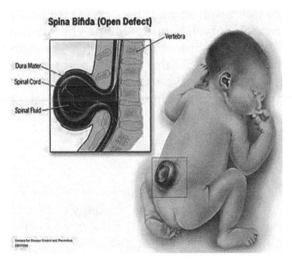

Figure 28.1. *Spina Bifida*

This chapter includes text excerpted from "Spina Bifida," Centers for Disease Control and Prevention (CDC), September 11, 2017.

Spina bifida might cause physical and intellectual disabilities that range from mild to severe. The severity depends on:

- The size and location of the opening in the spine

- Whether part of the spinal cord and nerves are affected

Types of Spina Bifida

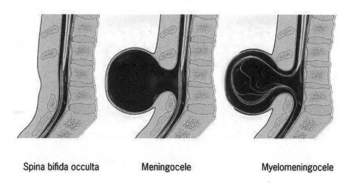

Spina bifida occulta   Meningocele   Myelomeningocele

Figure 28.2. *Types of Spina Bifida*

The three most common types of spina bifida are:

Myelomeningocele

When people talk about spina bifida, most often they are referring to myelomeningocele. Myelomeningocele is the most serious type of spina bifida. With this condition, a sac of fluid comes through an opening in the baby's back. Part of the spinal cord and nerves are in this sac and are damaged. This type of spina bifida causes moderate to severe disabilities, such as problems affecting how the person goes to the bathroom, loss of feeling in the person's legs or feet, and not being able to move the legs.

Meningocele

Another type of spina bifida is meningocele. With meningocele a sac of fluid comes through an opening in the baby's back. But, the spinal cord is not in this sac. There is usually little or no nerve damage. This type of spina bifida can cause minor disabilities.

Spina Bifida Occulta

Spina bifida occulta is the mildest type of spina bifida. It is sometimes called "hidden" spina bifida. With it, there is a small gap in the spine, but no opening or sac on the back. The spinal cord and the nerves usually are normal. Many times, spina bifida occulta is not discovered until late childhood or adulthood. This type of spina bifida usually does not cause any disabilities.

Causes and Prevention

We do not know all of the causes of spina bifida. The role that genetics and the environment play in causing spina bifida needs to be studied further.

However, we do know that there are ways for women to reduce the risk of having a baby with spina bifida both before and during her pregnancy.

If you are pregnant or could get pregnant, use the following tips to help prevent your baby from having spina bifida:

- Take 400 micrograms (mcg) of folic acid every day. If you have already had a pregnancy affected by spina bifida, you may need to take a higher dose of folic acid before pregnancy and during early pregnancy. Talk to your doctor to discuss what's best for you.

- Talk to your doctor or pharmacist about any prescription and over-the-counter (OTC) drugs, vitamins, and dietary or herbal supplements you are taking.

- If you have a medical condition—such as diabetes or obesity—be sure it is under control before you become pregnant.

- Avoid overheating your body, as might happen if you use a hot tub or sauna.

- Treat any fever you have right away with Tylenol® (or store brand acetaminophen).

Diagnosis

Spina bifida can be diagnosed during pregnancy or after the baby is born. Spina bifida occulta might not be diagnosed until late childhood or adulthood, or might never be diagnosed.

During Pregnancy

During pregnancy there are screening tests (prenatal tests) to check for spina bifida and other birth defects. Talk with your doctor about any questions or concerns you have about this prenatal testing.

- **AFP.** AFP stands for alpha-fetoprotein, a protein the unborn baby produces. This is a simple blood test that measures how much AFP has passed into the mother's bloodstream from the baby. A high level of AFP might mean that the baby has spina bifida. An AFP test might be part of a test called the "triple screen" that looks for neural tube defects and other issues.

- **Ultrasound.** An ultrasound is a type of picture of the baby. In some cases, the doctor can see if the baby has spina bifida or find other reasons that there might be a high level of AFP. Frequently, spina bifida can be seen with this test.

- **Amniocentesis.** For this test, the doctor takes a small sample of the amniotic fluid surrounding the baby in the womb. Higher than average levels of AFP in the fluid might mean that the baby has spina bifida.

After the Baby Is Born

In some cases, spina bifida might not be diagnosed until after the baby is born.

Sometimes there is a hairy patch of skin or a dimple on the baby's back that is first seen after the baby is born. A doctor can use an image scan, such as an, X-ray, magnetic resonance imaging (MRI), or computed tomography (CT), to get a clearer view of the baby's spine and the bones in the back.

Sometimes spina bifida is not diagnosed until after the baby is born because the mother did not receive prenatal care or an ultrasound did not show clear pictures of the affected part of the spine.

Treatments

Not all people born with spina bifida have the same needs, so treatment will be different for each person. Some people have problems that are more serious than others. People with myelomeningocele and meningocele will need more treatments than people with spina bifida occulta.

Remember!

Spina bifida happens in the first few weeks of pregnancy, often before a woman knows she's pregnant. Although folic acid is not a guarantee that a woman will have a healthy pregnancy, taking folic acid can help reduce a woman's risk of having a pregnancy affected by spina bifida. Because half of all pregnancies in the United States are unplanned, it is important that all women who can become pregnant take 400 mcg of folic acid daily one month before pregnancy and during early pregnancy.

Living with Spina Bifida

Spina bifida can range from mild to severe. Some people may have little to no disability. Other people may be limited in the way they move or function. Some people may even be paralyzed or unable to walk or move parts of their body.

Even so, with the right care, most people affected by spina bifida lead full, productive lives.

Chapter 29

Spinal Cord Injury and Disease

What Is a Spinal Cord Injury (SCI)?

The vertebrae normally protect the soft tissues of the spinal cord, but they can be broken or dislocated in a variety of ways that puts harmful pressure on the spinal cord. Injuries can occur at any level of the spinal cord. The segment of the cord that is injured, and the severity of the damage to the nervous tissue, will determine which body functions are compromised or lost. An injury to a part of the spinal cord causes physiological consequences to parts of the body controlled by nerves at and below the level of the injury.

Motor vehicle accidents and catastrophic falls are the most common causes of physical trauma that breaks, crushes, or presses on the vertebrae and can cause irreversible damage at the corresponding level of the spinal cord and below. Severe trauma to the cervical cord results in paralysis of most of the body, including the arms and legs, and is called tetraplegia (though the older term, quadriplegia, is still in common use). Trauma to the thoracic nerves in the upper, middle, or lower back results in paralysis of the trunk and lower extremities, called paraplegia.

This chapter includes text excerpted from "Spinal Cord Injury: Hope Through Research," National Institute of Neurological Disorders and Stroke (NINDS), July 2013. Reviewed January 2018.

Penetrating injuries, such as gunshot or knife wounds, damage the spinal cord; however, most traumatic injuries do not completely sever the spinal cord. Instead, an injury is more likely to cause fractures and compression of the vertebrae, which then crush and destroy the axons that carry signals up and down the spinal cord. A SCI can damage a few, many, or almost all of the axons that cross the site of injury. A variety of cells located in and around the injury site may also die. Some injuries in which there is little or no nerve cell death but only pressure induced blockage of nerve signaling or only demyelination without axonal damage will allow almost complete recovery. Others in which there is complete cell death across even a thin horizontal level of the spinal cord will result in complete paralysis.

What Happens When the Spinal Cord Is Injured?

Traumatic SCI usually begins with a sudden, mechanical blow or rupture to the spine that fractures or dislocates vertebrae. The damage begins at the moment of primary injury, when the cord is stretched or displaced by bone fragments or disc material. Nerve signaling stops immediately but may not return rapidly even if there is no structural damage to the cord. In severe injury, axons are cut or damaged beyond repair, and neural cell membranes are broken. Blood vessels may rupture and cause bleeding into the spinal cord's central tissue, or bleeding can occur outside the cord, causing pressure by the blood clot on the cord.

Within minutes, the spinal cord near the site of severe injury swells within the spinal canal. This may increase pressure on the cord and cut blood flow to spinal cord tissue. Blood pressure can drop, sometimes dramatically, as the body loses its ability to self-regulate. All these changes can cause a condition known as spinal shock that can last from several hours to several days.

There is some controversy among neurologists about the extent and impact of spinal shock, and even its definition in terms of physiological characteristics. It appears to occur in approximately half of the cases of SCI and is usually directly related to the size and severity of the injury. During spinal shock, the entire spinal cord below the lesion becomes temporarily disabled, causing complete paralysis, loss of all reflexes, and loss of sensation below the affected cord level.

The primary injury initiates processes that continue for days or weeks. It sets off a cascade of biochemical and cellular events that kills neurons, strips axons of their protective myelin covering, and triggers an inflammatory immune system response. This is the beginning of the secondary injury process. Days, or sometimes even weeks later, after this second wave of damage has passed, the area of destruction has increased—sometimes to several segments above and below the original injury.

- **Changes in blood flow cause ongoing damage.** The major reduction in blood flow to the site following the initial injury can last for as long as 24 hours and become progressively worse if there is continued compression of the cord due to swelling or bleeding. Because of the greater blood flow needs of gray matter, the impact is greater on the central cord than on the outlying white matter. Blood vessels in the gray matter also become leaky, sometimes as early as 5 minutes after injury, which initiates spinal cord swelling. Cells that line the still intact blood vessels in the spinal cord also begin to swell, and this further reduces blood flow to the injured area. The combination of leaking, swelling, and sluggish blood flow prevents the normal delivery of oxygen and nutrients to neurons, causing many of them to die.

- **Excessive release of neurotransmitters kills nerve cells.** After the injury, an excessive release of neurotransmitters (chemicals that allow neurons to signal each other) can cause additional damage by over stimulating nerve cells. The neurotransmitter glutamate is commonly used by axons in the spinal cord to stimulate activity in other neurons. But when spinal cells are injured, their axons flood the area with glutamate and trigger additional nerve cell damage. This process kills neurons near the injury site and the myelin forming oligodendrocytes at and beyond the injured area.

- **An invasion of immune system cells creates inflammation.** Under normal conditions, the blood-brain barrier keeps potentially destructive immune system cells from entering the brain or spinal cord. This barrier is a naturally occurring result of closely spaced cells along the blood vessels that prevent many substances from leaving the blood and entering brain tissues. But when the blood-brain barrier breaks down, immune system cells—primarily white blood cells—can invade the spinal cord tissue and trigger an inflammatory response. This inflammatory response can cause additional damage to some neurons and may kill others.

- **Free radicals attack nerve cells.** Another consequence of inflammation is the increased production of highly reactive forms of oxygen molecules called free radicals—chemicals that modify the chemical structure of other molecules in damaging ways, for example, damaging cell membranes. Free radicals are produced naturally as a byproduct of normal oxygen metabolism in small enough amounts that they cause no harm. But injury to the spinal cord causes cells to overproduce free radicals, which destroy critical molecules of the cell.

- **Nerve cells self-destruct.** For reasons that are still unclear, SCI sets off apoptosis—a normal process of cell death that helps the body get rid of old and unhealthy cells. Apoptosis kills oligo-dendrocytes in damaged areas of the spinal cord days to weeks after the injury. Apoptosis can strip myelin from intact axons in adjacent ascending and descending pathways, causing the axons to become dysfunctional and disrupting the spinal cord's ability to communicate with the brain.

- **Scarring occurs.** Following a SCI, astrocytes (star shaped glial cells that support the brain and spinal cord) wall off the injury site by forming a scar, which creates a physical and chemical barrier to any axons which could potentially regenerate and reconnect. Even if some intact myelinated axons remain, there may not be enough to convey any meaningful information to or from the brain.

Researchers are especially interested in studying the mechanisms of this wave of secondary damage because finding ways to stop it could save spinal cord tissue and thereby enable greater functional recovery.

What Immediate Treatments Are Available?

Injury to the spine isn't always obvious. Any injury that involves the head and neck, pelvic fractures, penetrating injuries in the area of the spine, or injuries that result from falling from heights should raise concerns regarding an unstable spinal column. Until imaging of the spine is done at an emergency or trauma center, people who might have spine injury should be cared for as if any significant movement of the neck or back could cause further damage.

At the accident scene, emergency personnel will immobilize the head and neck to prevent movement, put a rigid collar around the neck, and carefully place the person on a rigid backboard to prevent further damage to the spinal cord. Sedation may be given to relax the person and prevent movement. A breathing tube may be inserted if the injury is to the high cervical cord and the individual is at risk of respiratory arrest.

At the hospital or trauma center, realigning the spine using a rigid brace or axial traction (using a mechanical force to stretch the spine and relieve pressure on the spinal cord) is usually done as soon as possible to stabilize the spine and prevent additional damage. Fractured vertebrae, bone fragments, herniated discs, or other objects compressing the spinal column may need to be surgically removed. Spinal decompression surgery to relieve pressure within the spinal column also may be necessary in the days after injury. Results of a neurosurgical study show that, in some cases, earlier surgery is associated with better functional recovery.

How Are Spinal Cord Injuries Diagnosed?

The emergency room physician will test the individual to see if there is any movement or sensation at or below the level of injury. Methods to assess autonomic function also have been established (American Spinal Injury Association (ASIA), or, Autonomic Standards Classification). Emergency medical tests for a SCI include:

- **Magnetic resonance imaging (MRI),** which uses computer generated radio waves and a powerful magnetic field to produce detailed three dimensional images of body structures, including tissues, organs, bones, and nerves. It can document brain and spinal trauma from injury, as well as aid in diagnosing brain and spinal cord tumors, herniated disks, vascular (blood vessel) irregularities, bleeding and inflammation that might compress the spine and spinal cord, and injury to the ligaments that support the cervical spine.

- **Computerized tomography (CT)** provides rapid, clear two dimensional X-ray images of organs, bones, and tissues. Neurological CT scans are used to view the brain and spine. CT is excellent in detecting bone fractures, bleeding, and spinal stenosis (narrowing of the spinal canal), but CT has less ability to image the spinal cord or identify ligament injury associated with an unstable spine than MRI.

- **Plane X-rays** (which demonstrate the planes of bone on bone) of the person's chest and skull are often taken as part of a neurological workup. X-rays can be used to view most parts of the body, such as a joint or major organ system. In a conventional X-ray, a concentrated burst of low dose ionized radiation is passed through the body and onto a photographic plate. Since calcium in bones absorbs X-rays more easily than soft tissue or muscle, the bony structure appears white on the film. Vertebral misalignment or fracture can be seen within minutes. X-rays taken in different neck positions (i.e., flexion and extension views) detect instability of the cervical spine. Tissue masses such as injured ligaments or a bulging disc are not visible on conventional X-rays.

How Are Spinal Cord Injuries Classified?

Once the swelling from within and around the spinal cord has eased a bit—usually within a week to 10 days—physicians will conduct a complete neurological exam to classify the injury as complete or incomplete. An incomplete injury means that the ability of the spinal cord to convey messages to or from the brain is not completely lost. People with incomplete injuries retain some sensory function and may have voluntary motor activity below the injury site. A complete injury prevents nerve communications from the brain and spinal cord to parts of the body below the injury site. There is a total lack of sensory and motor function below the level of injury, even if the spinal cord was not completely severed. Studies have shown that people with incomplete injuries have a greater chance of recovering some function in the affected limbs than those with a complete injury.

Physicians use the International Standards of Neurologic Classification of Spinal Cord Injury (ISNCSCI) to measure the extent of neurologic injury following a SCI.

How Does an SCI Affect the Rest of the Body and How Is It Treated?

People who survive a SCI often have medical complications resulting in bladder, bowel, and sexual dysfunction. They may also develop chronic pain, autonomic dysfunction, and spasticity (increased tone in and contractions of muscles of the arms and legs), but this is highly variable and poorly understood. Higher levels of injury may have an increased susceptibility to respiratory and heart problems.

Breathing

A SCI high in the neck can affect the nerves and muscles in the neck and chest that are involved with breathing. Respiratory complications are often an indication of the severity of SCI. About one third of those with injury to the neck area will need help with breathing and require respiratory support via intubation, which involves inserting a tube connected to a machine that pushes oxygen into the lungs and removes carbon dioxide) through the nose or throat and into the airway. This may be temporary or permanent depending upon the severity and location of injury. Any injury to the spinal cord between the C1–C4 segments, which supply the phrenic nerves leading to the diaphragm, can stop breathing. (The phrenic nerves cause the diaphragm to move and the lungs to expand.) People with these injuries need immediate ventilatory support. People with high cervical cord injury may have trouble coughing and clearing secretions from their lungs. Special training regarding breathing and swallowing may be needed.

Pneumonia

Respiratory complications are the leading cause of death in people with SCI, commonly as a result of pneumonia. Intubation increases the risk of developing ventilator associated pneumonia; individuals with SCI who are intubated have to be carefully monitored and treated with antibiotics if symptoms of pneumonia appear. Attention to clearing secretions and preventing aspiration of mouth contents into the lungs can prevent pneumonia.

Circulatory Problems

Spinal cord injuries can cause a variety of changes in circulation, including blood pressure instability, abnormal heart rhythms (arrhythmias) that may appear days after the injury, and blood clots. Because the brain's control of the cardiac nerves is cut off, the heart can beat at a dangerously slow pace, or it can pound rapidly and irregularly. Arrhythmias are more common and severe in the most serious injuries. Low blood pressure also often occurs due to changes in nervous system control of blood vessels, which then widen, causing blood to pool in the small arteries far away from the heart. Blood pressure needs to be closely monitored to keep blood and oxygen flowing through the spinal cord tissue, with the understanding that baseline blood pressure can be significantly lower than usual in people living with spinal cord injuries. Since muscle movement contributes to moving blood back to the heart, people with spinal cord injuries are at triple the usual risk for blood clots due to stagnation of blood flow in the large veins in the legs. Treatment includes anticoagulant drugs and compression stockings to increase blood flow in the lower legs and feet.

Spasticity and Muscle Tone

When the spinal cord is damaged, information from the brain can no longer regulate reflex activity. Reflexes may become exaggerated over time, causing muscle spasticity. Muscles may waste away or diminish due to underuse. If spasms become severe enough, they may require medical treatment. For some, spasms can be as much of a help as they are a hindrance, since spasms can tone muscles that would otherwise waste away. Some people can even learn to use the increased tone in their legs to help them turn over in bed, propel them into and out of a wheelchair, or stand.

Autonomic Dysreflexia

The autonomic nervous system controls involuntary actions such as blood pressure, heartbeat, and bladder and bowel function. Autonomic dysreflexia (AD) is a life-threatening reflex action that primarily affects those with injuries to the neck or upper back. It happens when there is an irritation, pain, or stimulus to the nervous system below the level of injury. The irritated area tries to send a sensory signal to the brain, but the signal may be misdirected, causing a runaway reflex action in the spinal cord that has been disconnected from the brain's regulation. Unlike spasms that affect muscles, AD affects blood vessels and organ systems controlled by the sympathetic nervous system. Anything that causes pain or irritation can set off AD, including a full bladder, constipation, cuts, burns, bruises, sunburn, pressure of any kind on the body, or tight clothing. Symptoms of its onset may include flushing or sweating, a pounding headache, anxiety, sudden increase in blood pressure, vision changes, or goose bumps on the arms and legs. Emptying the bladder or bowels and removing or loosening tight clothing are just a few of the possibilities that should be tried to relieve whatever is causing the irritation. If possible, the person should be kept in a sitting position, rather than lying flat, to keep blood flowing to the lower extremities and help reduce blood pressure.

Pressure Sores (Pressure Ulcers)

Pressure sores are areas of skin tissue that have broken down because of continuous pressure on the skin and reduced blood flow to the area. People with paraplegia and tetraplegia are susceptible to pressure sores because they may lose all or part of skin sensations and cannot shift their weight. As a result, individuals must be shifted periodically by a caregiver if they cannot shift positions themselves.

Good nutrition and hygiene can also help prevent pressure sores by encouraging healthy skin. Special motorized rotating beds may be used to prevent and treat sores.

Pain

Some people who have spinal cord nerve are paralyzed often develop neurogenic pain—pain or an intense burning or stinging sensation may be unremitting due to hypersensitivity in some parts of the body. It can either be spontaneous or triggered by a variety of factors and can occur even in parts of the body that have lost normal sensation. Almost all people with SCI are prone to normal musculoskeletal pain as well, such as shoulder pain due to overuse of the shoulder joint from using a wheelchair. Treatments for chronic pain include medications, acupuncture, spinal, or brain electrical stimulation, and surgery. However, none of these treatments are completely effective at relieving neurogenic pain.

Bladder and Bowel Problems

Most spinal cord injuries affect bladder and bowel functions because the nerves that control the involved organs originate in the segments near the lower end of the spinal cord and lose normal brain input. Although the kidneys continue to produce urine, bladder control may be lost and the risk of bladder and urinary tract infections increases. Some people may need to use a catheter to empty their bladders. The digestive system may be unaffected, but people recovering from a SCI may need to learn ways to empty their bowels. A change in diet may be needed to help with control.

- **Sexual function.** Depending on the level of injury and recovery from the trauma, sexual function, and fertility may be affected. A urologist and other specialists can suggest different options for sexual functioning and health.

- **Depression.** Many people living with a SCI may develop depression as a result of lifestyle changes. Therapy and medicines may help treat depression.

Once someone has survived the injury and begins to cope psychologically and emotionally, the next concern is how to live with disabilities. Doctors are now able to predict with reasonable accuracy the likely long-term outcome of spinal cord injuries. This helps people experiencing SCI set achievable goals for themselves, and gives families and loved ones a realistic set of expectations for the future.

How Does Rehabilitation Help People Recover from SCIs?

No two people will experience the same emotions after surviving an SCI, but almost everyone will feel frightened, anxious, or confused about what has happened. It's common for people to have very mixed feelings: relief that they are still alive, but disbelief at the nature of their disabilities.

Rehabilitation programs combine physical therapies with skill building activities and counseling to provide social and emotional support. The education and active involvement of the newly injured person and his or her family and friends is crucial.

A rehabilitation team is usually led by a doctor specializing in physical medicine and rehabilitation (called a physiatrist), and often includes social workers, physical and occupational therapists, recreational therapists, rehabilitation nurses, rehabilitation psychologists, vocational counselors, nutritionists, a case worker, and other specialists.

In the initial phase of rehabilitation, therapists emphasize regaining communication skills and leg and arm strength. For some individuals, mobility will only be possible with the assistance of devices such as a walker, leg braces, or a wheelchair. Communication skills such as writing, typing, and using the telephone may also require adaptive devices for some people with tetraplegia.

Physical therapy includes exercise programs geared toward muscle strengthening. Occupational therapy helps redevelop fine motor skills, particularly those needed to perform activities of daily living such as getting in and out of a bed, self-grooming, and eating. Bladder and bowel management programs teach basic toileting routines. People acquire coping strategies for recurring episodes of spasticity, AD, and neurogenic pain.

Vocational rehabilitation includes identifying the person's basic work skills and physical and cognitive capabilities to determine the likelihood for employment; identifying potential workplaces and any assistive equipment that will be needed; and arranging for a user friendly workplace. If necessary, educational training is provided to develop skills for a new line of work that may be less dependent upon physical abilities and more dependent upon computer or communication skills. Individuals with disabilities that prevent them from returning to the workforce are encouraged to maintain productivity by participating in activities that provide a sense of satisfaction and self-esteem, such as educational classes, hobbies, memberships in special interest groups, and participation in family and community events.

Recreation therapy encourages people with SCI to participate in recreational sports or activities at their level of mobility, as well as achieve a more balanced and normal lifestyle that provides opportunities for socialization and self-expression.

Adaptive devices also may help people with SCI to regain independence and improve mobility and quality of life. Such devices may include a wheelchair, electronic stimulators, assisted gait training, neural prostheses, computer adaptations, and other computer-assisted technology.

Chapter 30

Spinal Muscular Atrophy (SMA)

What Is Spinal Muscular Atrophy (SMA)?

SMA is one of several hereditary diseases that progressively destroy lower motor neurons—nerve cells in the brainstem and spinal cord that control essential voluntary muscle activity such as speaking, walking, breathing, and swallowing. Lower motor neurons control movement in the arms, legs, chest, face, throat, and tongue.

When there are disruptions in the signals between lower motor neurons and muscles, the muscles gradually weaken and may begin wasting away and develop uncontrollable twitching (fasciculations). When there are disruptions in the signals between the upper motor neurons (located in the brain) and the lower motor neurons, the limb muscles develop stiffness (spasticity), movements become slow and effortful, and tendon reflexes such as knee and ankle jerks become overactive. Over time, the ability to control voluntary movement can be lost.

What Causes SMA?

SMA is caused by defects in the gene *SMN1*, which makes a protein that is important for the survival of motor neurons (SMN

This chapter includes text excerpted from "Spinal Muscular Atrophy Fact Sheet," National Institute of Neurological Disorders and Stroke (NINDS), July 2012. Reviewed January 2018.

protein). In SMA, insufficient levels of the SMN protein lead to degeneration of the lower motor neurons, producing weakness, and wasting of the skeletal muscles. This weakness is often more severe in the trunk and upper leg and arm muscles than in muscles of the hands and feet.

How Is It Inherited?

SMA disorders in children are inherited in an autosomal recessive manner. Autosomal recessive means the child must inherit a copy of the defective gene from both parents. These parents are likely to be asymptomatic (without symptoms of the disease). Autosomal recessive diseases often affect more than one person in the same generation (siblings or cousins).

Kennedy disease, an adult form of SMA is X-linked inherited, which means the mother carries the defective gene on one of her X chromosomes and passes the disorder along to her sons. Males inherit an X chromosome from their mother and a Y chromosome from their father, while females inherit an X chromosome from each parent. Daughters have a 50 percent chance of inheriting their mother's faulty X chromosome and a safe X chromosome from their father, which would make them asymptomatic carriers of the mutation.

What Are the Types of SMA?

SMA in children is classified into three types, based on ages of onset, severity, and progression of symptoms. All three types are caused by defects in the *SMN1* gene.

- **SMA type I, also called Werdnig-Hoffmann disease or infantile-onset SMA**, is evident by the time a child is 6 months old. Symptoms may include hypotonia (severely reduced muscle tone), diminished limb movements, lack of tendon reflexes, fasciculations, tremors, swallowing and feeding difficulties, and impaired breathing. Some children also develop scoliosis (curvature of the spine) or other skeletal abnormalities. Affected children never sit or stand and the vast majority usually die of respiratory failure before the age of 2. However, the survival rate in individuals with SMA type I has increased in recent years, in relation to the growing trend toward more proactive clinical care.

- Symptoms of **SMA type II, the intermediate form**, usually begin between 6–18 months of age. Children may be able to sit without support but are unable to stand or walk unaided, and may have respiratory difficulties, including an increased risk of respiratory infections. The progression of disease is variable. Life expectancy is reduced but some individuals live into adolescence or young adulthood.

- Symptoms of **SMA type III (Kugelberg-Welander disease)** appear between 2–17 years of age and include abnormal gait; difficulty running, climbing steps, or rising from a chair; and a fine tremor of the fingers. The lower extremities are most often affected. Complications include scoliosis and joint contractures— chronic shortening of muscles or tendons around joints, caused by abnormal muscle tone and weakness, which prevents the joints from moving freely. Individuals with SMA type III may be prone to respiratory infections, but with care may have a normal lifespan.

Other forms of SMA include:

- **Congenital SMA with arthrogryposis** (persistent contracture of joints with fixed abnormal posture of the limb) is a rare disorder. Manifestations include severe contractures, scoliosis, chest deformity, respiratory problems, unusually small jaws, and drooping of the upper eyelids.

- **Kennedy disease**, also known as progressive spinobulbar muscular atrophy (SBMA), may first be recognized between 15–60 years of age. The onset of symptoms varies and includes weakness and atrophy of the facial, jaw, and tongue muscles, leading to problems with chewing, swallowing, and changes in speech. Early symptoms may include muscle pain and fatigue. Weakness in arm and leg muscles closest to the trunk of the body develops over time, with muscle atrophy and fasciculations. Individuals with Kennedy disease also develop sensory loss in the feet and hands. Nerve conduction studies confirm that nearly all individuals have a sensory neuropathy (pain from sensory nerve inflammation or degeneration). Affected individuals may have enlargement of the male breasts or develop noninsulin-dependent diabetes mellitus.

How Is SMA Diagnosed?

A blood test is available that can indicate whether there are deletions or mutations of the *SMN1* gene. This test identifies at least 95 percent of SMA Types I, II, and III. Other diagnostic tests may include electromyography (which records the electrical activity from the brain and/or spinal cord to a peripheral nerve root found in the arms and legs that controls muscles during contraction and at rest), nerve conduction velocity studies (which measure electrical energy by assessing the nerve's ability to send a signal), muscle biopsy (used to diagnose neuromuscular disorders and may also reveal if a person is a carrier of a defective gene that could be passed on to children), and laboratory tests of blood, urine, and other substances.

Are There Treatments for SMA?

There is no cure for SMA. Treatment consists of managing the symptoms and preventing complications.

In December 2016, the U.S. Food and Drug Administration (FDA) approved nusinersen (Spinraza™) as the first drug approved to treat children and adults with spinal muscular atrophy. The drug is administered by intrathecal injection into the fluid surrounding the spinal cord. It is designed to increase production of the full-length SMN protein, which is critical for the maintenance of motor neurons.

Muscle relaxants such as baclofen, tizanidine, and the benzodiazepines (BZs) may reduce spasticity. Botulinum toxin may be used to treat jaw spasms or drooling. Excessive saliva can be treated with amitriptyline, glycopyolate, and atropine or by botulinum injections into the salivary glands. Antidepressants may be helpful in treating depression.

Physical therapy, occupational therapy, and rehabilitation may help to improve posture, prevent joint immobility, and slow muscle weakness and atrophy. Stretching and strengthening exercises may help reduce spasticity, increase range of motion, and keeps circulation flowing. Some individuals require additional therapy for speech, chewing, and swallowing difficulties. Applying heat may relieve muscle pain. Assistive devices such as supports or braces, orthotics, speech synthesizers, and wheelchairs may help some people retain independence.

Proper nutrition and a balanced diet are essential to maintaining weight and strength. People who cannot chew or swallow may require insertion of a feeding tube. Noninvasive ventilation at night can prevent apnea in sleep, and some individuals may also require assisted ventilation due to muscle weakness in the neck, throat, and chest during daytime.

What Is the Prognosis?

Prognosis varies depending on the type of SMA. Some forms of SMA are fatal.

The course of Kennedy disease varies but is generally slowly progressive. Individuals tend to remain ambulatory until late in the disease. The life expectancy for individuals with Kennedy disease is usually normal.

People with SMA may appear to be stable for long periods, but improvement should not be expected.

Chapter 31

Other Types of Hypokinetic Movement Disorders

Chapter Contents

Section 31.1

Corticobasal Degeneration

This section includes text excerpted from "Corticobasal
Degeneration," Genetic and Rare Diseases Information
Center (GARD), National Center for Advancing
Translational Sciences (NCATS), March 13, 2017.

Corticobasal degeneration (CBD) is characterized by the break
down (degeneration) of parts of the brain, including the cerebral
cortex and basal ganglia. The cerebral cortex is responsible for most
of the brain's processing of information, and the basal ganglia are
deep brain structures that help start and control movement. Signs
and symptoms of CBD include poor coordination, loss of movement,
rigidity, poor balance, unnatural posturing of the muscles, intellectual (cognitive) impairment, speech impairment, muscular jerks,
and difficulty swallowing. These symptoms develop and worsen over
time. Currently the cause of CBD is not known. Treatment depends
on the symptoms in each person. People with CBD usually do not
survive beyond an average of 7 years after symptoms begin. Aspiration pneumonia or other complications are usually the cause of
death.

Cause

The underlying cause of CBD is poorly understood. However,
researchers have found that a protein called tau plays a role in the
development of CBD. Tau is a specific type of protein that is normally found in the brain. In CBD, abnormal levels of tau accumulate in the brain cells, eventually leading to their deterioration and
causing symptoms of the condition. Exactly why this happens is
unknown. Tau also appears to play a role in other neurodegenerative
diseases such as Alzheimer disease, progressive supranuclear palsy,
and frontotemporal dementia. There is no evidence to suggest that
environmental exposure to toxic or infectious agents plays a role in
causing CBD.

Inheritance

CBD is almost always sporadic, developing by chance rather than being inherited. Rare familial cases have been reported, leading to the possibility that there may be a genetic basis for at least a pre-disposition to CBD. Some research has found associations with CBD and a specific form (variant) of the tau gene. However, not all people with CBD have the tau gene variant, and not all people with the gene variant develop CBD.

Treatment

Unfortunately, there is currently no treatment available to slow the course of corticobasal degeneration. Treatment of corticobasal degeneration is supportive.

Section 31.2

Multiple System Atrophy

This section includes text excerpted from "Multiple System Atrophy Fact Sheet," National Institute of Neurological Disorders and Stroke (NINDS), November 2014. Reviewed January 2018.

What Is Multiple System Atrophy (MSA)?

Multiple system atrophy (MSA) is a progressive neurodegenerative disorder characterized by a combination of symptoms that affect both the autonomic nervous system (the part of the nervous system that controls involuntary action such as blood pressure or digestion) and movement. The symptoms reflect the progressive loss of function and death of different types of nerve cells in the brain and spinal cord.

Symptoms of autonomic failure that may be seen in MSA include fainting spells and problems with heart rate, erectile dysfunction, and bladder control. Motor impairments (loss of or limited muscle control or movement, or limited mobility) may include tremor, rigidity, and/or loss of muscle coordination as well as difficulties with speech and gait (the way a person walks). Some of these features are similar to those seen in Parkinson disease (PD), and early in the disease course it often may be difficult to distinguish these disorders.

MSA is a rare disease, affecting potentially 15,000–50,000 Americans, including men and women and all racial groups. Symptoms tend to appear in a person's 50s and advance rapidly over the course of 5–10 years, with progressive loss of motor function and eventual confinement to bed. People with MSA often develop pneumonia in the later stages of the disease and may suddenly die from cardiac or respiratory issues.

While some of the symptoms of MSA can be treated with medications, currently there are no drugs that are able to slow disease progression and there is no cure.

MSA includes disorders that historically had been referred to as Shy-Drager syndrome, olivopontocerebellar atrophy, and striatonigral degeneration.

What Are the Common Signs or Symptoms?

The initial symptoms of MSA are often difficult to distinguish from the initial symptoms of Parkinson disease and include:

- slowness of movement, tremor, or rigidity (stiffness)

- clumsiness or incoordination

- impaired speech, a croaky, quivering voice

- fainting or lightheadedness due to orthostatic hypotension, a condition in which blood pressure drops when rising from a seated or lying down position

- bladder control problems, such as a sudden urge to urinate or difficulty emptying the bladder

Doctors divide MSA into two different types, depending on the most prominent symptoms at the time an individual is evaluated:

- the parkinsonian type (MSA-P), with primary characteristics similar to Parkinson disease (such as moving slowly, stiffness, and tremor) along with problems of balance, coordination, and autonomic nervous system dysfunction

- the cerebellar type (MSA-C), with primary symptoms featuring ataxia (problems with balance and coordination), difficulty swallowing, speech abnormalities or a quavering voice, and abnormal eye movements ("cerebellar" reflects a part of the brain involved with coordination)

MSA tends to progress more rapidly than PD, and most people with MSA will require an aid for walking, such as a cane or walker, within a few years after symptoms begin.

Additional symptoms of MSA include:

- contractures (chronic shortening of muscles or tendons around joints, which prevents the joints from moving freely) in the hands or limbs

- Pisa syndrome, an abnormal posture in which the body appears to be leaning to one side like the Leaning Tower of Pisa

- antecollis, in which the neck bends forward and the head drops down

- involuntary, uncontrollable sighing or gasping

- sleep disorders, including a tendency to act out dreams (called REM (rapid eye movement) sleep behavior disorder)

Some people with MSA may experience feelings of anxiety or depression.

What Causes MSA?

The cause of MSA is unknown. The vast majority of cases are sporadic, meaning they occur at random. A distinguishing feature of MSA is the accumulation of the protein alpha-synuclein in glia, the cells that support nerve cells in the brain. These deposits of alpha-synuclein particularly occur in oligodendroglia, a type of cell that makes myelin (a coating on nerve cells that lets them conduct electrical signals rapidly). This protein also accumulates in PD, but in nerve cells. Because they both have a buildup of alpha-synuclein in cells, MSA and PD are sometimes referred to as synucleinopathies. A possible risk factor for the disease is variations in the synuclein gene *SCNA*, which provides instructions for the production of alpha-synuclein.

How Is MSA Diagnosed?

Making a diagnosis of MSA can be difficult, particularly in the early stages, in part because many of the features are similar to those observed in PD.

After taking a clinical history and performing a brief neurological examination, a doctor may order a number of tests to help make the diagnosis. These tests might include autonomic testing (such as blood pressure control, heart rate control), assessment of bladder function, and/or neuroimaging such as an MRI (magnetic resonance imaging) or positron emission tomography (PET) scan. An MRI of the brain may identify changes which might suggest MSA or rule out other causes of the observed symptoms.

A PET scan (which allows doctors to see how organs and tissues are functioning) is sometimes used to see if metabolic function is reduced in specific parts of the brain. DaTscan can assess the dopamine transporter in a part of the brain called the striatum and can help physicians determine if the condition is caused by a dopamine system disorder; however this test cannot differentiate between MSA and PD. Individuals with MSA typically do not have sustained improvement in their symptoms with levodopa (a drug used to treat PD), a finding that often supports the diagnosis of MSA.

How Is It Treated?

There are no treatments to delay the progressive neurodegeneration of MSA, and there is no cure. There are treatments to help people cope with the symptoms of MSA.

In some individuals, levodopa may improve motor function; however, the benefit may not continue as the disease progresses.

The fainting and lightheadedness from orthostatic hypotension may be treated with simple interventions such as wearing compression stockings, adding extra salt and/or water to the diet, and avoiding heavy meals. The drugs fludrocortisone and midodrine sometimes are prescribed. In 2014, the U.S. Food and Drug Administration (FDA) approved the medication droxidopa for the treatment of orthostatic hypotension seen in MSA. Dihydroxyphenylserine helps to replace chemical signals called neurotransmitters which are decreased in the autonomic nervous system in MSA. Some medications used to treat orthostatic hypotension can be associated with high blood pressure when lying down, so affected individuals may be advised to sleep with the head of the bed tilted up.

Bladder control problems are treated according to the nature of the problem. Anticholinergic drugs, such as oxybutynin or tolteridine, may help reduce the sudden urge to urinate.

Fixed abnormal muscle postures (dystonia) may be controlled with injections of botulinum toxin.

Sleep problems such as REM sleep behavior disorder can be treated with medicines including clonazepam, melatonin, or some antidepressants.

Some individuals with MSA may have significant difficulties with swallowing and may need a feeding tube or nutritional support. Speech therapy may be helpful in identifying strategies to address swallowing difficulties.

Physical therapy helps maintain mobility, reduce contractures (chronic shortening of muscles or tendons around joints, which prevents the joints from moving freely), and decrease muscle spasms and abnormal posture.

Individuals may eventually need assistive devices such as walkers and wheelchairs. Occupational therapists help with home safety and learning new ways to address activities of daily living such as dressing and eating.

Section 31.3

Postpolio Syndrome

This section includes text excerpted from "Post-Polio Syndrome Fact Sheet," National Institute of Neurological Disorders and Stroke (NINDS), May 2012. Reviewed January 2018.

What Is Postpolio Syndrome (PPS)?

Polio, or poliomyelitis, is an infectious viral disease that can strike at any age and affects a person's nervous system. Between the late 1940s and early 1950s, polio crippled around 35,000 people each year in the United States alone, making it one of the most feared diseases of the twentieth century.

The polio vaccine was first introduced in 1955; its use since then has eradicated polio from the United States. The World Health Organization (WHO) reports polio cases have decreased by more than 99 percent since 1988, from an estimated 350,000 cases then, to 1,352 reported cases in 2010. As a result of the global effort to eradicate the disease, only three countries (Afghanistan, Nigeria, and Pakistan) remain polio-endemic as of February 2012, down from more than 125 in 1988.

PPS is a condition that affects polio survivors years after recovery from an initial acute attack of the poliomyelitis virus. Most often, polio survivors start to experience gradual new weakening in muscles that were previously affected by the polio infection. The most common symptoms include slowly progressive muscle weakness, fatigue (both generalized and muscular), and a gradual decrease in the size of muscles (muscle atrophy). Pain from joint degeneration and increasing skeletal deformities such as scoliosis (curvature of the spine) is common and may precede the weakness and muscle atrophy. Some individuals experience only minor symptoms while others develop visible muscle weakness and atrophy.

PPS is rarely life-threatening, but the symptoms can significantly interfere with an individual's ability to function independently. Respiratory muscle weakness, for instance, can result in trouble with proper breathing, affecting daytime functions and sleep. Weakness in swallowing muscles can result in aspiration of food and liquids into the lungs and lead to pneumonia.

Who Is at Risk?

While polio is a contagious disease, PPS cannot be caught from others having the disorder. Only a polio survivor can develop PPS.

The severity of weakness and disability after recovery from poliomyelitis tends to predict the relative risk of developing PPS. Individuals who had minimal symptoms from the original illness are more likely to experience only mild PPS symptoms. A person who was more acutely affected by the polio virus and who attained a greater recovery may experience a more severe case of PPS, with greater loss of muscle function and more severe fatigue.

The exact incidence and prevalence of PPS is unknown. The U.S. National Health Interview Survey (NHIS) in 1987 contained specific questions for persons given the diagnosis of poliomyelitis with or without paralysis. No survey since then has addressed the question. Results published in 1994–1995 estimated there were about 1 million polio survivors in the United States, with 443,000 reporting to have had paralytic polio. Accurate statistics do not exist today, as a percentage of polio survivors have died and new cases have been diagnosed. Researchers estimate that the condition affects 25–40 percent of polio survivors.

What Causes PPS?

The cause of PPS is unknown but experts have offered several theories to explain the phenomenon—ranging from the fatigue of over-worked nerve cells to possible brain damage from a viral infection to a combination of mechanisms. The new weakness of PPS appears to be related to the degeneration of individual nerve terminals in the motor units. A motor unit is formed by a nerve cell (or motor neuron) in the spinal cord or brain stem and the muscle fibers it activates. The polio virus attacks specific neurons in the brainstem and spinal cord. In an effort to compensate for the loss of these motor neurons, surviving cells sprout new nerve-end terminals and connect with other muscle fibers. These new connections may result in recovery of movement and gradual gain in power in the affected limbs.

Years of high use of these recovered but overly extended motor units adds stress to the motor neurons, which over time lose the ability to maintain the increased work demands. This results in the slow deterioration of the neurons, which leads to loss of muscle strength. Restoration of nerve function may occur in some fibers a second time, but eventually nerve terminals malfunction and permanent weakness occurs. This hypothesis explains why PPS occurs after a delay and has a slow and progressive course.

Through years of studies, scientists at the National Institute of Neurological Disorders and Stroke (NINDS) and at other institutions have shown that the weakness of PPS progresses very slowly. It is marked by periods of relative stability, interspersed with periods of decline.

How Is PPS Diagnosed?

The diagnosis of PPS relies nearly entirely on clinical information. There are no laboratory tests specific for this condition and symptoms vary greatly among individuals. Physicians diagnose PPS after completing a comprehensive medical history and physical examination, and by excluding other disorders that could explain the symptoms.

Physicians look for the following criteria when diagnosing PPS:

- Prior paralytic poliomyelitis with evidence of motor neuron loss. This is confirmed by history of the acute paralytic illness, signs of residual weakness and atrophy of muscles on neuromuscular examination, and signs of motor neuron loss on electromyography (EMG). Rarely, people had subtle paralytic polio where there was no obvious deficit. In such cases, prior polio should be confirmed with an EMG study rather than a reported history of nonparalytic polio.

- A period of partial or complete functional recovery after acute paralytic poliomyelitis, followed by an interval (usually 15 years or more) of stable neuromuscular function.

- Slowly progressive and persistent new muscle weakness or decreased endurance, with or without generalized fatigue, muscle atrophy, or muscle and joint pain. Onset may at times follow trauma, surgery, or a period of inactivity, and can appear to be sudden. Less commonly, symptoms attributed to PPS include new problems with breathing or swallowing.

- Symptoms that persist for at least a year.

- Exclusion of other neuromuscular, medical, and skeletal abnormalities as causes of symptoms.

PPS may be difficult to diagnose in some people because other medical conditions can complicate the evaluation. Depression, for example, is associated with fatigue and can be misinterpreted as PPS. A number of conditions may cause problems in persons with polio that are not due to additional loss of motor neuron function. For example, shoulder osteoarthritis from walking with crutches, a chronic rotator cuff tear leading to pain and disuse weakness, or progressive scoliosis causing breathing insufficiency can occur years after polio but are not indicators of PPS.

Polio survivors with new symptoms resembling PPS should consider seeking treatment from a physician trained in neuromuscular disorders. It is important to clearly establish the origin and potential causes for declining strength and to assess progression of weakness not explained by other health problems. Magnetic resonance imaging (MRI) and computed tomography (CT) of the spinal cord, electrophysiological studies, and other tests are frequently used to investigate the course of decline in muscle strength and exclude other diseases that could be causing or contributing to the new progressive symptoms. A muscle biopsy or a spinal fluid analysis can be used to exclude other, possibly treatable, conditions that mimic PPS. Polio survivors may acquire other illnesses and should always have regular check-ups and preventive diagnostic tests. However, there is no diagnostic test for PPS, nor is there one that can identify which polio survivors are at greatest risk.

How Is PPS Treated?

There are currently no effective pharmaceutical treatments that can stop deterioration or reverse the deficits caused by the syndrome itself. However, a number of controlled studies have demonstrated that nonfatiguing exercises may improve muscle strength and reduce tiredness. Most of the clinical trials in PPS have focused on finding safe therapies that could reduce symptoms and improve quality of life.

Researchers at the National Institutes of Health (NIH) have tried treating persons having PPS with high doses of the steroid prednisone and demonstrated a mild improvement in their condition, but the results were not statistically significant. Also, the side effects from the treatment outweighed benefits, leading researchers to conclude that prednisone should not be used to treat PPS.

Preliminary studies indicate that intravenous immunoglobulin may reduce pain and increase quality of life in postpolio survivors.

A small trial to treat fatigue using lamotrigine (an anticonvulsant drug) showed modest effect but this study was limited and larger, more controlled studies with the drug were not conducted to validate the findings.

Although there are no effective treatments, there are recommended management strategies. Patients should consider seeking medical advice from a physician experienced in treating neuromuscular disorders. Patients should also consider judicious use of exercise, preferably under the supervision of an experienced health professional. Physicians often advise patients on the use of mobility aids, ventilation equipment, revising daily living activities to avoid rapid muscle tiring and total body exhaustion, and avoiding activities that cause pain or fatigue lasting more than 10 minutes. Most importantly, patients should avoid the temptation to attribute all signs and symptoms to prior polio, thereby missing out on important treatments for concurrent conditions.

Learning about PPS is important for polio survivors and their families. Managing PPS can involve lifestyle changes. Support groups that encourage self-help, group participation, and positive action can be helpful. Counseling may be needed to help individuals and families adjust to the late effects of poliomyelitis. Experiencing new symptoms of weakness and using assistive devices may bring back distressing memories of the original illness.

What Is the Role of Exercise in the Treatment of PPS?

Pain, weakness, and fatigue can result from the overuse of muscles and joints. These same symptoms also can result from disuse of muscles and joints. This fact has caused a misunderstanding about whether to encourage or discourage exercise for polio survivors or individuals with PPS.

Exercise is safe and effective when carefully prescribed and monitored by experienced health professionals. Exercise is more likely to benefit those muscle groups that were least affected by polio. Cardiopulmonary endurance training is usually more effective than strengthening exercises, especially when activities are paced to allow for frequent breaks and strategies are used to conserve energy. Heavy or intense resistive exercise and weight-lifting using polio-affected muscles may be counterproductive, as this can further weaken rather than strengthen these muscles.

Exercise prescriptions should include:

• the specific muscle groups to be included,

• the specific muscle groups to be excluded, and

• the type of exercise, together with frequency and duration.

Exercise should be reduced or discontinued if it causes additional weakness, excessive fatigue, or unduly prolonged recovery time that is noted by either the individual with PPS or the professional monitoring the exercise. As a general rule, no muscle should be exercised to the point of causing ache, fatigue, or weakness.

Can PPS Be Prevented?

Polio survivors often ask if there is a way to prevent the development of PPS. Presently, no intervention has been found to stop the deterioration of surviving neurons. Physicians recommend that polio survivors get a good night's sleep, maintain a well-balanced diet, avoid unhealthy habits such as smoking and overeating, and follow a prescribed exercise program. Lifestyle changes, such as weight control, the use of assistive devices, and taking certain anti-inflammatory medications, may help with some of the symptoms of PPS.

Section 31.4

Stiff Person Syndrome (SPS)

This section includes text excerpted from "Stiff Person Syndrome," Genetic and Rare Diseases Information Center (GARD), National Center for Advancing Translational Sciences (NCATS), July 23, 2017.

Stiff person syndrome (SPS) is an autoimmune disease that affects the nervous system, specifically the brain and spinal cord. Symptoms may include muscle stiffness in the trunk and limbs and heightened sensitivity to noise, touch, and emotional distress, which can set off muscle spasms. People with SPS may also have abnormal postures, such as being hunched over. The syndrome affects twice as many women as men.

It is frequently associated with other autoimmune diseases such as diabetes, thyroiditis, vitiligo, and pernicious anemia. SPS may be diagnosed by a blood test for glutamic acid decarboxylase (GAD) antibodies because people with SPS usually have elevated levels of GAD antibodies. Treatment may involve high-dose diazepam, anticonvulsants, or intravenous immunoglobulin (IVIG).

Symptoms

SPS is characterized by episodes of muscle stiffness in the trunk and limbs. This muscle rigidity may cause abnormal postures such as being stiffened and hunched over. During episodes of muscle stiffness, affected individuals may also have muscle spasms. The spasms and muscle rigidity may cause people to fall when they are walking or standing. These spasms are especially likely during times of emotional distress or startle.

Age of onset of SPS can vary, but most people start experiencing symptoms between ages 30–60. Some people with this syndrome may have other clinical findings such as cerebral palsy or epilepsy.

Many people with stiff person syndrome suffer from anxiety and depression. This is caused in part by the symptoms of the syndrome affecting a person's daily life, but also because the cause of the syndrome is having low levels of neurotransmitters. Neurotransmitters help to maintain a person's mood.

Cause

Scientists don't yet understand the complete picture of what causes SPS, but research indicates that it is the result of an abnormal autoimmune response in the brain and spinal cord. Autoimmune responses occur when the immune system mistakenly attacks the body.

Most people with stiff person syndrome have antibodies that are made to attack GAD. GAD is a protein in some neurons that are involved in making a substance called gamma-aminobutyric acid (GABA), which is responsible for controlling muscle movement. The symptoms of stiff person syndrome may develop when the immune system mistakenly attacks the neurons that produce GAD. When GAD is not working properly, there is not enough GABA to help control muscle movement. The exact role that deficiency of GAD plays in the development of stiff person syndrome is not fully understood.

Some individuals with stiff person syndrome will have antibodies to amphiphysin, a protein involved in the transmission of signals from one neuron to another. Individuals with these antibodies have a higher risk for developing breast, lung, or colon cancer.

Inheritance

As is the case with most autoimmune diseases, genetic factors involved in causing SPS have not been established. While most cases appear to occur in an isolated manner, there have been reported cases of multiple people in the same family being affected by SPS. Although one specific genetic change (mutation) is not known to cause stiff person syndrome, it is thought that genetics in combination with other factors may play a role in causing SPS.

Diagnosis

A diagnosis of SPS is typically made based on the presence of the characteristic symptoms, a detailed medical history and clinical exam, and various tests. Specific tests are used to support or confirm the diagnosis, and to rule out conditions with overlapping symptoms. One commonly used diagnostic tool is a blood test to detect the presence of GAD antibodies. About 60–80 percent of affected people have antibodies against GAD that can be detected on a blood test. Therefore, the absence of GAD antibodies does not rule out SPS, but the presence of high levels of GAD antibodies in people with symptoms of SPS strongly supports the diagnosis.

Additionally, a doctor may recommend electromyography (EMG), which records electrical activity in skeletal muscles. The EMG of a person with SPS typically shows continuous motor activity in the skeletal muscles.

Other laboratory testing may also be used to determine if a person with SPS has other diseases that may be associated with the syndrome. This testing includes hemoglobin A1C levels to rule out diabetes mellitus, a complete blood count to rule out pernicious anemia, and thyroid-stimulating hormone (TSH) test to rule out thyroiditis. A lumbar puncture to analyze cerebral spinal fluid may also be obtained to rule out other causes of the symptoms associated with SPS. Proteins called oligoclonal bands indicate that the central nervous system is inflamed, and these bands can be seen in about two thirds of affected people who have GAD antibodies. Because the underlying genetic cause of SPS has not been established, genetic testing is not available.

Treatment

Treatment of SPS focuses on the specific symptoms present in each person. Benzodiazepines, diazepam, or baclofen may be used to treat muscle stiffness and spasms. Anti seizure medications and pain medications may also be effective for some people.

Studies have shown that intravenous immunoglobulin (IVIG) or plasmapheresis may be effective in improving some of the symptoms of SPS. For some people, autologous stem cell transplants have been shown to successfully treat SPS. Clinical trials are being completed to confirm if this may be an effective treatment. Physical and occupational therapy may help to slow the progression of stiff person syndrome, but should be completed by someone who is familiar with the condition so as not to make symptoms worse.

Prognosis

The long-term outlook for people affected by SPS can vary widely depending on the symptoms of each person. For some people with this syndrome, symptoms resolve with treatment, or symptoms only affect a particular area of the body. For other people, symptoms may progress to include the muscles of the face, and some of the muscles in the body may be constantly rigid. Progression of the symptoms related to SPS can lead to frequent falls, which can become dangerous.

Treatment may be helpful for some people with SPS, but for others current treatment options do not relieve the symptoms of the disorder. For these people, daily living can become very difficult due to symptoms of muscle rigidity, anxiety, and depression.

Part Four

Hyperkinetic Movement Disorders: Excessive or Unwanted Movements

Chapter 32

Dystonia

Chapter Contents

Section 32.1

Facts about Dystonias

This section includes text excerpted from "Dystonias
Fact Sheet," National Institute of Neurological Disorders and
Stroke (NINDS), January 2012. Reviewed January 2018.

What Is Dystonia?

Dystonia is a disorder characterized by involuntary muscle contractions that cause slow repetitive movements or abnormal postures. The movements may be painful, and some individuals with dystonia may have a tremor or other neurologic features. There are several different forms of dystonia that may affect only one muscle, groups of muscles, or muscles throughout the body. Some forms of dystonia are genetic but the cause for the majority of cases is not known.

What Are the Symptoms?

Dystonia can affect many different parts of the body, and the symptoms are different depending upon the form of dystonia. Early symptoms may include a foot cramp or a tendency for one foot to turn or drag—either sporadically or after running or walking some distance—or a worsening in handwriting after writing several lines. In other instances, the neck may turn or pull involuntarily, especially when the person is tired or under stress. Sometimes both eyes might blink rapidly and uncontrollably; other times, spasms will cause the eyes to close. Symptoms may also include tremor or difficulties speaking. In some cases, dystonia can affect only one specific action, while allowing others to occur unimpeded. For example, a musician may have dystonia when using her hand to play an instrument, but not when using the same hand to type. The initial symptoms can be very mild and may be noticeable only after prolonged exertion, stress, or fatigue. Over a period of time, the symptoms may become more noticeable or widespread; sometimes, however, there is little or no progression. Dystonia typically is not associated with problems thinking or understanding, but depression and anxiety may be present.

What Do Researchers Know about Dystonia?

The cause of dystonia is not known. Researchers believe that dystonia results from an abnormality in or damage to the basal ganglia or other brain regions that control movement. There may be abnormalities in the brain's ability to process a group of chemicals called neurotransmitters that help cells in the brain communicate with each other. There also may be abnormalities in the way the brain processes information and generates commands to move. In most cases, no abnormalities are visible using magnetic resonance imaging (MRI) or other diagnostic imaging.

The dystonias can be divided into three groups: idiopathic, genetic, and acquired.

- Idiopathic dystonia refers to dystonia that does not have a clear cause. Many instances of dystonia are idiopathic.

- There are several genetic causes of dystonia. Some forms appear to be inherited in a dominant manner, which means only one parent who carries the defective gene is needed to pass the disorder to their child. Each child of a parent having the abnormal gene will have a 50 percent chance of carrying the defective gene. It is important to note the symptoms may vary widely in type and severity even among members of the same family. In some instances, persons who inherit the defective gene may not develop dystonia. Having one mutated gene appears to be sufficient to cause the chemical imbalances that may lead to dystonia, but other genetic or even environmental factors may play a role. Knowing the pattern of inheritance can help families understand the risk of passing dystonia along to future generations.

- Acquired dystonia, also called secondary dystonia, results from environmental or other damage to the brain, or from exposure to certain types of medications. Some causes of acquired dystonia include birth injury (including hypoxia, a lack of oxygen to the brain, and neonatal brain hemorrhage), certain infections, reactions to certain drugs, heavy metal or carbon monoxide poisoning, trauma, or stroke. Dystonia can be a symptom of other diseases, some of which may be hereditary. Acquired dystonia often plateaus and does not spread to other parts of the body. Dystonia that occurs as a result of medications often ceases if the medications are stopped quickly.

When Do Symptoms Occur?

Dystonia can occur at any age, but is often described as either early, or childhood, onset versus adult onset.

Early-onset dystonia often begins with symptoms in the limbs and may progress to involve other regions. Some symptoms tend to occur after periods of exertion and/or fluctuate over the course of the day.

Adult-onset dystonia usually is located in one or adjacent parts of the body, most often involving the neck and/or facial muscles. Acquired dystonia can affect other regions of the body.

Dystonias often progress through various stages. Initially, dystonic movements may be intermittent and appear only during voluntary movements or stress. Later, individuals may show dystonic postures and movements while walking and ultimately even while they are relaxed. Dystonia can be associated with fixed postures and shortening of tendons.

How Are the Dystonias Classified?

One way to classify the dystonias is based upon the regions of the body which they affect:

- Generalized dystonia affects most or all of the body.

- Focal dystonia is localized to a specific part of the body.

- Multifocal dystonia involves two or more unrelated body parts.

- Segmental dystonia affects two or more adjacent parts of the body.

- Hemidystonia involves the arm and leg on the same side of the body.

There are several different forms of dystonia. Some of the more common focal forms are:

Cervical dystonia, also called spasmodic torticollis or torticollis, is the most common of the focal dystonias. In cervical dystonia, the muscles in the neck that control the position of the head are affected, causing the head to turn to one side or be pulled forward or backward. Sometimes the shoulder is pulled up. Cervical dystonia can occur at any age, although most individuals first experience symptoms in middle age. It often begins slowly and usually reaches a plateau over a few months or years. About 10 percent of those with torticollis may experience a spontaneous remission, but unfortunately the remission may not be lasting.

Blepharospasm, the second most common focal dystonia, is the involuntary, forcible contraction of the muscles controlling eye blinks. The first symptoms may be increased blinking, and usually both eyes are affected. Spasms may cause the eyelids to close completely, causing "functional blindness" even though the eyes are healthy and vision is normal.

Cranio-facial dystonia is a term used to describe dystonia that affects the muscles of the head, face, and neck (such as blepharospasm). The term Meige syndrome is sometimes applied to cranio-facial dystonia accompanied by blepharospasm. Oromandibular dystonia affects the muscles of the jaw, lips, and tongue. This dystonia may cause difficulties with opening and closing the jaw, and speech and swallowing can be affected. Spasmodic dysphonia, also called laryngeal dystonia, involves the muscles that control the vocal cords, resulting in strained or breathy speech.

Task-specific dystonias are focal dystonias that tend to occur only when undertaking a particular repetitive activity. Examples include writer's cramp that affects the muscles of the hand and sometimes the forearm, and only occurs during handwriting. Similar focal dystonias have also been called typist's cramp, pianist's cramp, and musician's cramp. Musician's dystonia is a term used to classify focal dystonias affecting musicians, specifically their ability to play an instrument or to perform. It can involve the hand in keyboard or string players, the mouth and lips in wind players, or the voice in singers.

In addition, there are forms of dystonia that may have a genetic cause:

- DYT1 dystonia is a rare form of dominantly inherited generalized dystonia that can be caused by a mutation in the *DYT1* gene. This form of dystonia typically begins in childhood, affects the limbs first, and progresses, often causing significant disability. Because the gene's effects are so variable, some people who carry a mutation in the *DYT1* gene may not develop dystonia.

- Dopa-responsive dystonia (DRD), also known as Segawa disease, is another form of dystonia that can have a genetic cause. Individuals with DRD typically experience onset during childhood and have progressive difficulty with walking. Symptoms characteristically fluctuate and are worse late in the day and after exercise. Some forms of DRD are due to mutations in the *DYT5* gene. Patients with this disorder have dramatic improvements in symptoms after treatment with levodopa, a medication commonly used to treat Parkinson disease (PD).

Researchers have identified another genetic cause of dystonia which is due to mutations in the *DYT6* gene. Dystonia caused by *DYT6* mutations often presents as cranio-facial dystonia, cervical dystonia, or arm dystonia. Rarely, a leg is affected at the onset.

Many other genes that cause dystonic syndromes have been found, and numerous genetic variants are known to date. Some important genetic causes of dystonia include mutations in the following genes: *DYT3*, which causes dystonia associated with parkinsonism; *DYT5* (GTP cyclohydrolase 1), which is associated with dopa-responsive dystonia (Segawa disease); *DYT6 (THAP1)*, associated with several clinical presentations of dystonia; *DYT11*, which causes dystonia associated with myoclonus (brief contractions of muscles); and *DYT12*, which causes rapid onset dystonia associated with parkinsonism.

What Treatments Are Available?

Currently, there are no medications to prevent dystonia or slow its progression. There are, however, several treatment options that can ease some of the symptoms of dystonia, so physicians can select a therapeutic approach based on each individual's symptoms.

- Botulinum toxin. Botulinum injections often are the most effective treatment for the focal dystonias. Injections of small amounts of this chemical into affected muscles prevents muscle contractions and can provide temporary improvement in the abnormal postures and movements that characterize dystonia. First used to treat blepharospasm, such injections are now widely used for treating other focal dystonias. The toxin decreases muscle spasms by blocking release of the neurotransmitter acetylcholine, which normally causes muscles to contract. The effect typically is seen a few days after the injections and can last for several months before the injections must be repeated. The details of the treatment will vary among individuals.

- Medications. Several classes of drugs that affect different neurotransmitters may be effective for various forms of dystonia. These medications are used "off-label," meaning they are approved by the U.S. Food and Drug Administration (FDA) to treat different disorders or conditions but have not been

specifically approved to treat dystonia. The response to drugs
varies among individuals and even in the same person over
time. These drugs include:

- Anticholinergic agents block the effects of the neurotransmitter
  acetylcholine. Drugs in this group include trihexyphenidyl and
  benztropine. Sometimes these medications can be sedating or
  cause difficulties with memory, especially at higher dosages
  and in older individuals. These side effects can limit their
  usefulness. Other side effects such as dry mouth and constipation can usually be managed with dietary changes or other
  medications.

- GABAergic agents are drugs that regulate the neurotransmitter
  GABA. These medications include the benzodiazepines such as
  diazepam, lorazepam, clonazepam, and baclofen. Drowsiness is
  their common side effect.

- Dopaminergic agents act on the dopamine system and the neurotransmitter dopamine, which helps control muscle movement.
  Some individuals may benefit from drugs that block the effects
  of dopamine, such as tetrabenazine. Side effects (such as weight
  gain and involuntary and repetitive muscle movements) can
  restrict the use of these medications. Dopa-responsive dystonia
  (DRD) is a specific form of dystonia that most commonly affects
  children, and often can be well managed with levodopa.

- Deep brain stimulation (DBS) may be recommended for some
  individuals with dystonia, especially when medications do
  not sufficiently alleviate symptoms or the side effects are too
  severe. DBS involves surgically implanting small electrodes
  that are connected to a pulse generator into specific brain
  regions that control movement. Controlled amounts of electricity are sent into the exact region of the brain that generates the
  dystonic symptoms and interfere with and block the electrical
  signals that cause the symptoms. DBS should be conducted
  by an interdisciplinary team involving neurologists, neurosur-
  geons, psychiatrists, and neuropsychologists, as there is intensive follow-up and adjustments to optimize an individual's DBS
  settings.

- Other surgeries aim to interrupt the pathways responsible for
  the abnormal movements at various levels of the nervous system. Some operations purposely damage small regions of the
  thalamus (thalamotomy), globus pallidus (pallidotomy), or other

deep centers in the brain. Other surgeries include cutting nerves leading to the nerve roots deep in the neck close to the spinal cord (anterior cervical rhizotomy) or removing the nerves at the point they enter the contracting muscles (selective peripheral denervation). Some patients report significant symptom reduction after surgery.

- Physical and other therapies may be helpful for individuals with dystonia and may be an adjunct to other therapeutic approaches. Speech therapy and/or voice therapy can be quite helpful for some affected by spasmodic dysphonia. Physical therapy, the use of splints, stress management, and biofeedback also may help individuals with certain forms of dystonia.

Section 32.2

Blepharospasm

This section contains text excerpted from the following sources:
Text under the heading "What Is Blepharospasm?" is excerpted from
"Benign Essential Blepharospasm," Genetics Home Reference (GHR),
National Institutes of Health (NIH), January 16, 2018; Text
beginning with the heading "What Causes Blepharospasm?"
is excerpted from "Facts about Blepharospasm," National Eye
Institute (NEI), August 2009. Reviewed January 2018.

What Is Blepharospasm?

Blepharospasm is a condition characterized by abnormal blinking or spasms of the eyelids. This condition is a type of dystonia, which is a group of movement disorders involving uncontrolled tensing of the muscles (muscle contractions), rhythmic shaking (tremors), and other involuntary movements.

What Causes Blepharospasm?

Blepharospasm is associated with an abnormal function of the basal ganglion from an unknown cause. The basal ganglion is the part of the brain responsible for controlling the muscles. In rare cases, heredity may play a role in the development of blepharospasm.

What Are the Symptoms of Blepharospasm?

Most people develop blepharospasm without any warning symptoms. It may begin with a gradual increase in blinking or eye irritation. Some people may also experience fatigue, emotional tension, or sensitivity to bright light. As the condition progresses, the symptoms become more frequent, and facial spasms may develop. Blepharospasm may decrease or cease while a person is sleeping or concentrating on a specific task.

How Is Blepharospasm Treated?

To date, there is no successful cure for blepharospasm, although several treatment options can reduce its severity.

In the United States and Canada, the injection of Oculinum (botulinum toxin, or Botox) into the muscles of the eyelids is an approved treatment for blepharospasm. Botulinum toxin, produced by the bacterium Clostridium botulinum, paralyzes the muscles of the eyelids.

Medications taken by mouth for blepharospasm are available but usually produce unpredictable results. Any symptom relief is usually short term and tends to be helpful in only 15 percent of the cases.

Myectomy, a surgical procedure to remove some of the muscles and nerves of the eyelids, is also a possible treatment option. This surgery has improved symptoms in 75–85 percent of people with blepharospasm.

Alternative treatments may include biofeedback, acupuncture, hypnosis, chiropractic, and nutritional therapy. The benefits of these alternative therapies have not been proven.

Section 32.3

Cervical Dystonia

This section includes text excerpted from "Cervical Dystonia," Genetic and Rare Diseases Information Center (GARD), National Center for Advancing Translational Sciences (NCATS), April 4, 2017.

Cervical dystonia is a neurological condition characterized by excessive pulling of the muscles of the neck and shoulder resulting in abnormal movements of the head (dystonia). Most commonly, the head turns to one side or the other. Tilting sideways, or to the back or front may also occur. The turning or tilting movements may be accompanied by shaking movement (tremor) and/or soreness of the muscles of the neck and shoulders. Cervical dystonia can occur at any age, but most cases occur in middle age. It often begins slowly and usually reaches a plateau over a few months or years. The cause of cervical dystonia is often unknown. In some cases there is a family history. Several genes have been associated with cervical dystonia, including GNAL, THAP1, CIZ1, and ANO3. Other cases may be linked to an underlying disease (e.g., Parkinson disease), neck trauma, or certain medications. Treatment may include local injections of botulinum toxin, pain medications, benzodiazepines (anti-anxiety medications), anticholinergics, physical therapy, or surgery.

Cause

Cervical dystonia may be classified as "primary" or "secondary." Primary dystonia refers to dystonia with no clear identifiable cause and is referred to as idiopathic. In primary dystonia, there is no known structural abnormality in the central nervous system, and no underlying disease present. Primary cervical dystonia is associated with a hereditary component in approximately 12 percent of cases, and it may possibly be linked to previous neck injury.

Secondary dystonia occurs as a consequence or symptom of an underlying abnormality or disease (e.g., Parkinson disease) and has a clear cause which can be inherited or acquired. It may be linked to the use of certain medications (e.g., neuroleptics), excessive toxin ingestion (e.g., in carbon monoxide poisoning), or structural lesions due to trauma (primarily of the basal ganglia).

Research

Research helps us better understand diseases and can lead to advances in diagnosis and treatment. This section provides resources to help you learn about medical research and ways to get involved.

Section 32.4

Hemifacial Spasm

This section includes text excerpted from "Hemifacial Spasm," National Institute of Neurological Disorders and Stroke (NINDS), January 5, 2018.

Hemifacial spasm is a neuromuscular disorder characterized by frequent involuntary contractions (spasms) of the muscles on one side (hemi-) of the face (facial). The disorder occurs in both men and women, although it more frequently affects middle-aged or elderly women. It is much more common in the Asian population. The first symptom is usually an intermittent twitching of the eyelid muscle that can lead to forced closure of the eye. The spasm may then gradually spread to involve the muscles of the lower face, which may cause the mouth to be pulled to one side. Eventually the spasms involve all of the muscles on one side of the face almost continuously. The condition may be caused by a facial nerve injury, or a tumor, or it may have no apparent cause. Rarely, doctors see individuals with spasm on both sides of the face. Most often hemifacial spasm is caused by a blood vessel pressing on the facial nerve at the place where it exits the brainstem.

Treatment

Surgical treatment in the form of microvascular decompression, which relieves pressure on the facial nerve, will relieve hemifacial spasm in many cases. This intervention has significant potential side-effects, so risks and benefits have to be carefully balanced. Other treatments include injections of botulinum toxin into the affected areas, which is the most effective therapy and the only one used in most cases. Drug therapy is generally not effective.

Prognosis

The prognosis for an individual with hemifacial spasm depends on the treatment and their response. Some individuals will become relatively free from symptoms with injection therapy. Some may require surgery. In most cases, a balance can be achieved, with tolerable residual symptoms.

Section 32.5

Laryngeal Spasm

"Laryngeal Spasm," © 2018 Omnigraphics.
Reviewed January 2018.

Laryngeal spasm is a sudden spasm of the vocal cords that makes it difficult to speak or breathe temporarily. The spasm happens for less than a minute and may cause a person to get alarmed. When a breath is taken in, the vocal cord closes up, blocking air into the lungs. Though the condition is not fatal or serious, a person may not be able to speak or breathe momentarily during a spasm. Laryngeal spasm can result due to certain underlying conditions such as anxiety or stress. Asthma, allergies, exercise, irritants, vocal cord dysfunction, or gastroesophageal reflux disease (GERD) are few other conditions that trigger laryngeal spasm.

Causes of Laryngospasm

Recurring laryngospasm are usually symptoms of other health conditions that may exist. Some of them are discussed below.

Gastrointestinal Reaction

GERD is a chronic condition that happens when stomach acids or undigested food comes back to the esophagus. The lining of the esophagus and tissue of the larynx is delicate; hence, regular exposure to stomach acids can cause injury. A gastrointestinal reaction such as this can cause laryngeal spasm.

Vocal Cord Dysfunction

When the inhalation and exhalation process happens and the vocal cords behave abnormally, a vocal cord dysfunction may occur. This may trigger laryngospasms. Asthma is also similar to vocal cord dysfunction and happens due to air pollutants.

Stress or Emotional Anxiety

If a person is undergoing intense feelings of anxiety or stress, laryngospasm can occur as a physical reaction in the body. In addition to the regular doctor, a mental healthcare provider needs to be consulted.

Sleep-Related Laryngospasm

Some people can be woken from a deep sleep when experiencing sleep-related laryngospasm. It can be a frightening experience as a person may feel disoriented and unable to breathe. However, this condition lasts for only a few seconds. Repeated laryngospasms during sleep can be a result of vocal cord dysfunction or acid reflux. A laryngospasm can also happen during surgery when general anesthesia is given.

Symptoms

- People who experience laryngospasm may have a sensation of choking or may find it difficult to breathe.
- The episode may happen at night during sleep.
- During the spasm, the vocal cords stop in a closed position.
- During the spasm, if the person is able to breathe a little bit, a hoarse whistling sound called stridor can be heard, which refers to the air moving through the small opening.

Treatment

- Laryngospasms can be frightening and, hence, the feeling of shock from such an experience can make the symptoms worse.

Breathing exercises can help a person keep calm if there are recurrent laryngospasm episodes.

- If a person experiences tension in the vocal cords during a spasm, drinking small sips of water can bring quick relief as it helps wash down anything that irritates the vocal cords.

- If GERD is the cause of the problem, treatment for GERD can help manage the condition. Healthcare providers recommend proton pump inhibitors (PPIs) such as Lansoprazole or Dexlansoprazole that help reduce production of stomach acids. Some patients are recommended surgery such as fundoplication to strengthen the valves between stomach and esophagus, thereby allowing food and liquid to go through.

Prevention

Laryngospasms are hard to predict and prevent unless the cause is known. The condition caused by digestion or acid reflux can be treated by treating digestive problems. Some lifestyle changes can help relieve GERD, thereby preventing laryngospasms.

- Heartburn triggers such as caffeine, fruit and fruit juices, fatty foods, and peppermint can be avoided.

- Eating smaller meals 2–3 hours before bedtime is advised.

- Avoid allergy triggers.

- Breathing techniques can help the person stay calm and relaxed, thereby preventing laryngospasms.

- Quitting smoking and limiting alcoholic drinks can help prevent the spasm.

- Raising the head level of the bed by a few inches can help prevent the spasm.

References

1. Robinson, Jennifer. "Laryngospasm," WebMD, January 2016.

2. Rosenow 111, Edward.C. "Laryngospasm: What Causes It?" Mayo Clinic, November 18, 2014.

3. Watson, Kathryn, Weatherspoon, Deborah. "Laryngospasm," Healthline, March 24, 2017.

Section 32.6

Myoclonus-Dystonia

This section includes text excerpted from "Myoclonus-Dystonia,"
Genetics Home Reference (GHR), National Institutes of
Health (NIH), October 2017.

Myoclonus-dystonia is a movement disorder that typically affects
the neck, torso, and arms. Individuals with this condition experience
quick, involuntary muscle jerks or twitches (myoclonus). About half of
individuals with myoclonus-dystonia develop dystonia, which is involuntary tensing of various muscles that causes unusual positioning. In
myoclonus-dystonia, dystonia often affects one or both hands, causing
writer's cramp, or the neck, causing the head to turn (torticollis).

The movement problems usually first appear in childhood or early
adolescence with the development of myoclonus. In most cases, the
movement problems remain stable throughout life. In some adults,
myoclonus improves with alcohol consumption, which can lead to
affected individuals self-medicating and becoming alcohol-dependent.

People with myoclonus-dystonia often develop psychological disorders such as depression, anxiety, panic attacks, and obsessive-compulsive disorder (OCD).

Frequency

The prevalence of myoclonus-dystonia in Europe is estimated to
be 1 in 500,000 individuals. Its prevalence elsewhere in the world is
unknown.

Genetic Changes

Mutations in the *SGCE* gene cause 30–50 percent of cases of myoclonus-dystonia. The *SGCE* gene provides instructions for making a
protein called epsilon (ε)-sarcoglycan, whose function is unknown. The
ε-sarcoglycan protein is located within the outer membrane of cells in
many tissues, but it is most abundant in nerve cells (neurons) in the
brain and in muscle cells.

SGCE gene mutations that cause myoclonus-dystonia result in a shortage (deficiency) of functional ε-sarcoglycan protein. This lack of functional protein seems to affect the regions of the brain involved in coordinating and controlling movements (the cerebellum and basal ganglia, respectively). It is unknown why *SGCE* gene mutations seem to affect only these areas of the brain.

Mutations in multiple other genes are associated with myoclonus-dystonia. Mutations in each of these genes cause a small percentage of cases. These genes are primarily active (expressed) in the brain and mutations likely lead to impairment of normal movement.

Some people with myoclonus-dystonia do not have an identified mutation in any of the known associated genes. The cause of the condition in these individuals is unknown.

Inheritance Pattern

In cases in which the genetic cause is known, myoclonus-dystonia is inherited in an autosomal dominant pattern, which means one copy of the altered gene in each cell is sufficient to cause the disorder. In cases in which the cause of the condition is unknown, the inheritance is unclear.

When caused by *SGCE* gene mutations, myoclonus-dystonia occurs only when the mutation is inherited from a person's father. People normally inherit one copy of each gene from their mother and one copy from their father. For most genes, both copies are active, or "turned on," in all cells. For a small subset of genes, however, only one of the two copies is active. For some of these genes, only the copy inherited from a person's father (the paternal copy) is active, while for other genes, only the copy inherited from a person's mother (the maternal copy) is active. These differences in gene activation based on the gene's parent of origin are caused by a phenomenon called genomic imprinting.

Because only the paternal copy of the *SGCE* gene is active, myoclonus-dystonia occurs when mutations affect the paternal copy of the *SGCE* gene. Mutations in the maternal copy of the gene typically do not cause any health problems. Rarely, individuals who inherit an *SGCE* gene mutation from their mothers will develop features of myoclonus-dystonia. It is unclear why a gene that is supposed to be turned off is active in these rare cases.

Other genes associated with myoclonus-dystonia are not imprinted, and mutations that cause the condition can be inherited from either parent.

Chapter 33

Tremor Disorders

Chapter Contents

Section 33.1

Facts about Tremors

This section includes text excerpted from "Tremor
Fact Sheet," National Institute of Neurological Disorders and
Stroke (NINDS), May 2017.

What Is Tremor?

Tremor is an involuntary, rhythmic muscle contraction leading to
shaking movements in one or more parts of the body. It is a common
movement disorder that most often affects the hands but can also
occur in the arms, head, vocal cords, torso, and legs. Tremor may be
intermittent (occurring at separate times, with breaks) or constant.
It can occur sporadically (on its own) or happen as a result of another
disorder.

Tremor is most common among middle-aged and older adults,
although it can occur at any age. The disorder generally affects men
and women equally. Tremor is not life threatening. However, it can be
embarrassing and even disabling, making it difficult or even impossible
to perform work and daily life tasks.

What Causes Tremor?

Generally, tremor is caused by a problem in the deep parts of the
brain that control movements. Most types of tremor have no known
cause, although there are some forms that appear to be inherited and
run in families.

Tremor can occur on its own or be a symptom associated with a
number of neurological disorders, including:

- multiple sclerosis (MS)

- stroke

- traumatic brain injury (TBI)

- neurodegenerative diseases that affect parts of the brain (e.g.,
  Parkinson disease (PD)).

Some other known causes can include:

- the use of certain medicines (particular asthma medication, amphetamines, caffeine, corticosteroids, and drugs used for certain psychiatric and neurological disorders)

- alcohol abuse or withdrawal

- mercury poisoning

- overactive thyroid

- liver or kidney failure

- anxiety or panic

What Are the Symptoms of Tremor?

Symptoms of tremor may include:

- a rhythmic shaking in the hands, arms, head, legs, or torso

- shaky voice

- difficulty writing or drawing

- problems holding and controlling utensils, such as a spoon

Some tremor may be triggered by or become worse during times of stress or strong emotion, when an individual is physically exhausted, or when a person is in certain postures or makes certain movements.

How Is Tremor Classified?

Tremor can be classified into two main categories:

1. Resting tremor occurs when the muscle is relaxed, such as when the hands are resting on the lap. With this disorder, a person's hands, arms, or legs may shake even when they are at rest. Often, the tremor only affects the hand or fingers. This type of tremor is often seen in people with Parkinson disease and is called a "pillrolling" tremor because the circular finger and hand movements resemble rolling of small objects or pills in the hand.

2. Action tremor occurs with the voluntary movement of a muscle. Most types of tremor are considered action tremor. There are several sub-classifications of action tremor, many of which overlap.

- Postural tremor occurs when a person maintains a position against gravity, such as holding the arms outstretched.

- Kinetic tremor is associated with any voluntary movement, such as moving the wrists up and down or closing and opening the eyes.

- Intention tremor is produced with purposeful movement toward a target, such as lifting a finger to touch the nose. Typically the tremor will become worse as an individual gets closer to their target.

- Task-specific tremor only appears when performing highly-skilled, goal-oriented tasks such as handwriting or speaking.

- Isometric tremor occurs during a voluntary muscle contraction that is not accompanied by any movement such as holding a heavy book or a dumbbell in the same position.

What Are the Different Categories or Types of Tremor?

Tremor is most commonly classified by its appearance and cause or origin. There are more than 20 types of tremor. Some of the most common forms of tremor include:

Essential Tremor

Essential tremor (previously also called benign essential tremor or familial tremor) is one of the most common movement disorders. The exact cause of essential tremor is unknown. For some people this tremor is mild and remains stable for many years. The tremor usually appears on both sides of the body, but is often noticed more in the dominant hand because it is an action tremor.

The key feature of essential tremor is a tremor in both hands and arms, which is present during action and when standing still. Additional symptoms may include head tremor (e.g., a "yes" or "no" motion) without abnormal posturing of the head and a shaking or quivering sound to the voice if the tremor affects the voice box. The action tremor in both hands in essential tremor can lead to problems with writing, drawing, drinking from a cup, or using tools or a computer.

Tremor frequency (how "fast" the tremor shakes) may decrease as the person ages, but the severity may increase, affecting the person's ability to perform certain tasks or activities of daily living. Heightened emotion, stress, fever, physical exhaustion, or low blood sugar may trigger tremor and/or increase its severity. Though the tremor can start at any age, it most often appears for the first time during adolescence or in middle age (between ages 40–50). Small amounts of alcohol may help decrease essential tremor, but the mechanism behind this is unknown.

About 50 percent of the cases of essential tremor are thought to be caused by a genetic risk factor (referred to as familial tremor). Children of a parent who has familial tremor have greater risk of inheriting the condition. Familial forms of essential tremor often appear early in life.

For many years essential tremor was not associated with any known disease. However, some scientists think essential tremor is accompanied by a mild degeneration of certain areas of the brain that control movement. This is an ongoing debate in the research field.

Dystonic Tremor

Dystonic tremor occurs in people who are affected by dystonia—a movement disorder where incorrect messages from the brain cause muscles to be overactive, resulting in abnormal postures or sustained, unwanted movements. Dystonic tremor usually appears in young or middle-aged adults and can affect any muscle in the body. Symptoms may sometimes be relieved by complete relaxation.

Although some of the symptoms are similar, dystonic tremor differs from essential tremor in some ways. The dystonic tremor:

- is associated with abnormal body postures due to forceful muscle spasms or cramps.

- can affect the same parts of the body as essential tremor, but also—and more often than essential tremor—the head, without any other movement in the hands or arms.

- can also mimic resting tremor, such as the one seen in Parkinson disease.

- Also, the severity of dystonic tremor may be reduced by touching the affected body part or muscle, and tremor movements are "jerky" or irregular instead of rhythmic.

Cerebellar Tremor

Cerebellar tremor is typically a slow, high-amplitude (easily visible) tremor of the extremities (e.g., arm, leg) that occurs at the end of a purposeful movement such as trying to press a button. It is caused by damage to the cerebellum and its pathways to other brain regions resulting from a stroke or tumor. Damage also may be caused by disease such as multiple sclerosis or an inherited degenerative disorder such as ataxia (in which people lose muscle control in the arms and legs) and Fragile X syndrome (a disorder marked by a range of intellectual and developmental problems). It can also result from chronic damage to the cerebellum due to alcoholism.

Psychogenic Tremor

Psychogenic tremor (also called functional tremor) can appear as any form of tremor. It symptoms may vary but often start abruptly and may affect all body parts. The tremor increases in times of stress and decreases or disappears when distracted. Many individuals with psychogenic tremor have an underlying psychiatric disorder such as depression or posttraumatic stress disorder (PTSD).

Physiologic Tremor

Physiologic tremor occurs in all healthy individuals. It is rarely visible to the eye and typically involves a fine shaking of both of the hands and also the fingers. It is not considered a disease but is a normal human phenomenon that is the result of physical properties in the body (for example, rhythmical activities such as heartbeat and muscle activation).

Enhanced Physiologic Tremor

Enhanced physiological tremor is a more noticeable case of physiologic tremor that can be easily seen. It is generally not caused by a neurological disease but by reaction to certain drugs, alcohol withdrawal, or medical conditions including an overactive thyroid and hypoglycemia. It is usually reversible once the cause is corrected.

Parkinsonian Tremor

Parkinsonian tremor is a common symptom of PD, although not all people with PD have tremor. Generally, symptoms include shaking in one or both hands at rest. It may also affect the chin, lips, face, and legs. The tremor may initially appear in only one limb or on just one side of the body. As the disease progresses, it may spread to both sides of the body. The tremor is often made worse by stress or strong emotions. More than 25 percent of people with PD also have an associated action tremor.

Orthostatic Tremor

Orthostatic tremor is a rare disorder characterized by rapid muscle contractions in the legs that occur when standing. People typically experience feelings of unsteadiness or imbalance, causing them to immediately attempt to sit or walk. Because the tremor has such a high frequency (very fast shaking) it may not visible to the naked eye but can be felt by touching the thighs or calves or can be detected by a doctor examining the muscles with a stethoscope. In some cases the tremor can become more severe over time. The cause of orthostatic tremor is unknown.

How Is Tremor Diagnosed and Treated?

Tremor is diagnosed based on a physical and neurological examination and an individual's medical history. During the physical evaluation, a doctor will assess the tremor based on:

- whether the tremor occurs when the muscles are at rest or in action

- the location of the tremor on the body (and if it occurs on one or both sides of the body)

- the appearance of the tremor (tremor frequency and amplitude)

The doctor will also check other neurological findings such as impaired balance, speech abnormalities, or increased muscle stiffness. Blood or urine tests can rule out metabolic causes such as thyroid malfunction and certain medications that can cause tremor. These tests may also help to identify contributing causes such as drug interactions, chronic alcoholism, or other conditions or diseases. Diagnostic imaging may help determine if the tremor is the result of damage in the brain.

Additional tests may be administered to determine functional limitations such as difficulty with handwriting or the ability to hold a fork or cup. Individuals may be asked to perform a series of tasks or exercises such as placing a finger on the tip of their nose or drawing a spiral.

The doctor may order an electromyogram to diagnose muscle or nerve problems. This test measures involuntary muscle activity and muscle response to nerve stimulation.

Although there is no cure for most forms of tremor, treatment options are available to help manage symptoms. In some cases, a person's symptoms may be mild enough that they do not require treatment.

Section 33.2

Essential Tremor: The Most Common Form of Tremor

This section includes text excerpted from "Essential Tremor," Genetics Home Reference (GHR), National Institutes of Health (NIH), January 16, 2018.

What Is Essential Tremor?

Essential tremor is a movement disorder that causes involuntary, rhythmic shaking (tremor), especially in the hands. It is distinguished from tremor that results from other disorders or known causes, such as Parkinson disease (PD) or head trauma. Essential tremor usually occurs alone, without other neurological signs or symptoms. However, some experts think that essential tremor can include additional features, such as mild balance problems.

Essential tremor usually occurs with movements and can occur during many different types of activities, such as eating, drinking, or writing. Essential tremor can also occur when the muscles are opposing gravity, such as when the hands are extended. It is usually not evident at rest.

In addition to the hands and arms, muscles of the trunk, face, head, and neck may also exhibit tremor in this disorder; the legs and feet are less often involved. Head tremor may appear as a "yes-yes" or "no-no" movement while the affected individual is seated or standing. In some people with essential tremor, the tremor may affect the voice (vocal tremor).

Essential tremor does not shorten the lifespan. However, it may interfere with fine motor skills such as using eating utensils, writing, shaving, or applying makeup, and in some cases these and other activities of daily living can be greatly impaired. Symptoms of essential tremor may be aggravated by emotional stress, anxiety, fatigue, hunger, caffeine, cigarette smoking, or temperature extremes.

Essential tremor may appear at any age but is most common in the elderly. Some studies have suggested that people with essential tremor have a higher than average risk of developing neurological conditions including PD or sensory problems such as hearing loss, especially in individuals whose tremor appears after age 65.

How Common Is Essential Tremor?

Essential tremor is a common disorder, affecting up to 10 million people in the United States. Estimates of its prevalence vary widely because several other disorders, as well as other factors such as certain medications, can result in similar tremors. In addition, mild cases are often not brought to medical attention, or may not be detected in clinical exams that do not include the particular circumstances in which an individual's tremor occurs. Severe cases are often misdiagnosed as PD.

What Genes Are Related to Essential Tremor?

The causes of essential tremor are unknown. Researchers are studying several areas (loci) on particular chromosomes that may be linked to essential tremor, but no specific genetic associations have been confirmed. Several genes as well as environmental factors likely help determine an individual's risk of developing this complex condition. The specific changes in the nervous system that account for the signs and symptoms of essential tremor are unknown.

How Do People Inherit Essential Tremor?

Essential tremor can be passed through generations in families, but the inheritance pattern varies. In most affected families, essential tremor appears to be inherited in an autosomal dominant pattern, which means one copy of an altered gene in each cell is sufficient to cause the disorder, although no genes that cause essential tremor have been identified. In other families, the inheritance pattern is unclear. Essential tremor may also appear in people with no history of the disorder in their family.

In some families, some individuals have essential tremor while others have other movement disorders, such as involuntary muscle tensing (dystonia). The potential genetic connection between essential tremor and other movement disorders is an active area of research.

Section 33.3

Fragile X Syndrome Causes Tremors

This section includes text excerpted from "Fragile X-Associated
Tremor and Ataxia Syndrome (FXTAS)—Condition Information,"
Eunice Kennedy Shriver National Institute of Child Health and
Human Development (NICHD), December 1, 2016.

What Is Fragile X-Associated Tremor and Ataxia Syndrome (FXTAS)?

FXTAS is a condition that develops in some men and women who
have an altered form of a specific gene. People with FXTAS have a
change or mutation in a gene called the **Fragile X Mental Retarda-
tion 1 (FMR1)** gene. This gene is found on the X chromosome.

FXTAS occurs later in life (in people older than age 50) and is
characterized by tremors when making purposeful movements, balance problems, Parkinson disease (PD)-like symptoms such as muscle
stiffness or rigidity, and memory loss. Most people have no symptoms
until the onset of the condition later in life.

How Is a Change in the FMR1 gene Related to Fragile X-Associated Tremor and Ataxia Syndrome (FXTAS)?

People with FXTAS have a change or mutation in the *FMR1* gene
found on the X chromosome.

In the gene, the information for making a protein has two parts:
the introduction, and the instructions for making the protein itself.
Researchers call the introduction the **promoter** because of how it
helps to start the process of building the protein.

The promoter part of the *FMR1* gene includes many **repeats**—
repeated instances of a specific deoxyribonucleic acid (DNA) sequence
called the cytosine-guanine-guanine (CGG) sequence. A normal *FMR1*
gene has between 6–40 repeats in the promoter; the average is 30
repeats.

People with between 55–200 repeats have a **premutation** of the
gene. The premutation causes the gene to not work properly, but it

does not cause intellectual and developmental disability (IDD). FXTAS occurs in some people who have the premutation.

The premutation is also related to fragile X-associated primary ovarian insufficiency (FXPOI).

People with 200 or more repeats in the promoter part of the gene have a full mutation, meaning the gene might not work at all. People with a full mutation often have fragile X syndrome, the most common inherited form of IDD. Individuals with the full mutation are not at risk for FXTAS.

Inheriting FXTAS

Anyone with the *FMR1* gene mutation can pass it to their children. However, a person who inherits the gene may not develop FXTAS. Males will pass it down to all of their daughters and not their sons. Females have a 50/50 chance to pass it along to both their sons and daughters. In addition, parents can have children with a condition associated with fragile X even if the parents do not have that condition themselves.

What Causes FXTAS?

Because FXTAS occurs only in those who have the premutation on the *FMR1* gene, the premutation is related to the condition.

If the premutation was the only cause of FXTAS, then everyone with the premutation would develop FXTAS after age 50. However, it is still not clear why some people with the premutation develop FXTAS while others do not. This topic is an active area of study.

What Are the Symptoms of FXTAS?

Although FXTAS affects individuals differently, the symptoms of the disorder are similar to those of PD or Alzheimer disease (AD), including memory loss, slowed speech, tremors, and a shuffling gait. Some people will have many symptoms that appear quickly and get worse over time. Others have only a few mild symptoms.

Men have slightly different symptoms of FXTAS than women do. Symptoms of FXTAS in men include:

- Balance problems, called ataxia

- Intention tremor (shaking when trying to perform purposeful movements, such as touching one's nose or grabbing something)

- Parkinson-like symptoms, such as muscle stiffness or rigidity, a shuffling gait or walk, and slowed speech

- Memory loss, including forgetting how to do things that were once done easily (such as balancing a checkbook), getting lost going to familiar places, or forgetting the names of everyday objects

- Irritability and moodiness

- Low blood pressure

- Numbness or burning in the hands and feet

- Incontinence

- Impotence

- Loss of reading skills and math skills

- Difficulty learning new things

Women with FXTAS may have the following symptoms:

- High blood pressure

- Balance problems, called ataxia

- Premature ovarian failure, in about 20 percent of women

- Intention tremors

- Seizure disorders

- Thyroid problems (usually an underactive thyroid gland, called hypothyroidism) in about 50 percent of women

- Muscle pain such as fibromyalgia, in about 40 percent of women

Symptoms of FXTAS usually develop after age 50. The average age of people newly diagnosed with FXTAS is about 61.

How Many People Are Affected by or at Risk of FXTAS?

The exact number of people with a premutation is unknown. Research shows that about 1 in 151 females and 1 in 468 males may have an *FMR1* gene premutation, which puts them at risk for FXTAS. But not everyone with a premutation will show symptoms.

FXTAS is less common among women, and their symptoms are generally milder.

In people with a premutation, 30–40 percent of men older than 50, 3–8 percent of women older than age 50 will develop FXTAS.

How Do Healthcare Providers Diagnose FXTAS?

Healthcare providers can order a blood test to determine if a person who has symptoms of FXTAS is a carrier. A laboratory will conduct the tests to determine what form of the *FMR1* gene is present.

However, FXTAS is often misdiagnosed. The similarity of symptoms can lead some healthcare providers to pursue those conditions before considering FXTAS. Many of the FXTAS symptoms, such as memory problems and balance problems, may also be seen as natural parts of aging.

A healthcare provider may use a combination of a blood test, symptoms, and information from brain imaging, such as magnetic resonance imaging (MRI), to confirm a FXTAS diagnosis. In about 60 percent of men and 13 percent of women with FXTAS, the MRI will show white matter lesions (areas of dead cells) in the middle cerebellar peduncle of the brain. This is called the middle cerebellar peduncle (MCP) sign.

What Are the Treatments for FXTAS?

Certain medications and therapies are helpful for treating symptoms of FXTAS and may help slow its progression. However, no treatment can stop FXTAS from progressing and none is considered a cure.

Symptoms of FXTAS differ from person to person, and treatment should address a person's individual needs. Healthcare providers may work as a team to provide appropriate treatment, such as physical therapy for difficulty with movement and balance, medication for tremors, and psychological counseling and support services for the individual and family. Other therapies may include rehabilitative treatments such as speech and occupational therapy and gait training. A urologist may be consulted regarding sexual health.

In addition, the children of FXTAS patients may want to confirm their *FMR1* gene status and to discuss their situation with a genetic counselor.

FXTAS: Other FAQs

Are There Disorders or Conditions Associated with FXTAS?

Some medical conditions are reported to be associated with the *FMR1* premutation, but only in men. These include:

- Abnormal heart rhythm (arrhythmia)
- Balance disorders

- Congestive heart failure

- High blood sugar

- Sleep apnea

- Mood disorders, including major depressive disorder, anxiety disorder, and posttraumatic stress disorder

High blood pressure is also associated with FXTAS in both men and women, but it seems to be more common among women with the *FMR1* premutation.

How Can the FMR1 *Gene Change When Passed from Parent to Child?*

Premutation genes—the kind associated with FXTAS and characterized by 55–199 extra CGG sequences in the *FMR1* gene—can grow spontaneously from generation to generation. That is, the gene's CGG sequences can increase in number on their own. They can even expand to the level of full mutation (200 or more CGG sequences), making fragile X syndrome more likely.

The *FMR1* premutation form is more likely to expand depending on the number of CGG repeats it has. The greater the number, the greater the risk of expansion. Risk also increases with each passing generation.

Why Is FXTAS *Often Misdiagnosed?*

Before *Eunice Kennedy Shriver* National Institute of Child Health and Human Development (NICHD)-supported researchers discovered FXTAS in 2001, it was often misdiagnosed. The symptoms of FXTAS— memory loss, tremors, muscle stiffness or rigidity, a shuffling gait or walk, and slowed speech—are similar to AD and PD symptoms.

A characteristic of FXTAS is also ataxia, which means clumsiness of movement or loss of coordination that is not due to muscle weakness. Ataxia is most often caused by loss of function in the cerebellum, the part of the brain that controls the body's coordination. It can also be caused by problems with the motor sensory pathways leading in and out of the cerebellum. Although symptoms of FXTAS are similar to those of other conditions, its diagnosis is unique due to the white matter lesions (areas of dead cells) in the cerebellum.

Chapter 34

Choreatic Disorders

Chapter Contents

Section 34.1

What Is Chorea?

This section includes text excerpted from "Chorea Information Page," National Institute of Neurological Disorders and Stroke (NINDS), January 5, 2018.

Chorea is an abnormal involuntary movement disorder, one of a group of neurological disorders called dyskinesias, which are caused by overactivity of the neurotransmitter dopamine in the areas of the brain that control movement. Chorea is characterized by brief, irregular contractions that are not repetitive or rhythmic, but appear to flow from one muscle to the next. Chorea often occurs with athetosis, which adds twisting and writhing movements. Chorea is a primary feature of Huntington's disease, a progressive, hereditary movement disorder that appears in adults, but it may also occur in a variety of other conditions. Sydenham's chorea occurs in a small percentage (20 percent) of children and adolescents as a complication of rheumatic fever. Chorea can also be induced by drugs (levodopa, anti-convulsants, and anti-psychotics) metabolic and endocrine disorders, and vascular incidents.

Treatment

There is no standard course of treatment for chorea. Treatment depends on the type of chorea and the associated disease. Treatment for Huntington's disease is supportive, while treatment for Sydenham's chorea usually involves antibiotic drugs to treat the infection, followed by drug therapy to prevent recurrence. Adjusting medication dosages can treat drug-induced chorea. Metabolic and endocrine-related choreas are treated according to the cause(s) of symptoms.

Prognosis

The prognosis for individuals with chorea varies depending on the type of chorea and the associated disease. Huntington's disease is a progressive, and ultimately, fatal disease. Sydenham's chorea is treatable and curable.

Section 34.2

Sydenham Chorea

This section includes text excerpted from "Sydenham's Chorea,"
Genetic and Rare Diseases Information Center (GARD), National
Center for Advancing Translational Sciences (NCATS), July 10, 2015.

Sydenham chorea is a neurological disorder characterized by rapid, jerky, irregular, and involuntary movements (chorea), especially of the face and limbs.

Symptoms

Symptoms may include muscle weakness, slurred speech, headaches, and seizures. Children with Sydenham chorea often have emotional or behavioral problems such as obsessive-compulsive disorder (OCD), distractibility, irritability, and inappropriate outbursts of laughing or crying. Sydenham chorea mostly affects children and adolescents and usually follows a Streptococcal infection by anywhere from 1–8 months. Sydenham chorea is one of the major clinical signs of acute rheumatic fever. The uncontrolled movements are often worse during periods of stress, fatigue, or excitement. In some cases, only one side of the body is affected. Sydenham chorea usually resolves within 3 weeks–3 months. However, symptoms may last longer in some cases.

Treatment

In most cases, patients with Sydenham chorea recover fully with no treatment. Drugs that have been used to treat patients with significant movement problems include corticosteroids, valproic acid, diazepam, chlorpromazine, and carbamazepine. In patients who do not respond to these drugs, haloperidol or pimozide may be used. In addition, patients with Sydenham chorea are usually treated with antibiotics to prevent another Streptococcal infection and to minimize the risk of rheumatic heart disease. Sydenham chorea usually resolves within 12–15 months, though symptoms may persist for two years or more. Up to 30 percent of patients experience a recurrence of Sydenham chorea within a few years. Some believe that treatment with an antibiotic reduces the risk of recurrence.

Section 34.3

Paroxysmal Choreoathetosis Disease

This section includes text excerpted from "Paroxysmal Choreoathetosis Information Page," National Institute of Neurological Disorders and Stroke (NINDS), January 5, 2018.

Paroxysmal choreoathetosis is a movement disorder characterized by episodes or attacks of involuntary movements of the limbs, trunk, and facial muscles. The disorder may occur in several members of a family, or in only a single family member. Prior to an attack some individuals experience tightening of muscles or other physical symptoms. Involuntary movements precipitate some attacks, and other attacks occur when the individual has consumed alcohol or caffeine, or is tired or stressed. Attacks can last from 10 seconds to over an hour. Some individuals have lingering muscle tightness after an attack. Paroxysmal choreoathetosis frequently begins in early adolescence. A gene associated with the disorder has been discovered. The same gene is also associated with epilepsy.

Treatment

Drug therapy, particularly carbamazepine, has been very successful in reducing or eliminating attacks of paroxysmal choreoathetosis. While carbamazepine is not effective in every case, other drugs have been substituted with good effect.

Prognosis

Generally, paroxysmal choreoathetosis lessens with age, and many adults have a complete remission. Because drug therapy is so effective, the prognosis for the disorder is good.

Section 34.4

Tardive Dyskinesia

This section contains text excerpted from the following sources: Text
in this section begins with excerpts from "Press Announcements—
FDA Approves First Drug to Treat Tardive Dyskinesia," U.S. Food
and Drug Administration (FDA), April 11, 2017; Text beginning with
the heading "Cause" is excerpted from "Tardive Dyskinesia," Genetic
and Rare Diseases Information Center (GARD), National Center
for Advancing Translational Sciences (NCATS), December 19, 2014.
Reviewed January 2018.

Tardive dyskinesia is a neurological disorder characterized by repetitive involuntary movements, usually of the jaw, lips and tongue, such as grimacing, sticking out the tongue, and smacking the lips. Some affected people also experience involuntary movement of the extremities or difficulty breathing. "Tardive dyskinesia can be disabling and can further stigmatize patients with mental illness," said Mitchell Mathis, M.D., director of the Division of Psychiatry Products (DPP) in the U.S. Food and Drug Administration's (FDA) Center for Drug Evaluation and Research (CDER). "Approving the first drug for the treatment of tardive dyskinesia is an important advance for patients suffering with this condition." Tardive dyskinesia is a serious side effect sometimes seen in patients who have been treated with antipsychotic medications, especially the older medications, for long periods to treat chronic conditions, such as schizophrenia and bipolar disorder. Tardive dyskinesia can also occur in patients taking antipsychotic medications for depression and certain medications for gastrointestinal disorders and other conditions. It is unclear why some people who take these medications develop tardive dyskinesia yet others do not.

Cause

Tardive dyskinesia is caused by the long-term use of certain types of medications called neuroleptics. Neuroleptic drugs are usually prescribed for psychiatric conditions; less commonly, they may be used to treat gastrointestinal or neurological conditions. Tardive dyskinesia usually develops in people who have taken these medications

291

for many years, although some cases may occur with shorter use of the drugs. It is unclear why some people who take neuroleptic medications develop the signs and symptoms of tardive dyskinesia while others do not.

Diagnosis

A diagnosis of tardive dyskinesia is typically made in people who have taken neuroleptic medications for at least three months, have signs and symptoms that are suggestive of the condition, and have undergone testing to rule out other conditions that cause similar features. This testing may include specialized laboratory tests and imaging studies such as computed tomography (CT) scan, magnetic resonance imaging (MRI) scan, positron emission tomography (PET) scan and single-photon emission computerized tomography (SPECT) scan.

Treatment

The treatment for tardive dyskinesia varies from person to person. Initial treatment usually consists of discontinuing the use of neuroleptic medications if it is safe for the affected person. In people with severe psychiatric conditions, this may not be an option, although the neuroleptic drug can sometimes be replaced with an alternative medication.

Other medications can be prescribed to specifically treat the signs and symptoms of tardive dyskinesia. In some affected people, these drugs help reduce the severity of involuntary movements. For example, a medication called tetrabenazine has been approved by the FDA for the treatment of tardive dyskinesia. Other drugs such as benzodiazepines, clozapine, or botulinum toxin (Botox) injections also may be tried.

Prognosis

The long-term outlook (prognosis) for people with tardive dyskinesia varies. When diagnosed early, the condition may resolve by simply stopping the medication that caused the symptoms. However, some affected people continue to have symptoms long after the neuroleptic drug is discontinued. In these cases, the symptoms can sometimes become permanent and/or worsen over time.

Chapter 35

Huntington Disease (HD)

Chapter Contents

Section 35.1

All about Huntington Disease

This section contains text excerpted from the following sources: Text in this section begins with excerpts from "Huntington's Disease: Hope through Research," National Institute of Neurological Disorders and Stroke (NINDS), January 4, 2018; Text beginning with the heading "What Is Huntington Disease?" is excerpted from "Huntington Disease," Genetics Home Reference (GHR), National Institutes of Health (NIH), January 16, 2018.

In 1872, the American physician George Huntington wrote about an illness that he called "an heirloom from generations away back in the dim past." He was not the first to describe the disorder, which has been traced back to the Middle Ages at least. One of its earliest names was chorea,* which, as in "choreography," is the Greek word for dance. The term chorea describes how people affected with the disorder writhe, twist, and turn in a constant, uncontrollable dance-like motion. Later, other descriptive names evolved. "Hereditary chorea" emphasizes how the disease is passed from parent to child. "Chronic progressive chorea" stresses how symptoms of the disease worsen over time. Today, physicians commonly use the simple term Huntington's disease (HD) to describe this highly complex disorder that causes untold suffering for thousands of families.

More than 15,000 Americans have HD. At least 150,000 others have a 50 percent risk of developing the disease and thousands more of their relatives live with the possibility that they, too, might develop HD.

What Is Huntington Disease?

Huntington disease (HD) is a progressive brain disorder that causes uncontrolled movements, emotional problems, and loss of thinking ability (cognition).

Adult-onset HD, the most common form of this disorder, usually appears in a person's thirties or forties. Early signs and symptoms can include irritability, depression, small involuntary movements, poor coordination, and trouble learning new information or making decisions. Many people with Huntington disease develop involuntary jerking or twitching movements known as chorea. As the disease progresses, these movements become more pronounced. Affected individuals may have trouble walking, speaking, and swallowing. People with this disorder also experience changes in personality and a decline in thinking and reasoning abilities. Individuals with the adult-onset form of Huntington disease usually live about 15–20 years after signs and symptoms begin.

A less common form of Huntington disease known as the juvenile form begins in childhood or adolescence. It also involves movement problems and mental and emotional changes. Additional signs of the juvenile form include slow movements, clumsiness, frequent falling, rigidity, slurred speech, and drooling. School performance declines as thinking and reasoning abilities become impaired. Seizures occur in 30–50 percent of children with this condition. Juvenile HD tends to progress more quickly than the adult-onset form; affected individuals usually live 10–15 years after signs and symptoms appear.

How Common Is HD?

HD affects an estimated 3–7 per 100,000 people of European ancestry. The disorder appears to be less common in some other populations, including people of Japanese, Chinese, and African descent.

What Are the Genetic Changes Related to HD?

Mutations in the *HTT* gene cause HD. The *HTT* gene provides instructions for making a protein called huntingtin. Although the function of this protein is unknown, it appears to play an important role in nerve cells (neurons) in the brain.

The *HTT* mutation that causes HD involves a deoxyribonucleic acid (DNA) segment known as a cytosine-adenine-guanine (CAG) trinucleotide repeat. This segment is made up of a series of three DNA building blocks (cytosine, adenine, and guanine) that appear multiple times in a row. Normally, the CAG segment is repeated 10–35 times within the gene. In people with HD, the CAG segment is repeated 36 to more than 120 times. People with 36–39 CAG repeats may or may not develop the signs and symptoms of HD, while people with 40 or more repeats almost always develop the disorder.

An increase in the size of the CAG segment leads to the production of an abnormally long version of the huntingtin protein. The elongated protein is cut into smaller, toxic fragments that bind together and accumulate in neurons, disrupting the normal functions of these cells. The dysfunction and eventual death of neurons in certain areas of the brain underlie the signs and symptoms of HD.

Can HD Be Inherited?

This condition is inherited in an autosomal dominant pattern, which means one copy of the altered gene in each cell is sufficient to cause the disorder. An affected person usually inherits the altered gene from one affected parent. In rare cases, an individual with HD does not have a parent with the disorder.

As the altered *HTT* gene is passed from one generation to the next, the size of the CAG trinucleotide repeat often increases in size. A larger number of repeats is usually associated with an earlier onset of signs and symptoms. This phenomenon is called anticipation. People with the adult-onset form of HD typically have 40–50 CAG repeats in the *HTT* gene, while people with the juvenile form of the disorder tend to have more than 60 CAG repeats.

Individuals who have 27–35 CAG repeats in the *HTT* gene do not develop HD, but they are at risk of having children who will develop the disorder. As the gene is passed from parent to child, the size of the CAG trinucleotide repeat may lengthen into the range associated with HD (36 repeats or more).

Section 35.2

First Drug Treatment Approved for HD

This section contains text excerpted from the following sources: Text in this section begins with excerpts from "Huntington's Disease: Hope Through Research," National Institute of Neurological Disorders and Stroke (NINDS), January 4, 2018; Text under the heading "Tetrabenazine" is excerpted from "Tetrabenazine," LiverTox®, National Institutes of Health (NIH), March 13, 2017.

Physicians may prescribe a number of medications to help control emotional and movement problems associated with Huntington disease (HD). It is important to remember however, that while medicines may help keep these clinical symptoms under control, there is no treatment to stop or reverse the course of the disease.

In August 2008, the U.S. Food and Drug Administration (FDA) approved tetrabenazine to treat Huntington's chorea, making it the first drug approved for use in the United States to treat the disease. Antipsychotic drugs, such as haloperidol, or other drugs, such as clonazepam, may help to alleviate choreic movements and may also be used to help control hallucinations, delusions, and violent outbursts. Antipsychotic drugs, however, are not prescribed for another form of muscle contraction associated with HD, called dystonia, and may in fact worsen the condition, causing stiffness and rigidity. These medications may also have severe side effects, including sedation, and for that reason should be used in the lowest possible doses.

For depression, physicians may prescribe fluoxetine, sertraline, nortriptyline, or other compounds. Tranquilizers can help control anxiety and lithium may be prescribed to combat pathological excitement and severe mood swings. Medications may also be needed to treat the severe obsessive-compulsive rituals of some individuals with HD.

Most drugs used to treat the symptoms of HD have side effects such as fatigue, restlessness, or hyperexcitability. Sometimes it may be difficult to tell if a particular symptom, such as apathy or incontinence, is a sign of the disease or a reaction to medication.

Tetrabenazine

Tetrabenazine is a potent, selective inhibitor of the monoamine transporter 2 that causes a depletion of neuroactive peptides in nerve terminals and is used to treat chorea associated with Huntington disease. Tetrabenazine has not been associated with serum enzyme elevations during therapy or linked to instances of clinically apparent liver injury.

Tetrabenazine is an inhibitor of the synaptic vesicular monoamine transporter 2 (VMAT2), the inhibition of which causes a depletion of neuroactive monoamines (serotonin, norepinephrine and particularly dopamine) in nerve terminals. The reduction in these active neurotransmitters results in a decrease in spontaneous jerk-like movements of the extremities, trunk, face and neck (chorea) that are typical of patients with degenerative neurologic conditions such as Huntington disease. Tetrabenazine, however, does not prevent the progression or alter the outcome of these diseases. Tetrabenazine is used off-label to treat other forms of chorea, tetrabenazine is not formally approved for those indications. Tetrabenazine is available as tablets of 12.5

and 25 mg generically and under the brand name Xenazine. The recommended initial dose is 12.5 mg once daily, with subsequent careful increase to a maximum of 25 mg twice daily. Because of the variable metabolism of tetrabenazine (by CYP 2D6), the maintenance dose varies by individual, and inducers or inhibitors of CYP 2D6 should be avoided. Common side effects include fatigue, sedation, somnolence, insomnia, depression, restlessness (akathisia), agitation, and nausea. Less common, but potentially serious adverse events include severe depression, suicidality, symptomatic hypotension, and neuroleptic malignant syndrome.

Tetrabenazine has not been associated with serum enzyme elevations greater than occurs with placebo therapy, but information on liver test results during therapy is limited and occasional instances of asymptomatic alanine transaminase (ALT) elevations leading to drug discontinuation or dose modification have been reported. In prelicensure pivotal registration trials in several hundred patients, tetrabenazine was not associated with cases of jaundice or hepatitis. Since licensure, there have been no published reports of clinically apparent liver injury, jaundice or hepatitis attributed to tetrabenazine. Thus, clinically apparent liver injury with jaundice due to tetrabenazine must be very rare, if it occurs at all.

Chapter 36

Neuroacanthocytosis and Neurodegeneration

Chapter Contents

Section 36.1

Neuroacanthocytosis

This section includes text excerpted from "Neuroacanthocytosis
Information Page," National Institute of Neurological Disorders
and Stroke (NINDS), January 5, 2018.

Neuroacanthocytosis refers to a group of genetic conditions that
are characterized by movement disorders and acanthocytosis (abnormal, spiculated red blood cells). Four syndromes are classified as neuroacanthocytosis: Chorea acanthocytosis, McLeod syndrome (MLS),
Huntington disease (HD) like 2 (HDL2), and panthothenate kinase
associated neurodegeneration (PKAN). Acanthocytosis may not always
be observed in HDL2 and PKAN. These disorders are caused by different genetic mutations, and the signs and symptoms vary, but usually
include chorea (involuntary, dance like movements), parkinsonism
(slowness of movement), dystonia (abnormal body postures), and problems walking. There may also be muscle weakness, involuntary movements of the face and tongue, tongue/lip biting (which is mostly characteristic of Chorea acanthocytosis), as well as difficulty with speech
and eating, cognitive impairment, psychiatric symptoms, and seizures.
Individuals with McLeod syndrome often have cardiac problems.

Many features of these disorders are due to degeneration of the
basal ganglia, a part of the brain that controls movement. Additional
disorders that are also known have neurologic symptoms, acanthocytosis, and either lipoprotein disorders or systemic findings. The diagnosis
of neuroacanthocytosis is typically based on the symptoms and clinical
observation, a review of family history, and the evaluation of specific
laboratory and imaging studies.

Treatment

There are no treatments to prevent or slow the progression of
neuroacanthocytosis and treatment is symptomatic and supportive.
Medications that block dopamine, such as some of the antipsychotics,
may decrease the involuntary movements. Botulinum toxin injections
usually improve symptoms of dystonia. A feeding tube may be needed

for individuals with feeding difficulties to maintain proper nutrition. Seizures may be treated with a variety of anticonvulsants, and anti-depressants may also be appropriate for some individuals. Speech, occupational, and physical therapy may also be beneficial.

Prognosis

Neuroacanthocytosis is a progressive disease, and in some cases may be complicated by poor nutritional status, cardiac abnormalities, and pneumonia.

Section 36.2

Neurodegeneration with Brain Iron Accumulation

This section includes text excerpted from "Neurodegeneration with Brain Iron Accumulation Information Page," National Institute of Neurological Disorders and Stroke (NINDS), January 31, 2016.

Neurodegeneration with brain iron accumulation (NBIA) is a rare, inherited, neurological movement disorder characterized by an abnormal accumulation of iron in the brain and progressive degeneration of the nervous system. Symptoms, which vary greatly among patients and usually develop during childhood, may include dystonia (slow writhing, distorting muscle contractions of the limbs, face, or trunk), dysarthria (slurred or slow speech) choreoathetosis (involuntary, purposeless jerky muscle movements), muscle rigidity (uncontrolled tightness of the muscles), spasticity (sudden, involuntary muscle spasms), and/or ataxia (inability to coordinate movements), confusion, disorientation, seizures, stupor, and dementia. Visual changes are also common, most often due to atrophy of the optic nerve (optic atrophy) or degeneration of the retinal layer in the back of the eye (retinal degeneration, cognitive decline occurs in some forms of NBIA; the majority of individuals with NBIA do not have cognitive impairment. Several genes have been found that cause NBIA.

Treatment

There is no cure for NBIA, nor is there a standard course of treatment. Treatment is symptomatic and supportive, and may include physical or occupational therapy, exercise physiology, and/or speech pathology. Many medications are available to treat the primary symptoms of dystonia and spasticity, including oral medications, intrathecal baclofen pump (in which a small pump is implanted under the skin and is programmed to deliver a specific amount of medication on a regular basis), deep brain stimulation, and botulinum toxin injection.

Prognosis

NBIA is a progressive condition. Most individuals experience periods of rapid decline lasting weeks to months, with relatively stable periods in between. The rate of progression correlates with the age at onset, meaning that children with early symptoms tend to fare more poorly. For those with early onset, dystonia and spasticity can eventually limit the ability to walk, usually leading to use of a wheelchair by the mid-teens. Life expectancy is variable, although premature death does occur in NBIA. Premature death usually occurs due to secondary complications such as impaired swallowing or confinement to a bed or wheelchair, which can lead to poor nutrition or aspiration pneumonia. With improved medical care, however, a greater number of affected individuals reach adulthood. For those with atypical, late onset NBIA, many are diagnosed as adults and live well into adulthood.

Chapter 37

Movement Disorders during Sleep

Chapter Contents

Section 37.1

Restless Legs Syndrome (RLS)

This section includes text excerpted from "Restless Legs
Syndrome Fact Sheet," National Institute of Neurological
Disorders and Stroke (NINDS), May 2017.

What Is Restless Legs Syndrome?

Restless legs syndrome (RLS), also called Willis-Ekbom disease, causes unpleasant or uncomfortable sensations in the legs and an irresistible urge to move them. Symptoms commonly occur in the late afternoon or evening hours, and are often most severe at night when a person is resting, such as sitting or lying in bed. They also may occur when someone is inactive and sitting for extended periods (for example, when taking a trip by plane or watching a movie). Since symptoms can increase in severity during the night, it could become difficult to fall asleep or return to sleep after waking up. Moving the legs or walking typically relieves the discomfort but the sensations often recur once the movement stops. RLS is classified as a sleep disorder since the symptoms are triggered by resting and attempting to sleep, and as a movement disorder, since people are forced to move their legs in order to relieve symptoms. It is, however, best characterized as a neurological sensory disorder with symptoms that are produced from within the brain itself.

RLS is one of several disorders that can cause exhaustion and daytime sleepiness, which can strongly affect mood, concentration, job and school performance, and personal relationships. Many people with RLS report they are often unable to concentrate, have impaired memory, or fail to accomplish daily tasks. Untreated moderate to severe RLS can lead to about a 20 percent decrease in work productivity and can contribute to depression and anxiety. It also can make traveling difficult.

It is estimated that up to 7–10 percent of the U.S. population may have RLS. RLS occurs in both men and women, although women are more likely to have it than men. It may begin at any age. Many individuals who are severely affected are middle-aged or older, and the symptoms typically become more frequent and last longer with age.

More than 80 percent of people with RLS also experience periodic limb movement of sleep (PLMS). PLMS is characterized by involuntary leg (and sometimes arm) twitching or jerking movements during sleep that typically occur every 15–40 seconds, sometimes throughout the night. Although many individuals with RLS also develop PLMS, most people with PLMS do not experience RLS.

Fortunately, most cases of RLS can be treated with nondrug therapies and if necessary, medications.

What Are Common Signs and Symptoms of RLS?

People with RLS feel the irresistible urge to move, which is accompanied by uncomfortable sensations in their lower limbs that are unlike normal sensations experienced by people without the disorder. The sensations in their legs are often difficult to define but may be described as aching throbbing, pulling, itching, crawling, or creeping. These sensations less commonly affect the arms, and rarely the chest or head. Although the sensations can occur on just one side of the body, they most often affect both sides. They can also alternate between sides. The sensations range in severity from uncomfortable to irritating to painful.

Because moving the legs (or other affected parts of the body) relieves the discomfort, people with RLS often keep their legs in motion to minimize or prevent the sensations. They may pace the floor, constantly move their legs while sitting, and toss and turn in bed.

A classic feature of RLS is that the symptoms are worse at night with a distinct symptom-free period in the early morning, allowing for more refreshing sleep at that time. Some people with RLS have difficulty falling asleep and staying asleep. They may also note a worsening of symptoms if their sleep is further reduced by events or activity.

RLS symptoms may vary from day to day, in severity and frequency, and from person to person. In moderately severe cases, symptoms occur only once or twice a week but often result in significant delay of sleep onset, with some disruption of daytime function. In severe cases of RLS, the symptoms occur more than twice a week and result in burdensome interruption of sleep and impairment of daytime function.

People with RLS can sometimes experience remissions—spontaneous improvement over a period of weeks or months before symptoms reappear—usually during the early stages of the disorder. In general, however, symptoms become more severe over time.

People who have both RLS and an associated medical condition tend to develop more severe symptoms rapidly. In contrast, those who have RLS that is not related to any other condition show a very slow progression of the disorder, particularly if they experience onset at an early age; many years may pass before symptoms occur regularly.

What Causes RLS?

In most cases, the cause of RLS is unknown (called primary RLS). However, RLS has a genetic component and can be found in families where the onset of symptoms is before age 40. Specific gene variants have been associated with RLS. Evidence indicates that low levels of iron in the brain also may be responsible for RLS.

Considerable evidence also suggests that RLS is related to a dysfunction in one of the sections of the brain that control movement (called the basal ganglia) that use the brain chemical dopamine. Dopamine is needed to produce smooth, purposeful muscle activity and movement. Disruption of these pathways frequently results in involuntary movements. Individuals with Parkinson disease (PD), another disorder of the basal ganglia's dopamine pathways, have increased chance of developing RLS.

RLS also appears to be related to or accompany the following factors or underlying conditions:

- end-stage renal disease and hemodialysis

- iron deficiency

- certain medications that may aggravate RLS symptoms, such as antinausea drugs (e.g. prochlorperazine or metoclopramide), antipsychotic drugs (e.g., haloperidol or phenothiazine derivatives), antidepressants that increase serotonin (e.g., fluoxetine or sertraline), and some cold and allergy medications that contain older antihistamines (e.g., diphenhydramine)

- use of alcohol, nicotine, and caffeine

- pregnancy, especially in the last trimester; in most cases, symptoms usually disappear within 4 weeks after delivery

- neuropathy (nerve damage)

Sleep deprivation and other sleep conditions like sleep apnea also may aggravate or trigger symptoms in some people. Reducing or completely eliminating these factors may relieve symptoms.

How Is RLS Diagnosed?

Since there is no specific test for RLS, the condition is diagnosed by a doctor's evaluation. The five basic criteria for clinically diagnosing the disorder are:

- A strong and often overwhelming need or urge to move the legs that is often associated with abnormal, unpleasant, or uncomfortable sensations.

- The urge to move the legs starts or get worse during rest or inactivity.

- The urge to move the legs is at least temporarily and partially or totally relieved by movements.

- The urge to move the legs starts or is aggravated in the evening or night.

- The above four features are not due to any other medical or behavioral condition.

A physician will focus largely on the individual's descriptions of symptoms, their triggers and relieving factors, as well as the presence or absence of symptoms throughout the day. A neurological and physical exam, plus information from the person's medical and family history and list of current medications, may be helpful. Individuals may be asked about frequency, duration, and intensity of symptoms; if movement helps to relieve symptoms; how much time it takes to fall asleep; any pain related to symptoms; and any tendency toward daytime sleep patterns and sleepiness, disturbance of sleep, or daytime function. Laboratory tests may rule out other conditions such as kidney failure, iron deficiency anemia (which is a separate condition related to iron deficiency), or pregnancy that may be causing symptoms of RLS. Blood tests can identify iron deficiencies as well as other medical disorders associated with RLS.

In some cases, sleep studies such as polysomnography (a test that records the individual's brain waves, heartbeat, breathing, and leg movements during an entire night) may identify the presence of other causes of sleep disruption (e.g., sleep apnea), which may impact management of the disorder. Periodic limb movement of sleep during a sleep study can support the diagnosis of RLS but, again, is not exclusively seen in individuals with RLS.

Diagnosing RLS in children may be especially difficult, since it may be hard for children to describe what they are experiencing, when and how often the symptoms occur, and how long symptoms last. Pediatric

RLS can sometimes be misdiagnosed as "growing pains" or attention deficit disorder.

How Is RLS Treated?

RLS can be treated, with care directed toward relieving symptoms. Moving the affected limb(s) may provide temporary relief. Sometimes RLS symptoms can be controlled by finding and treating an associated medical condition, such as peripheral neuropathy, diabetes, or iron deficiency anemia.

Iron supplementation or medications are usually helpful but no single medication effectively manages RLS for all individuals. Trials of different drugs may be necessary. In addition, medications taken regularly may lose their effect over time or even make the condition worse, making it necessary to change medications.

Treatment options for RLS include:

Lifestyle changes. Certain lifestyle changes and activities may provide some relief in persons with mild to moderate symptoms of RLS. These steps include avoiding or decreasing the use of alcohol and tobacco, changing or maintaining a regular sleep pattern, a program of moderate exercise, and massaging the legs, taking a warm bath, or using a heating pad or ice pack. There are new medical devices that have been cleared by the U.S. Food and Drug Administration (FDA), including a foot wrap that puts pressure underneath the foot and another that is a pad that delivers vibration to the back of the legs. Aerobic and leg-stretching exercises of moderate intensity also may provide some relief from mild symptoms.

Iron. For individuals with low or low-normal blood tests called ferritin and transferrin saturation, a trial of iron supplements is recommended as the first treatment. Iron supplements are available over-the-counter. A common side effect is upset stomach, which may improve with use of a different type of iron supplement. Because iron is not well-absorbed into the body by the gut, it may cause constipation that can be treated with a stool softeners such as polyethylene glycol. In some people, iron supplementation does not improve a person's iron levels. Others may require iron given through an IV line in order to boost the iron levels and relieve symptoms.

Anti-seizure drugs. Anti-seizure drugs are becoming the first-line prescription drugs for those with RLS. The FDA has approved gabapentin enacarbil for the treatment of moderate to severe RLS, This drug appears to be as effective as dopaminergic treatment (discussed below) and, at least to date, there have been no reports of problems with a progressive worsening of symptoms due to medication (called augmentation). Other medications may be prescribed "off-label" to relieve some of the symptoms of the disorder.

Other anti-seizure drugs such as the standard form of gabapentin and pregabalin can decrease such sensory disturbances as creeping and crawling as well as nerve pain. Dizziness, fatigue, and sleepiness are among the possible side effects. Recent studies have shown that pregabalin is as effective for RLS treatment as the dopaminergic drug pramipexole, suggesting this class of drug offers equivalent benefits.

Dopaminergic agents. These drugs, which increase dopamine effect, are largely used to treat Parkinson disease. They have been shown to reduce symptoms of RLS when they are taken at nighttime. The FDA has approved ropinirole, pramipexole, and rotigotine to treat moderate to severe RLS. These drugs are generally well tolerated but can cause nausea, dizziness, or other short-term side effects. Levodopa plus carbidopa may be effective when used intermittently, but not daily.

Although dopamine-related medications are effective in managing RLS symptoms, long-term use can lead to worsening of the symptoms in many individuals. With chronic use, a person may begin to experience symptoms earlier in the evening or even earlier until the symptoms are present around the clock. Over time, the initial evening or bedtime dose can become less effective, the symptoms at night become more intense, and symptoms could begin to affect the arms or trunk. Fortunately, this apparent progression can be reversed by removing the person from all dopamine-related medications.

Another important adverse effect of dopamine medications that occurs in some people is the development of impulsive or obsessive behaviors such as obsessive gambling or shopping. Should they occur, these behaviors can be improved or reversed by stopping the medication.

Opioids. Drugs such as methadone, codeine, hydrocodone, or oxycodone are sometimes prescribed to treat individuals with more severe symptoms of RLS who did not respond well to other medications. Side effects include constipation, dizziness, nausea, exacerbation of sleep apnea, and the risk of addiction; however, very low doses are often effective in controlling symptoms of RLS.

Benzodiazepines. These drugs can help individuals obtain a more restful sleep. However, even if taken only at bedtime they can sometimes cause daytime sleepiness, reduce energy, and affect concentration. Benzodiazepines such as clonazepam and lorazepam are generally prescribed to treat anxiety, muscle spasms, and insomnia. Because these drugs also may induce or aggravate sleep apnea in some cases, they should not be used in people with this condition. These are last-line drugs due to their side effects.

What Is the Prognosis for People with RLS?

RLS is generally a lifelong condition for which there is no cure. However, current therapies can control the disorder, minimize symptoms, and increase periods of restful sleep. Symptoms may gradually worsen with age, although the decline may be somewhat faster for individuals who also suffer from an associated medical condition. A diagnosis of RLS does not indicate the onset of another neurological disease, such as PD. In addition, some individuals have remissions—periods in which symptoms decrease or disappear for days, weeks, months, or years—although symptoms often eventually reappear. If RLS symptoms are mild, do not produce significant daytime discomfort, or do not affect an individual's ability to fall asleep, the condition does not have to be treated.

Section 37.2

Periodic Limb Movement Disorder

"Periodic Limb Movement Disorder," © 2016 Omnigraphics.
Reviewed January 2018.

Periodic limb movement disorder (PLMD) is a type of sleep disorder in which patients experience repetitive, rhythmic jerking or twitching movements in the legs or other limbs during sleep. The movements typically occur in a regular pattern every 20–40 seconds. Episodes most commonly take place in the early part of the night and last for less than an hour. Although the patient is usually not aware of them, the movements often disrupt sleep, resulting in such symptoms as daytime drowsiness and memory or attention problems.

PLMD is often confused with restless leg syndrome. In this condition, patients experience uncomfortable sensations in their legs while awake that create an irresistible urge to move the affected limbs. Although approximately 80 percent of people with restless legs syndrome also have PLMD, PLMD is considered a separate condition and does not appear to increase the risk of restless leg syndrome.

Symptoms

- The main symptom of PLMD is tightening or flexing of muscles in the lower legs—including the big toe, foot, ankle, knee, or hip—during sleep. Although PLMD can also affect the arms or occur while awake, this is uncommon. The movements are usually concentrated during non-Rapid Eye Movement (REM) sleep in the first half of the night. Each movement typically lasts around 2 seconds, and they tend to recur every 20–40 seconds, although the pattern can vary from night to night. The movements can range from slight twitches to strenuous kicks.

- Most people with PLMD are unaware of the movements and only learn about them from another person who shares the same bed. For some patients, however, the repetitive movements can disrupt sleep and cause such symptoms as not feeling well rested after a good night's sleep, feeling tired or falling asleep during the day, having trouble remembering or paying attention, or becoming depressed.

Causes and Risk Factors

Researchers have not uncovered the cause of primary PLMD, although some believe that it may be linked to abnormalities in the regulation of nerve impulses from the brain to the limbs. PLMD affects males and females equally, and it can affect people of any age. The incidence of PLMD increases with age, however, and affects 34 percent of people over the age of 60.

Secondary PLMD is caused by underlying medical conditions, including the following:

- diabetes
- iron deficiency anemia
- spinal cord injury

- restless leg syndrome

- sleep apnea

- narcolepsy

- REM sleep behavior disorder

- sleep-related eating disorder

- multiple-system atrophy

Certain types of medications have also been found to increase the risk or worsen symptoms of PLMD, including antidepressants such as amitriptyline (Elavil) and lithium; dopamine-receptor antagonists like Haldol; and withdrawal from sedatives like Valium.

Diagnosis

- Diagnosis of PLMD begins with a visit to a sleep specialist. Patients are typically asked to keep a sleep diary for several weeks, to evaluate their sleep using a rating system such as the Epworth Sleepiness Scale, and to provide a complete medical history, including any medications taken. In most cases, patients will then undergo an overnight sleep study, during which a polysomnogram keeps track of brain activity, heartbeat, breathing, and limb movement. In addition to diagnosing PLMD and other sleep disorders, the sleep specialist can help identify other potential causes of sleep problems, such as medical conditions, medications, substance abuse, or mental health disorders.

- Other medical tests can be used to detect underlying causes of PLMD, such as diabetes, anemia, or metabolic disorders. Doctors may take blood samples to check hormone levels, organ function, and blood chemistry. They may also look for infections or traces of drugs that can contribute to secondary PLMD. If no underlying cause can be found, the patient may be referred to a neurologist to rule out nervous system disorders and confirm the diagnosis of PLMD.

Treatment

- Many people with PLMD do not experience symptoms or require treatment. When sleep disruption makes treatment necessary, however, there are several medications available to help reduce the movements or help the patient sleep through them. Some of the medications commonly prescribed to treat PLMD include:

- Benzodiazepines like clonazepam (Klonopin), which suppress muscle contractions;

- Anticonvulsant agents like gabapentin (Neurontin), which also reduce muscle contractions;

- Dopaminergic agents like levodopa/carbidopa (Sinemet) and pergolide (Permax), which increase the levels of the neurotransmitter dopamine in the brain and are also used to treat restless leg syndrome and Parkinson disease;

- GABA agonists like baclofen (Lioresal), which inhibit the release of neurotransmitters in the brain that stimulate muscle contractions.

References

1. "Periodic Limb Movement Disorder," WebMD, 2016.
2. "Sleep Education: Periodic Limb Movements," American Academy of Sleep Medicine, 2014.

Chapter 38

Hereditary Spastic Paraplegia (HSP)

Hereditary spastic paraplegia (HSP) is a group of hereditary, degenerative, neurological disorders that primarily affect the upper motor neurons. Upper motor neurons in the brain and spinal cord deliver signals to the lower motor neurons, which in turn, carry messages to the muscles. In hereditary spastic paraplegia, upper motor neurons slowly degenerate so the muscles do not receive the correct messages, causing progressive spasticity (increased muscle tone/stiffness) and weakness of the legs. This leads to difficulty walking. As degeneration continues, symptoms worsen. If only the lower body is affected, HSP is classified as uncomplicated or pure. HSP is classified as complicated or complex if other systems are involved. In these cases, additional symptoms, including impaired vision, ataxia, epilepsy, cognitive impairment, peripheral neuropathy, and/or deafness, occur. The different forms of HSP are caused by mutations in different genes. Inheritance varies. There are no specific treatments to prevent, slow, or reverse HSP. Individual symptoms may be treated with medications and/or physical therapy.

This chapter includes text excerpted from "Hereditary Spastic Paraplegia," Genetic and Rare Diseases Information Center (GARD), National Center for Advancing Translational Sciences (NCATS), November 1, 2017.

Symptoms

The hallmark feature of HSP is progressive weakness and spasticity (stiffness) of the legs. Symptoms typically develop between the second and fourth decades (although earlier and later presentation has been described). Early in the disease course, there may be mild gait difficulties and stiffness. These symptoms typically slowly progress so that eventually, individuals with HSP may require the assistance of a cane, walker, or wheelchair. In some cases, additional symptoms may occur. These can include:

- impaired vision
- ataxia
- urinary urgency and frequency
- hyperactive reflexes
- Babinski sign
- difficulty with balance
- epilepsy
- cognitive impairment
- peripheral neuropathy
- deafness

Inheritance

At this point, over 70 different types of HSP have been described. The different patterns of inheritance are autosomal dominant, autosomal recessive, and X-linked recessive.

Diagnosis

HSP is diagnosed on the basis of the following:

- **Characteristic clinical symptoms** of slowly progressive weakness and stiffness in the legs often accompanied by urinary urgency

- **Neurologic examination** demonstrating damage to the nerve paths connecting the spinal cord and the brain (corticospinal tract), such as spastic weakness, exaggerated reflexes, typically associated with bilateral extensor plantar responses; often accompanied by a mild inability to sense vibration in the lower part of the legs and muscle changes of the urinary bladder

- **Family history** shows a pattern of inheritance that is either autosomal dominant, autosomal recessive, or X-linked recessive

- **Exclusion** of other disorders that cause spasticity and weakness in the legs

- **Identification of a disease causing mutation in an HSP causing gene**; such testing is increasingly available and can confirm the diagnosis of HSP.

Treatment

There are no specific treatments to prevent, slow, or reverse HSP. Treatment is symptomatic and supportive. Medications may be considered for spasticity and urinary urgency. Regular physical therapy is important for muscle strength and to preserve range of motion.

Prognosis

The prognosis for individuals with HSP varies. Some individuals are very disabled and others have only mild disability. The majority of individuals with uncomplicated HSP have a normal life expectancy.

Chapter 39

Tourette Syndrome (TS)

Tourette syndrome (TS) is a condition of the nervous system. TS causes people to have "tics."

Tics are sudden twitches, movements, or sounds that people do repeatedly. People who have tics cannot stop their body from doing these things. For example, a person might keep blinking over and over again. Or, a person might make a grunting sound unwillingly.

Having tics is a little bit like having hiccups. Even though you might not want to hiccup, your body does it anyway. Sometimes people can stop themselves from doing a certain tic for awhile, but it's hard. Eventually the person has to do the tic.

Types of Tics

There are two types of tics—motor and vocal:

Motor Tics

Motor tics are movements of the body. Examples of motor tics include blinking, shrugging the shoulders, or jerking an arm.

Vocal Tics

Vocal tics are sounds that a person makes with his or her voice. Examples of vocal tics include humming, clearing the throat, or yelling out a word or phrase.

This chapter includes text excerpted from "Facts about Tourette Syndrome," Centers for Disease Control and Prevention (CDC), May 11, 2017.

Tics can be either simple or complex:

Simple Tics

Simple tics involve just a few parts of the body. Examples of simple tics include squinting the eyes or sniffing.

Complex Tics

Complex tics usually involve several different parts of the body and can have a pattern. An example of a complex tic is bobbing the head while jerking an arm, and then jumping up.

Risk Factors and Causes

Doctors and scientists do not know the exact cause of TS. Research suggests that it is an inherited genetic condition. That means it is passed on from parent to child through genes.

Who Is Affected?

In the United States, 1 of every 360 children 6-17 years of age have been diagnosed with TS. TS can affect people of all racial and ethnic groups. Boys are affected 3–5 times more often than girls.

Symptoms

The main symptoms of TS are tics. Symptoms usually begin when a child is 5–10 years of age. The first symptoms often are motor tics that occur in the head and neck area. Tics usually are worse during times that are stressful or exciting. They tend to improve when a person is calm or focused on an activity.

The types of tics and how often a person has tics changes a lot over time. Even though the symptoms might appear, disappear, and reappear, these conditions are considered chronic.

In most cases, tics decrease during adolescence and early adulthood, and sometimes disappear entirely. However, many people with TS experience tics into adulthood and, in some cases, tics can become worse during adulthood.

Although the media often portray people with TS as involuntarily shouting out swear words (called coprolalia) or constantly repeating the words of other people (called echolalia), these symptoms are rare, and are not required for a diagnosis of TS.

Diagnosis

The American Psychiatric Association's (APA) *Diagnostic and Statistical Manual of Mental Disorders*, Fifth Edition (DSM-5) is used by health professionals to help diagnose tic disorders.

Tics are sudden twitches, movements, or sounds that people do repeatedly. People who have tics cannot stop their body from doing these things. For example, a person with a motor tic might keep blinking over and over again. Or, a person with a vocal tic might make a grunting sound unwillingly.

Three tic disorders are included in the DSM-5:

1.   Tourette disorder (also called TS)

2.   Persistent (also called chronic) motor or vocal tic disorder

3.   Provisional tic disorder

The tic disorders differ from each other in terms of the type of tic present (motor or vocal, or a combination of both), and how long the symptoms have lasted. People with TS have both motor and vocal tics, and have had tic symptoms for at least 1 year. People with persistent motor or vocal tic disorders have either motor or vocal tics, and have had tic symptoms for at least 1 year. People with provisional tic disorders can have motor or vocal tics, or both, but have had their symptoms less than 1 year.

Here are the criteria in shortened form. Please note that they are presented for your information only and should not be used for self-diagnosis. If you are concerned about any of the symptoms listed, you should consult a trained healthcare provider with experience in diagnosing and treating tic disorders.

Tourette Syndrome (TS)

For a person to be diagnosed with TS—he or she must:

* have two or more motor tics (for example, blinking or shrugging the shoulders) and at least one vocal tic (for example, humming, clearing the throat, or yelling out a word or phrase), although they might not always happen at the same time.

* have had tics for at least a year. The tics can occur many times a day (usually in bouts) nearly every day, or off and on.

* have tics that begin before he or she is 18 years of age.

- have symptoms that are not due to taking medicine or other drugs or due to having another medical condition (for example, seizures, Huntington disease (HD), or postviral encephalitis).

Persistent (Chronic) Motor or Vocal Tic Disorder

For a person to be diagnosed with a persistent tic disorder, he or she must:

- have one or more motor tics (for example, blinking or shrugging the shoulders) or vocal tics (for example, humming, clearing the throat, or yelling out a word or phrase), but not both.

- have tics that occur many times a day nearly every day or on and off throughout a period of more than a year.

- have tics that start before he or she is 18 years of age.

- have symptoms that are not due to taking medicine or other drugs, or due to having a medical condition that can cause tics (for example, seizures, HD, or postviral encephalitis).

- not have been diagnosed with TS.

Provisional Tic Disorder

For a person to be diagnosed with this disorder, he or she must:

- have one or more motor tics (for example, blinking or shrugging the shoulders) or vocal tics (for example, humming, clearing the throat, or yelling out a word or phrase).

- have been present for no longer than 12 months in a row.

- have tics that start before he or she is 18 years of age.

- have symptoms that are not due to taking medicine or other drugs, or due to having a medical condition that can cause tics (for example, HD or postviral encephalitis).

- not have been diagnosed with TS or persistent motor or vocal tic disorder.

Treatment

Although there is no cure for TS, there are treatments to help manage the tics caused by TS. Many people with TS have tics that do not get in the way of living their daily life and, therefore, do not need any treatment. However, medication and behavioral treatments are available if tics cause pain or injury; interfere with school, work, or social life; or cause stress. A promising new behavioral treatment is the Comprehensive Behavioral Intervention for Tics (CBIT)

Educating the community (for example, peers, educators, and coworkers) about TS can increase understanding of the symptoms, reduce teasing, and decrease stress for people living with TS. People with TS cannot help having tics, and are not being disruptive on purpose. When others understand these facts, people with TS might receive more support, which might, in turn, help lessen some tic symptoms.

It is common for people with TS to have co-occurring conditions, particularly attention deficit hyperactivity disorder (ADHD) and obsessive-compulsive disorder (OCD). People with additional conditions will require different treatments based on the symptoms. Sometimes treating these other conditions can help reduce tics. To develop the best treatment plan, people with tics, parents, and healthcare providers should work closely with one another, and with everyone involved in treatment and support—which may include teachers, child care providers, coaches, therapists, and other family members. Taking advantage of all the resources available will help guide success.

Medications

Medications can be used to reduce severe or disruptive tics that might have led to problems in the past with family and friends, other students, or coworkers. Medications also can be used to reduce symptoms of related conditions, such as ADHD or OCD.

Medications do not eliminate tics completely. However, they can help some people with TS in their everyday life. There is no one medication that is best for all people. Most medications prescribed for TS have not been approved by the U.S. Food and Drug Administration (FDA) for treating tics.

Medications affect each person differently. One person might do well with one medication, but not another. When deciding the best treatment, a doctor might try different medications and doses, and it may take time to find the treatment plan that works best. The doctor will want to find the medication and dose that have the best results and the fewest side effects. Doctors often start with small doses and slowly increase as needed.

As with all medications, those used to treat tics can have side effects. Side effects can include weight gain, stiff muscles, tiredness, restlessness, and social withdrawal. The side effects need to be considered carefully when deciding whether or not to use any medication to treat tics. In some cases, the side effects can be worse than the tics.

Even though medications often are used to treat the symptoms of TS, they might not be helpful for everyone. Two common reasons for not using medications to treat TS are unpleasant side effects and failure of the medications to work as well as expected.

Behavioral Therapy

Behavioral therapy is a treatment that teaches people with TS ways to manage their tics. Behavioral therapy is not a cure for tics. However, it can help reduce the number of tics, the severity of tics, the impact of tics, or a combination of all of these. It is important to understand that even though behavioral therapies might help reduce the severity of tics, this does not mean that tics are just psychological or that anyone with tics should be able to control them.

Habit Reversal

Habit reversal is one of the most studied behavioral interventions for people with tics. It has two main parts: awareness training and competing response training. In the awareness training part, people identify each tic out loud. In the competing response part, people learn to do a new behavior that cannot happen at the same time as the tic. For example, if the person with TS has a tic that involves head rubbing, a new behavior might be for that person to place his or her hands on his or her knees, or to cross his or her arms so that the head rubbing cannot take place.

Comprehensive Behavioral Intervention for Tics (CBIT)

CBIT is a new, evidence-based type of behavioral therapy for TS and chronic tic disorders. CBIT includes habit reversal in addition to other strategies, including education about tics and relaxation techniques. CBIT has been shown to be effective at reducing tic symptoms and tic-related impairment among children and adults.

In CBIT, a therapist will work with a child (and his or her parents) or an adult with TS to better understand the types of tics the person is having and to understand the situations in which the tics are at their worst. Changes to the surroundings may be made, if possible, and the person with TS will also learn to do a new behavior instead of the tic (habit reversal). For example, if a child with TS often has a certain tic during math class, the math teacher can be educated about TS, and perhaps the child's seat can be changed so that the tics are not as visible. In addition, the child also can work with a psychologist to learn habit reversal techniques. This helps to decrease how often the tic occurs by doing a new behavior (like putting his or her hands on his or her knees when an urge to perform the tic happens). CBIT skills can be learned with practice, with the help of an experienced therapist, and with the support and encouragement of those close to the person with TS.

Many health professionals have recognized that behavioral therapy can be very effective in managing the symptoms of TS. Unfortunately, very few clinicians have been trained in these types of treatments specifically for TS and tic disorders.

Other Concerns and Conditions

TS often occurs with other related conditions (also called co-occurring conditions). These conditions can include ADHD, OCD, and other behavioral or conduct problems. People with TS and related conditions can be at higher risk for learning, behavioral, and social problems.

The symptoms of other disorders can complicate the diagnosis and treatment of TS and create extra challenges for people with TS and their families, educators, and health professionals.

Findings from a national Centers for Disease Control and Prevention (CDC) study indicated that 86 percent of children who had been diagnosed with TS also had been diagnosed with at least one additional mental health, behavioral, or developmental condition based on parent report.

Among children with TS:

- 63 percent had ADHD.

- 26 percent had behavioral problems, such as oppositional defiant disorder (ODD) or conduct disorder (CD).

- 49 percent had anxiety problems.

- 25 percent had depression.

- 35 percent had an autism spectrum disorder

- 47 percent had a learning disability

- 29 percent had a speech or language problem.

- 30 percent had a developmental delay.

- 12 percent had an intellectual disability

Because co-occurring conditions are so common among people with TS, it is important for doctors to assess every child with TS for other conditions and problems.

ADHD

In a national CDC study, ADHD was the most common co-occurring condition among children with TS. Of children who had been diagnosed with TS, 63 percent also had been diagnosed with ADHD.

Children with ADHD have trouble paying attention and controlling impulsive behaviors. They might act without thinking about what the result will be and, in some cases, they are also overly active. It is normal for children to have trouble focusing and behaving at one time or another. However, these behaviors continue beyond early childhood (0–5 years of age) among children with ADHD. Symptoms of ADHD can continue and can cause difficulty at school, at home, or with friends.

Obsessive-Compulsive Behaviors

People with obsessive-compulsive behaviors have unwanted thoughts (obsessions) that they feel a need to respond to (compulsions). Obsessive-compulsive behaviors and OCD have been shown to occur among more than one-third of people with TS. Sometimes it is difficult to tell the difference between complex tics that a child with TS may have and obsessive-compulsive behaviors.

Behavior or Conduct Problems

Findings from the CDC study indicated that behavior or conduct problems, such as oppositional defiant disorder (ODD) or conduct disorder (CD), had been diagnosed among 26 percent of children with TS.

ODD

People with ODD show negative, defiant and hostile behaviors toward adults or authority figures. ODD usually starts before a child is 8 years of age, but no later than early adolescence. Symptoms might occur most often with people the individual knows well, such as family members or a regular care provider. The behaviors associated with

ODD are present beyond what might be expected for the person's age, and result in major problems in school, at home, or with peers.

Examples of ODD behaviors include:

- Losing one's temper a lot.

- Arguing with adults or refusing to comply with adults' rules or requests.

- Getting angry or being resentful or vindictive often.

- Annoying others on purpose or easily becoming annoyed with others.

- Blaming other people often for one's own mistakes or misbehavior.

CD

People with CD have aggression toward others and break rules, laws, and social norms. Increased injuries and difficulty with friends also are common among people with CD. In addition, the symptoms of CD happen in more than one area in the person's life (for example, at home, in the community, and at school).

CD is severe and highly disruptive to a person's life and to others in his or her life. It also is very challenging to treat. If a person has CD it is important to get a diagnosis and treatment plan from a mental health professional as soon as possible.

Rage

Some people with TS have anger that is out of control, or episodes of "rage." Rage is not a disorder that can be diagnosed. Symptoms of rage might include extreme verbal or physical aggression. Examples of verbal aggression include extreme yelling, screaming, and cursing. Examples of physical aggression include extreme shoving, kicking, hitting, biting, and throwing objects. Rage symptoms are more likely to occur among those with other behavioral disorders such as ADHD, ODD, or CD.

Among people with TS, symptoms of rage are more likely to occur at home than outside the home. Treatment of rage can include learning how to relax, social skills training, and therapy. Some of these methods will help individuals and families better understand what can cause the rage, how to avoid encouraging these behaviors, and how to use appropriate discipline for these behaviors. In addition, treating other behavioral disorders that the person might have, such as ADHD, ODD, or CD can help to reduce symptoms of rage.

Anxiety

There are many different types of anxiety disorders with many different causes and symptoms. These include generalized anxiety disorder, OCD, panic disorder, posttraumatic stress disorder (PTSD), separation anxiety, and different types of phobias. Separation anxiety is most common among young children. These children feel very worried when they are apart from their parents.

Depression

Everyone feels worried, anxious, sad, or stressed from time to time. However, if these feelings do not go away and they interfere with daily life (for example, keeping a child home from school or other activities, or keeping an adult from working or attending social activities), a person might have depression. Having either a depressed mood or a loss of interest or pleasure for at least 2 weeks might mean that someone has depression. Children and teens with depression might be irritable instead of sad.

To be diagnosed with depression, other symptoms also must be present, such as:

- Changes in eating habits or weight gain or loss.

- Changes in sleep habits.

- Changes in activity level (others notice increased activity or that the person has slowed down).

- Less energy.

- Feelings of worthlessness or guilt.

- Difficulty thinking, concentrating, or making decisions.

- Repeated thoughts of death.

- Thoughts or plans about suicide, or a suicide attempt.

- Depression can be treated with counseling and medication.

Other Health Concerns

Children with TS can also have other health conditions that require care. Findings from the recent CDC study found that 43 percent of children who had been diagnosed with TS also had been diagnosed with at least one additional chronic health condition.

Among children with TS:

- 28 percent had asthma.

- 13 percent had hearing or vision problems.

- 12 percent had a bone, joint, or muscle problems.

- 9 percent had suffered a brain injury or concussion.

The rates of asthma and hearing or vision problems were similar to children with TS, but bone, joint, or muscle problems as well as brain injury or concussion were higher for children with TS. Children with TS were also less likely to receive effective coordination of care or have a medical home, which means a primary care setting where a team of providers provides healthcare and preventive services.

Educational Concerns

As a group, people with TS have levels of intelligence similar to those of people without TS. However, people with TS might be more likely to have learning differences, a learning disability, or a developmental delay that affects their ability to learn.

Many people with TS have problems with writing, organizing, and paying attention. People with TS might have problems processing what they hear or see. This can affect the person's ability to learn by listening to or watching a teacher. Or, the person might have problems with their other senses (such as how things feel, smell, taste, and movement) that affects learning and behavior. Children with TS might have trouble with social skills that affect their ability to interact with others.

As a result of these challenges, children with TS might need extra help in school. Many times, these concerns can be addressed with accommodations and behavioral interventions (for example, help with social skills).

Accommodations can include things such as providing a different testing location or extra testing time, providing tips on how to be more organized, giving the child less homework, or letting the child use a computer to take notes in class. Children also might need behavioral interventions, therapy, or they may need to learn strategies to help with stress, paying attention, or other symptoms.

Chapter 40

Other Hyperkinetic Movement Disorders

Chapter Contents

Section 40.1

Angelman Syndrome

This section includes text excerpted from "Angelman Syndrome," Genetics Home Reference (GHR), National Institutes of Health (NIH), May 2015.

What Is Angelman Syndrome?

Angelman syndrome is a complex genetic disorder that primarily affects the nervous system. Characteristic features of this condition include delayed development, intellectual disability, severe speech impairment, and problems with movement and balance (ataxia). Most affected children also have recurrent seizures (epilepsy) and a small head size (microcephaly). Delayed development becomes noticeable by the age of 6–12 months, and other common signs and symptoms usually appear in early childhood.

Children with Angelman syndrome typically have a happy, excitable demeanor with frequent smiling, laughter, and hand-flapping movements. Hyperactivity, a short attention span, and a fascination with water are common. Most affected children also have difficulty sleeping and need less sleep than usual.

With age, people with Angelman syndrome become less excitable, and the sleeping problems tend to improve. However, affected individuals continue to have intellectual disability, severe speech impairment, and seizures throughout their lives. Adults with Angelman syndrome have distinctive facial features that may be described as "coarse." Other common features include unusually fair skin with light-colored hair and an abnormal side-to-side curvature of the spine (scoliosis). The life expectancy of people with this condition appears to be nearly normal.

How Common Is Angelman Syndrome?

Angelman syndrome affects an estimated 1 in 12,000–20,000 people.

What Are the Genetic Changes Related to Angelman Syndrome?

Many of the characteristic features of Angelman syndrome result from the loss of function of a gene called *UBE3A*. People normally inherit one copy of the *UBE3A* gene from each parent. Both copies of this gene are turned on (active) in many of the body's tissues. In certain areas of the brain, however, only the copy inherited from a person's mother (the maternal copy) is active. This parent-specific gene activation is caused by a phenomenon called genomic imprinting. If the maternal copy of the *UBE3A* gene is lost because of a chromosomal change or a gene mutation, a person will have no active copies of the gene in some parts of the brain.

Several different genetic mechanisms can inactivate or delete the maternal copy of the *UBE3A* gene. Most cases of Angelman syndrome (about 70%) occur when a segment of the maternal chromosome 15 containing this gene is deleted. In other cases (about 11%), Angelman syndrome is caused by a mutation in the maternal copy of the *UBE3A* gene.

In a small percentage of cases, Angelman syndrome results when a person inherits two copies of chromosome 15 from his or her father (paternal copies) instead of one copy from each parent. This phenomenon is called paternal uniparental disomy. Rarely, Angelman syndrome can also be caused by a chromosomal rearrangement called a translocation, or by a mutation or other defect in the region of deoxyribonucleic acid (DNA) that controls activation of the *UBE3A* gene. These genetic changes can abnormally turn off (inactivate) *UBE3A* or other genes on the maternal copy of chromosome 15.

The causes of Angelman syndrome are unknown in 10–15 percent of affected individuals. Changes involving other genes or chromosomes may be responsible for the disorder in these cases.

In some people who have Angelman syndrome, the loss of a gene called *OCA2* is associated with light-colored hair and fair skin. The *OCA2* gene is located on the segment of chromosome 15 that is often deleted in people with this disorder. However, loss of the *OCA2* gene does not cause the other signs and symptoms of Angelman syndrome. The protein produced from this gene helps determine the coloring (pigmentation) of the skin, hair, and eyes.

Can Angelman Syndrome Be Inherited?

Most cases of Angelman syndrome are not inherited, particularly those caused by a deletion in the maternal chromosome 15 or by paternal uniparental disomy. These genetic changes occur as random events during the formation of reproductive cells (eggs and sperm) or in early embryonic development. Affected people typically have no history of the disorder in their family.

Rarely, a genetic change responsible for Angelman syndrome can be inherited. For example, it is possible for a mutation in the *UBE3A* gene or in the nearby region of DNA that controls gene activation to be passed from one generation to the next.

Section 40.2

Wilson Disease

This section includes text excerpted from "Wilson Disease," Genetics Home Reference (GHR), National Institutes of Health (NIH), January 16, 2018.

What Is Wilson Disease?

Wilson disease is an inherited disorder in which excessive amounts of copper accumulate in the body, particularly in the liver, brain, and eyes. The signs and symptoms of Wilson disease usually first appear between the ages of 6–45, but they most often begin during the teenage years. The features of this condition include a combination of liver disease and neurological and psychiatric problems.

Liver disease is typically the initial feature of Wilson disease in affected children and young adults; individuals diagnosed at an older age usually do not have symptoms of liver problems, although they may have very mild liver disease. The signs and symptoms of liver disease include yellowing of the skin or whites of the eyes (jaundice), fatigue, loss of appetite, and abdominal swelling.

Nervous system or psychiatric problems are often the initial features in individuals diagnosed in adulthood and commonly occur in young adults with Wilson disease. Signs and symptoms of these problems can include clumsiness, tremors, difficulty walking, speech problems, impaired thinking ability, depression, anxiety, and mood swings.

In many individuals with Wilson disease, copper deposits in the front surface of the eye (the cornea) form a green-to-brownish ring, called the Kayser-Fleischer ring, that surrounds the colored part of the eye. Abnormalities in eye movements, such as a restricted ability to gaze upwards, may also occur.

How Common Is Wilson Disease?

Wilson disease is a rare disorder that affects approximately 1 in 30,000 individuals.

What Genes Are Related to Wilson Disease?

Wilson disease is caused by mutations in the *ATP7B* gene. This gene provides instructions for making a protein called copper-transporting ATPase 2, which plays a role in the transport of copper from the liver to other parts of the body. Copper is necessary for many cellular functions, but it is toxic when present in excessive amounts. The copper-transporting ATPase 2 protein is particularly important for the elimination of excess copper from the body. Mutations in the *ATP7B* gene prevent the transport protein from functioning properly. With a shortage of functional protein, excess copper is not removed from the body. As a result, copper accumulates to toxic levels that can damage tissues and organs, particularly the liver and brain.

Research indicates that a normal variation in the *PRNP* gene may modify the course of Wilson disease. The *PRNP* gene provides instructions for making prion protein, which is active in the brain and other tissues and appears to be involved in transporting copper. Studies have focused on the effects of a *PRNP* gene variation that affects position 129 of the prion protein. At this position, people can have either the protein building block (amino acid) methionine or the amino acid valine. Among people who have mutations in the *ATP7B* gene, it appears that having methionine instead of valine at position 129 of the prion protein is associated with delayed onset of symptoms and an increased occurrence of neurological symptoms, particularly tremors. Larger studies are needed, however, before the effects of this *PRNP* gene variation on Wilson disease can be established.

How Do People Inherit Wilson Disease?

This condition is inherited in an autosomal recessive pattern, which means both copies of the gene in each cell have mutations. The parents of an individual with an autosomal recessive condition each carry one copy of the mutated gene, but they typically do not show signs and symptoms of the condition.

Part Five

Diagnosis and Treatment of Movement Disorders

Chapter 41

Neurological Tests and Procedures Used to Diagnose Movement Disorders

Diagnostic tests and procedures are vital tools that help physicians confirm or rule out the presence of a neurological disorder or other medical condition. A century ago, the only way to make a positive diagnosis for many neurological disorders was by performing an autopsy after a patient had died. But decades of basic research into the characteristics of disease, and the development of techniques that allow scientists to see inside the living brain and monitor nervous system activity as it occurs, have given doctors powerful and accurate tools to diagnose disease and to test how well a particular therapy may be working.

Perhaps the most significant changes in diagnostic imaging over the past 20 years are improvements in spatial resolution (size, intensity, and clarity) of anatomical images and reductions in the time needed to send signals to and receive data from the area being imaged. These advances allow physicians to simultaneously see the structure of the brain and the changes in brain activity as they occur. Scientists

This chapter includes text excerpted from "Patient and Caregiver Education—Neurological Diagnostic Tests and Procedures Fact Sheet," National Institute of Neurological Disorders and Stroke (NINDS), December 1, 2016.

continue to improve methods that will provide sharper anatomical images and more detailed functional information.

Researchers and physicians use a variety of diagnostic imaging techniques and chemical and metabolic analyses to detect, manage, and treat neurological disease. Some procedures are performed in specialized settings, conducted to determine the presence of a particular disorder or abnormality. Many tests that were previously conducted in a hospital are now performed in a physician's office or at an outpatient testing facility, with little if any risk to the patient. Depending on the type of procedure, results are either immediate or may take several hours to process.

What Are Some of the More Common Screening Tests?

Laboratory screening tests of blood, urine, or other substances are used to help diagnose disease, better understand the disease process, and monitor levels of therapeutic drugs. Certain tests, ordered by the physician as part of a regular check-up, provide general information, while others are used to identify specific health concerns. For example, blood and blood product tests can detect brain and/or spinal cord infection, bone marrow disease, hemorrhage, blood vessel damage, toxins that affect the nervous system, and the presence of antibodies that signal the presence of an autoimmune disease. Blood tests are also used to monitor levels of therapeutic drugs used to treat epilepsy and other neurological disorders. Genetic testing of DNA (deoxyribonucleic acid) extracted from white cells in the blood can help diagnose Huntington disease and other congenital diseases. Analysis of the fluid that surrounds the brain and spinal cord can detect meningitis, acute and chronic inflammation, rare infections, and some cases of multiple sclerosis. Chemical and metabolic testing of the blood can indicate protein disorders, some forms of muscular dystrophy and other muscle disorders, and diabetes. Urinalysis can reveal abnormal substances in the urine or the presence or absence of certain proteins that cause diseases including the mucopolysaccharidoses.

Genetic testing or counseling can help parents who have a family history of a neurological disease determine if they are carrying one of the known genes that cause the disorder or find out if their child is affected. Genetic testing can identify many neurological disorders, including spina bifida, in utero (while the child is inside the mother's womb). Genetic tests include the following:

- Amniocentesis, usually done at 14–16 weeks of pregnancy, tests a sample of the amniotic fluid in the womb for genetic defects (the fluid and the fetus have the same DNA). Under local anesthesia, a thin needle is inserted through the woman's abdomen and into the womb. About 20 milliliters of fluid (roughly 4 teaspoons) is withdrawn and sent to a lab for evaluation. Test results often take 1–2 weeks.

- Chorionic villus sampling, or CVS, is performed by removing and testing a very small sample of the placenta during early pregnancy. The sample, which contains the same DNA as the fetus, is removed by catheter or fine needle inserted through the cervix or by a fine needle inserted through the abdomen. It is tested for genetic abnormalities and results are usually available within 2 weeks. CVS should not be performed after the tenth week of pregnancy.

- Uterine ultrasound is performed using a surface probe with gel. This noninvasive test can suggest the diagnosis of conditions such as chromosomal disorders.

What Is a Neurological Examination?

A neurological examination assesses motor and sensory skills, the functioning of one or more cranial nerves, hearing and speech, vision, coordination and balance, mental status, and changes in mood or behavior, among other abilities. Items including a tuning fork, flashlight, reflex hammer, ophthalmoscope, and needles are used to help diagnose brain tumors, infections such as encephalitis and meningitis, and diseases such as Parkinson disease, Huntington disease, amyotrophic lateral sclerosis (ALS), and epilepsy. Some tests require the services of a specialist to perform and analyze results.

X-rays of the patient's chest and skull are often taken as part of a neurological work-up. X-rays can be used to view any part of the body, such as a joint or major organ system. In a conventional X-ray, also called a radiograph, a technician passes a concentrated burst of low-dose ionized radiation through the body and onto a photographic plate. Since calcium in bones absorbs X-rays more easily than soft tissue or muscle, the bony structure appears white on the film. Any vertebral misalignment or fractures can be seen within minutes. Tissue masses such as injured ligaments or a bulging disc are not visible on conventional X-rays. This fast, noninvasive, painless procedure is usually performed in a doctor's office or at a clinic.

Fluoroscopy is a type of X-ray that uses a continuous or pulsed beam of low-dose radiation to produce continuous images of a body part in motion. The fluoroscope (X-ray tube) is focused on the area of interest and pictures are either videotaped or sent to a monitor for viewing. A contrast medium may be used to highlight the images. Fluoroscopy can be used to evaluate the flow of blood through arteries.

What Are Some Diagnostic Tests Used to Diagnose Neurological Disorders?

Based on the result of a neurological exam, physical exam, patient history, X-rays of the patient's chest and skull, and any previous screening or testing, physicians may order one or more of the following diagnostic tests to determine the specific nature of a suspected neurological disorder or injury. These diagnostics generally involve either nuclear medicine imaging, in which very small amounts of radioactive materials are used to study organ function and structure, or diagnostic imaging, which uses magnets and electrical charges to study human anatomy.

The following list of available procedures—in alphabetical rather than sequential order—includes some of the more common tests used to help diagnose a neurological condition.

Angiography is a test used to detect blockages of the arteries or veins. A cerebral angiogram can detect the degree of narrowing or obstruction of an artery or blood vessel in the brain, head, or neck. It is used to diagnose stroke and to determine the location and size of a brain tumor, aneurysm, or vascular malformation. This test is usually performed in a hospital outpatient setting and takes up to 3 hours, followed by a 6- to 8-hour resting period. The patient, wearing a hospital or imaging gown, lies on a table that is wheeled into the imaging area. While the patient is awake, a physician anesthetizes a small area of the leg near the groin and then inserts a catheter into a major artery located there. The catheter is threaded through the body and into an artery in the neck. Once the catheter is in place, the needle is removed and a guide wire is inserted. A small capsule containing a radiopaque dye (one that is highlighted on X-rays) is passed over the guide wire to the site of release. The dye is released and travels through the bloodstream into the head and neck. A series of X-rays is taken and any obstruction is noted. Patients may feel a warm to hot sensation or slight discomfort as the dye is released.

Biopsy involves the removal and examination of a small piece of tissue from the body. Muscle or nerve biopsies are used to diagnose neuromuscular disorders and may also reveal if a person is a carrier of a defective gene that could be passed on to children. A small sample of muscle or nerve is removed under local anesthetic and studied under a microscope. The sample may be removed either surgically, through a slit made in the skin, or by needle biopsy, in which a thin hollow needle is inserted through the skin and into the muscle. A small piece of muscle or nerve remains in the hollow needle when it is removed from the body. The biopsy is usually performed at an outpatient testing facility. A brain biopsy, used to determine tumor type, requires surgery to remove a small piece of the brain or tumor. Performed in a hospital, this operation is riskier than a muscle biopsy and involves a longer recovery period.

Brain scans are imaging techniques used to diagnose tumors, blood vessel malformations, or hemorrhage in the brain. These scans are used to study organ function or injury or disease to tissue or muscle. Types of brain scans include computed tomography, magnetic resonance imaging, and positron emission tomography.

Cerebrospinal fluid analysis involves the removal of a small amount of the fluid that protects the brain and spinal cord. The fluid is tested to detect any bleeding or brain hemorrhage, diagnose infection to the brain and/or spinal cord, identify some cases of multiple sclerosis and other neurological conditions, and measure intracranial pressure.

The procedure is usually done in a hospital. The sample of fluid is commonly removed by a procedure known as a lumbar puncture, or spinal tap. The patient is asked to either lie on one side, in a ball position with knees close to the chest, or lean forward while sitting on a table or bed. The doctor will locate a puncture site in the lower back, between two vertebrate, then clean the area and inject a local anesthetic. The patient may feel a slight stinging sensation from this injection. Once the anesthetic has taken effect, the doctor will insert a special needle into the spinal sac and remove a small amount of fluid (usually about three teaspoons) for testing. Most patients will feel a sensation of pressure only as the needle is inserted.

A common after-effect of a lumbar puncture is headache, which can be lessened by having the patient lie flat. Risk of nerve root injury or infection from the puncture can occur but it is rare. The entire procedure takes about 45 minutes.

Computed tomography, also known as a CT scan, is a noninvasive, painless process used to produce rapid, clear two-dimensional images of organs, bones, and tissues. Neurological CT scans are used to view the brain and spine. They can detect bone and vascular

343

irregularities, certain brain tumors and cysts, herniated discs, epilepsy, encephalitis, spinal stenosis (narrowing of the spinal canal), a blood clot or intracranial bleeding in patients with stroke, brain damage from head injury, and other disorders. Many neurological disorders share certain characteristics and a CT scan can aid in proper diagnosis by differentiating the area of the brain affected by the disorder.

Scanning takes about 20 minutes (a CT of the brain or head may take slightly longer) and is usually done at an imaging center or hospital on an outpatient basis. The patient lies on a special table that slides into a narrow chamber. A sound system built into the chamber allows the patient to communicate with the physician or technician. As the patient lies still, X-rays are passed through the body at various angles and are detected by a computerized scanner. The data is processed and displayed as cross-sectional images, or "slices," of the internal structure of the body or organ. A light sedative may be given to patients who are unable to lie still and pillows may be used to support and stabilize the head and body. Persons who are claustrophobic may have difficulty taking this imaging test.

Occasionally a contrast dye is injected into the bloodstream to highlight the different tissues in the brain. Patients may feel a warm or cool sensation as the dye circulates through the bloodstream or they may experience a slight metallic taste.

Although very little radiation is used in CT, pregnant women should avoid the test because of potential harm to the fetus from ionizing radiation.

Discography is often suggested for patients who are considering lumbar surgery or whose lower back pain has not responded to conventional treatments. This outpatient procedure is usually performed at a testing facility or a hospital. The patient is asked to put on a metal-free hospital gown and lie on an imaging table. The physician numbs the skin with anesthetic and inserts a thin needle, using X-ray guidance, into the spinal disc. Once the needle is in place, a small amount of contrast dye is injected and CT scans are taken. The contrast dye outlines any damaged areas. More than one disc may be imaged at the same time. Patient recovery usually takes about an hour. Pain medicine may be prescribed for any resulting discomfort.

An intrathecal contrast-enhanced CT scan (also called cisternography) is used to detect problems with the spine and spinal nerve roots. This test is most often performed at an imaging center. The patient is asked to put on a hospital or imaging gown. Following application of a topical anesthetic, the physician removes a small sample of the spinal fluid via lumbar puncture. The sample is mixed with a contrast dye and injected into the spinal sac located at the base of the lower back. The patient is then asked to move to a position that will allow the contrast fluid to travel to the area to be studied. The dye allows the spinal canal and nerve roots to be seen more clearly on a CT scan. The scan may take up to an hour to complete. Following the test, patients may experience some discomfort and/or headache that may be caused by the removal of spinal fluid.

Electroencephalography, or EEG, monitors brain activity through the skull. EEG is used to help diagnose certain seizure disorders, brain tumors, brain damage from head injuries, inflammation of the brain and/or spinal cord, alcoholism, certain psychiatric disorders, and metabolic and degenerative disorders that affect the brain. EEGs are also used to evaluate sleep disorders, monitor brain activity when a patient has been fully anesthetized or loses consciousness, and confirm brain death.

This painless, risk-free test can be performed in a doctor's office or at a hospital or testing facility. Prior to taking an EEG, the person must avoid caffeine intake and prescription drugs that affect the nervous system. A series of cup-like electrodes are attached to the patient's scalp, either with a special conducting paste or with extremely fine needles. The electrodes (also called leads) are small devices that are attached to wires and carry the electrical energy of the brain to a machine for reading. A very low electrical current is sent through the electrodes and the baseline brain energy is recorded. Patients are then exposed to a variety of external stimuli—including bright or flashing light, noise or certain drugs—or are asked to open and close the eyes, or to change breathing patterns. The electrodes transmit the resulting changes in brain wave patterns. Since movement and nervousness can change brain wave patterns, patients usually recline in a chair or on a bed during the test, which takes up to an hour. Testing for certain disorders requires performing an EEG during sleep, which takes at least 3 hours.

In order to learn more about brain wave activity, electrodes may be inserted through a surgical opening in the skull and into the brain to reduce signal interference from the skull.

Electromyography, or EMG, is used to diagnose nerve and muscle dysfunction and spinal cord disease. It records the electrical activity from the brain and/or spinal cord to a peripheral nerve root (found in the arms and legs) that controls muscles during contraction and at rest.

During an EMG, very fine wire electrodes are inserted into a muscle to assess changes in electrical voltage that occur during movement and when the muscle is at rest. The electrodes are attached through a series of wires to a recording instrument. Testing usually takes place at a testing facility and lasts about an hour but may take longer, depending on the number of muscles and nerves to be tested. Most patients find this test to be somewhat uncomfortable.

An EMG is usually done in conjunction with a nerve conduction velocity (NCV) test, which measures electrical energy by assessing the nerve's ability to send a signal. This two-part test is conducted most often in a hospital. A technician tapes two sets of flat electrodes on the skin over the muscles. The first set of electrodes is used to send small pulses of electricity (similar to the sensation of static electricity) to stimulate the nerve that directs a particular muscle. The second set of electrodes transmits the responding electrical signal to a recording machine. The physician then reviews the response to verify any nerve damage or muscle disease. Patients who are preparing to take an EMG or NCV test may be asked to avoid caffeine and not smoke for 2-3 hours prior to the test, as well as to avoid aspirin and nonsteroidal anti-inflammatory drugs for 24 hours before the EMG. There is no discomfort or risk associated with this test.

Electronystagmography (ENG) describes a group of tests used to diagnose involuntary eye movement, dizziness, and balance disorders, and to evaluate some brain functions. The test is performed at an imaging center. Small electrodes are taped around the eyes to record eye movements. If infrared photography is used in place of electrodes, the patient wears special goggles that help record the information. Both versions of the test are painless and risk-free.

Evoked potentials (also called evoked response) measure the electrical signals to the brain generated by hearing, touch, or sight. These tests are used to assess sensory nerve problems and confirm neurological conditions including multiple sclerosis, brain tumor, acoustic neuroma (small tumors of the inner ear), and spinal cord injury. Evoked potentials are also used to test sight and hearing (especially in infants and young children), monitor brain activity among coma patients, and confirm brain death.

Testing may take place in a doctor's office or hospital setting. It is painless and risk-free. Two sets of needle electrodes are used to test for nerve damage. One set of electrodes, which will be used to measure the electrophysiological response to stimuli, is attached to the patient's scalp using conducting paste. The second set of electrodes is attached to the part of the body to be tested. The physician then records the amount of time it takes for the impulse generated by stimuli to reach the brain. Under normal circumstances, the process of signal transmission is instantaneous.

Auditory evoked potentials (also called brain stem auditory evoked response) are used to assess high-frequency hearing loss, diagnose any damage to the acoustic nerve and auditory pathways in the brainstem, and detect acoustic neuromas. The patient sits in a soundproof room and wears headphones. Clicking sounds are delivered one at a time to one ear while a masking sound is sent to the other ear. Each ear is usually tested twice, and the entire procedure takes about 45 minutes.

Visual evoked potentials detect loss of vision from optic nerve damage (in particular, damage caused by multiple sclerosis). The patient sits close to a screen and is asked to focus on the center of a shifting checkerboard pattern. Only one eye is tested at a time; the other eye is either kept closed or covered with a patch. Each eye is usually tested twice. Testing takes 30–45 minutes.

Somatosensory evoked potentials measure response from stimuli to the peripheral nerves and can detect nerve or spinal cord damage or nerve degeneration from multiple sclerosis and other degenerating diseases. Tiny electrical shocks are delivered by electrode to a nerve in an arm or leg. Responses to the shocks, which may be delivered for more than a minute at a time, are recorded. This test usually lasts less than an hour.

Magnetic resonance imaging (MRI) uses computer-generated radio waves and a powerful magnetic field to produce detailed images of body structures including tissues, organs, bones, and nerves. Neurological uses include the diagnosis of brain and spinal cord tumors, eye disease, inflammation, infection, and vascular irregularities that may lead to stroke. Magnetic resonance imaging (MRI) can also detect and monitor degenerative disorders such as multiple sclerosis and can document brain injury from trauma.

The equipment houses a hollow tube that is surrounded by a very large cylindrical magnet. The patient, who must remain still during the test, lies on a special table that is slid into the tube. The patient will be asked to remove jewelry, eyeglasses, removable dental work, or other items that might interfere with the magnetic imaging. The patient should wear a sweatshirt and sweatpants or other clothing free of metal eyelets or buckles. MRI scanning equipment creates a magnetic field around the body strong enough to temporarily realign water molecules in the tissues. Radio waves are then passed through the body to detect the "relaxation" of the molecules back to a random alignment and trigger a resonance signal at different angles within the body. A computer processes this resonance into either a three-dimensional picture or a two-dimensional "slice" of the tissue being scanned, and differentiates between bone, soft tissues and fluid-filled spaces by their water content and structural properties. A contrast dye may be used to enhance visibility of certain areas or tissues. The patient may hear grating or knocking noises when the magnetic field is turned on and off. (Patients may wear special earphones to block out the sounds.) Unlike CT scanning, MRI does not use ionizing radiation to produce images. Depending on the part(s) of the body to be scanned, MRI can take up to an hour to complete. The test is painless and risk-free, although persons who are obese or claustrophobic may find it somewhat uncomfortable. (Some centers also use open MRI machines that do not completely surround the person being tested and are less confining. However, open MRI does not currently provide the same picture quality as standard MRI and some tests may not be available using this equipment). Due to the incredibly strong magnetic field generated by an MRI, patients with implanted medical devices such as a pacemaker should avoid the test.

Functional MRI (fMRI) uses the blood's magnetic properties to produce real-time images of blood flow to particular areas of the brain. An fMRI can pinpoint areas of the brain that become active and note how long they stay active. It can also tell if brain activity within a region occurs simultaneously or sequentially. This imaging process is used to assess brain damage from head injury or degenerative disorders such as Alzheimer disease and to identify and monitor other neurological disorders, including multiple sclerosis, stroke, and brain tumors.

Myelography involves the injection of a water- or oil-based contrast dye into the spinal canal to enhance X-ray imaging of the spine. Myelograms are used to diagnose spinal nerve injury, herniated discs, fractures, back or leg pain, and spinal tumors.

The procedure takes about 30 minutes and is usually performed in a hospital. Following an injection of anesthesia to a site between two vertebrae in the lower back, a small amount of the cerebrospinal fluid is removed by spinal tap and the contrast dye is injected into the spinal canal. After a series of X-rays is taken, most or all of the contrast dye is removed by aspiration. Patients may experience some pain during the spinal tap and when the dye is injected and removed. Patients may also experience headache following the spinal tap. The risk of fluid leakage or allergic reaction to the dye is slight.

Positron emission tomography (PET) scans provide two- and three-dimensional pictures of brain activity by measuring radioactive isotopes that are injected into the bloodstream. PET scans of the brain are used to detect or highlight tumors and diseased tissue, measure cellular and/or tissue metabolism, show blood flow, evaluate patients who have seizure disorders that do not respond to medical therapy and patients with certain memory disorders, and determine brain changes following injury or drug abuse, among other uses. PET may be ordered as a follow-up to a CT or MRI scan to give the physician a greater understanding of specific areas of the brain that may be involved with certain problems. Scans are conducted in a hospital or at a testing facility, on an outpatient basis. A low-level radioactive isotope, which binds to chemicals that flow to the brain, is injected into the bloodstream and can be traced as the brain performs different functions. The patient lies still while overhead sensors detect gamma rays in the body's tissues. A computer processes the information and displays it on a video monitor or on film. Using different compounds, more than one brain function can be traced simultaneously. PET is painless and relatively risk-free. Length of test time depends on the part of the body to be scanned. PET scans are performed by skilled technicians at highly sophisticated medical facilities.

A polysomnogram measures brain and body activity during sleep. It is performed over one or more nights at a sleep center. Electrodes are pasted or taped to the patient's scalp, eyelids, and/or chin. Throughout the night and during the various wake/sleep cycles, the electrodes record brain waves, eye movement, breathing, leg and skeletal muscle activity, blood pressure, and heart rate. The patient may be videotaped to note any movement during sleep. Results are then used to identify any characteristic patterns of sleep disorders, including restless legs syndrome, periodic limb movement disorder, insomnia, and breathing disorders such as obstructive sleep apnea. Polysomnograms are noninvasive, painless, and risk-free.

Single photon emission computed tomography (SPECT), a nuclear imaging test involving blood flow to tissue, is used to evaluate certain brain functions. The test may be ordered as a follow-up to an MRI to diagnose tumors, infections, degenerative spinal disease, and stress fractures. As with a PET scan, a radioactive isotope, which binds to chemicals that flow to the brain, is injected intravenously into the body. Areas of increased blood flow will collect more of the isotope. As the patient lies on a table, a gamma camera rotates around the head and records where the radioisotope has traveled. That information is converted by computer into cross-sectional slices that are stacked to produce a detailed three-dimensional image of blood flow and activity within the brain. The test is performed at either an imaging center or a hospital.

Thermography uses infrared sensing devices to measure small temperature changes between the two sides of the body or within a specific organ. Also known as digital infrared thermal imaging, thermography may be used to detect vascular disease of the head and neck, soft tissue injury, various neuromusculoskeletal disorders, and the presence or absence of nerve root compression. It is performed at an imaging center, using infrared light recorders to take thousands of pictures of the body from a distance of 5-8 feet. The information is converted into electrical signals which results in a computer-generated two-dimensional picture of abnormally cold or hot areas indicated by color or shades of black and white. Thermography does not use radiation and is safe, risk-free, and noninvasive.

Ultrasound imaging, also called ultrasound scanning or sonography, uses high-frequency sound waves to obtain images inside the body. Neurosonography (ultrasound of the brain and spinal column) analyzes blood flow in the brain and can diagnose stroke, brain tumors, hydrocephalus (build-up of cerebrospinal fluid in the brain), and vascular problems. It can also identify or rule out inflammatory processes causing pain. It is more effective than an X-ray in displaying soft tissue masses and can show tears in ligaments, muscles, tendons, and other soft tissue masses in the back. Transcranial Doppler ultrasound is used to view arteries and blood vessels in the neck and determine blood flow and risk of stroke.

During ultrasound, the patient lies on an imaging table and removes clothing around the area of the body to be scanned. A jelly-like lubricant is applied and a transducer, which both sends and receives high-frequency sound waves, is passed over the body. The sound wave echoes are recorded and displayed as a computer-generated real-time visual image of the structure or tissue being examined. Ultrasound is painless, noninvasive, and risk-free. The test is performed on an outpatient basis and takes 15–30 minutes to complete.

Chapter 42

Working with Your Doctor

Talking with Your Doctor—Make the Most of Your Appointment

Patients and healthcare providers share a very personal relationship. Doctors need to know a lot about you, your family, and your lifestyle to give you the best medical care. And you need to speak up and share your concerns and questions. Clear and honest communication between you and your physician can help you both make smart choices about your health.

Begin with some preparation. Before your health exam, make a list of any concerns and questions you have. Bring this list to your appointment, so you won't forget anything.

Do you have a new symptom? Have you noticed side effects from your medicines? Do you want to know the meaning of a certain word? Don't wait for the doctor to bring up a certain topic, because he or she may not know what's important to you. Speak up with your concerns.

This chapter contains text excerpted from the following sources: Text under the heading "Talking with Your Doctor—Make the Most of Your Appointment" is excerpted from "Talking with Your Doctor," *NIH News in Health*, National Institutes of Health (NIH), June 2015; Text under the heading "Five Ways to Make the Most of Your Time at the Doctor's Office" is excerpted from "5 Ways to Make the Most of Your Time at the Doctor's Office," National Institute on Aging (NIA), National Institutes of Health (NIH), May 18, 2017.

351

"There's no such thing as a dumb question in the doctor's office," says Dr. Matthew Memoli, an infectious disease doctor at National Institutes of Health (NIH). "I try very hard to make my patients feel comfortable so that they feel comfortable asking questions, no matter how dumb they think the question is."

Even if the topic seems sensitive or embarrassing, it's best to be honest and upfront with your healthcare provider. You may feel uncomfortable talking about sexual problems, memory loss, or bowel issues, but these are all important to your health. It's better to be thorough and share a lot of information than to be quiet or shy about what you're thinking or feeling. Remember, your doctor is used to talking about all kinds of personal matters.

Consider taking along a family member or friend when you visit the doctor. Your companion can help if there are language or cultural differences between you and your doctor. If you feel unsure about a topic, the other person can help you describe your feelings or ask questions on your behalf. It also helps to have someone else's perspective. Your friend may think of questions or raise concerns that you hadn't considered.

Many people search online for health information. They use web-based tools to research symptoms and learn about different illnesses. But you can't diagnose your own condition or someone else's based on a Web search.

"As a physician, I personally have no problem with people looking on the Web for information, but they should use that information not as a way to self-diagnose or make decisions, but as a way to plan their visit with the doctor," says Memoli. Ask your doctor to recommend specific websites or resources, so you know you're getting your facts from a trusted source. Federal agencies are among the most reliable sources of online health information.

Many healthcare providers now use electronic health records. Ask your doctor how to access your records, so you can keep track of test results, diagnoses, treatment plans, and medicines. These records can also help you prepare for your next appointment.

After your appointment, if you're uncertain about any instructions or have other questions, call or E-mail your healthcare provider. Don't wait until your next visit to make sure you understand your diagnosis, treatment plan, or anything else that might affect your health.

Your body is complicated and there's a lot to consider, so make sure you do everything you can to get the most out of your medical visits.

Five Ways to Make the Most of Your Time at the Doctor's Office

1. Be Honest

It is tempting to say what you think the doctor wants to hear, for example, that you smoke less or eat a more balanced diet than you really do. While this is natural, it's not in your best interest. Your doctor can suggest the best treatment only if you say what is really going on. For instance, you might say: *"I have been trying to quit smoking, as you recommended, but I am not making much headway."*

2. Decide What Questions Are Most Important

Pick three or four questions or concerns that you most want to talk about with the doctor. You can tell him or her what they are at the beginning of the appointment, and then discuss each in turn. If you have time, you can then go on to other questions.

3. Stick to the Point

Although your doctor might like to talk with you at length, each patient is given a limited amount of time. To make the best use of your time, stick to the point. For instance, give the doctor a brief description of the symptom, when it started, how often it happens, and if it is getting worse or better.

4. Share Your Point of View About the Visit

Tell the doctor if you feel rushed, worried, or uncomfortable. If necessary, you can offer to return for a second visit to discuss your concerns. Try to voice your feelings in a positive way. For example, you could say something like: *"I know you have many patients to see, but I'm really worried about this. I'd feel much better if we could talk about it a little more."*

5. Remember, the Doctor May Not Be Able to Answer All Your Questions

Even the best doctor may be unable to answer some questions. Most doctors will tell you when they don't have answers. They also may help you find the information you need or refer you to a specialist. If a doctor regularly brushes off your questions or symptoms as simply a part of aging, think about looking for another doctor.

Chapter 43

Managing Spasticity

Spasticity is a condition in which there is an abnormal increase in muscle tone or stiffness of muscle, which might interfere with movement, speech, or be associated with discomfort or pain. Spasticity is usually caused by damage to nerve pathways within the brain or spinal cord that control muscle movement. It may occur in association with spinal cord injury, multiple sclerosis, cerebral palsy, stroke, brain or head trauma, amyotrophic lateral sclerosis, hereditary spastic paraplegias, and metabolic diseases such as adrenoleukodystrophy, phenylketonuria, and Krabbe disease. Symptoms may include *hypertonicity* (increased muscle tone), *clonus* (a series of rapid muscle contractions), exaggerated deep tendon reflexes, muscle spasms, *scissoring* (involuntary crossing of the legs), and fixed joints (contractures). The degree of spasticity varies from mild muscle stiffness to severe, painful, and uncontrollable muscle spasms. Spasticity can interfere with rehabilitation in patients with certain disorders, and often interferes with daily activities.

This chapter contains text excerpted from the following sources: Text in this chapter begins with excerpts from "Spasticity Information Page," National Institute of Neurological Disorders and Stroke (NINDS), December 19, 2016; Text beginning with the heading "Why Is It Important to Get Help?" is excerpted from "Spasticity—Stiff Muscles and Limited Movement," U.S. Department of Veterans Affairs (VA), November 20, 2010. Reviewed January 2018.

Why Is It Important to Get Help?

Spasticity develops slowly over weeks or months. It ranges from slight muscle stiffness to muscle shortening. When the muscles shorten, the joints can "freeze" into position. This is a painful condition called a contracture. Contractures prevent normal movement and interfere with doing daily tasks. Properly positioning spastic limbs helps prevent contractures.

Symptoms of spasticity include:

- Stiffness or tightness of muscles and joints

- Painful muscle spasms or cramping of muscles

- Involuntary (uncontrollable) jerking motions

- Exaggerated deep-tendon reflexes (knee-jerk reflex)

- Abnormal position of the arm; tight fist, bent elbow and arm pressed against the chest

- Abnormal position of the legs; crossing the legs as the tips of scissors would close (scissoring)

What Do You Need to Know?

Spasticity is out of your loved one's control. Things that trigger spasticity or make it worse are:

- Pain (pressure sores)

- Infections (bladder, toenail, ear)

- Cold temperatures

- Constipation

- Fatigue or stress

What Treatments Should You Discuss with Your Healthcare Team?

Your loved one's needs determine the type of treatment. Often, treatment involves a mix of therapy and medicine. The goals are to relieve symptoms, reduce pain, and improve movement.

Physical exercise and stretching—This will help loosen stiff muscles. A physical therapist works with your loved one. Often, this includes full range of motion exercises several times a week. Gentle stretching of tight muscles may be needed. The physical therapist may suggest constraint-induced movement therapy (CIMT). CIMT involves restricting movement in the unaffected arm to force the use of the affected arm.

Braces and splints—These assistive devices hold the muscles in a more normal position. This helps to prevent contractures and improve comfort.

Oral medicines—There are medicines to treat the effects of spasticity. Some work to temporarily block nerve impulses. Others work to relax the muscles. Talk to your healthcare team about medicines for your loved one.

Injections of a medicine—Medicines, such as Botox® help to block nerve activity. This loosens the muscles. Intrathecal baclofen therapy (ITB) is used to treat severe spasticity. A surgically placed pump delivers baclofen into the spinal fluid. Baclofen is a medicine that relaxes the muscles.

Surgery—This is often the last choice for treating severe, chronic spasticity. It involves operating on the bones, muscles or nerves. Surgery works to block pain and restore some movement.

Helpful Tips

Encourage your loved one to remain active—Exercise and stretching can help ease symptoms and maintain movement. Reinforce using the affected arm as much as possible for daily tasks.

Properly position spastic limbs to prevent contractures—Proper positioning can keep affected limbs from becoming fixed into a set position. The physical therapist can teach you proper positioning.

Watch for skin breakdown—Spasticity in the fingers can cause the nails to tear into the skin. Spastic limbs may rub against each other. Check the skin regularly for any redness or sores. A good time to do this is during bath time. Talk to your healthcare team about any concerns.

Listen and be supportive—Spasticity can be mentally and physically stressful. Allow your loved one to express his or her feelings.

Remember

- Spasticity develops slowly over weeks or months. Tell your healthcare team if your loved one shows signs of spasticity.

- Check the skin regularly for skin breakdown. Talk to your healthcare team about any concerns.

- Talk to the physical therapist about how to properly position spastic limbs to prevent contractures.

Chapter 44

Treating Spasticity in Children and Adolescents

Chapter Contents

Section 44.1

Surgical and Nonsurgical Treatment Options for Spasticity

This section contains text excerpted from the following sources: Text in this section begins with excerpts from "Comparative Efficacy of Three Preparations of Botox-A in Treating Spasticity," ClinicalTrials. gov, National Institutes of Health (NIH), January 9, 2014. Reviewed January 2018; Text beginning with the heading "Drug Treatments" is excerpted from "Cerebral Palsy: Hope Through Research," National Institute of Neurological Disorders and Stroke (NINDS), July 2013. Reviewed January 2018.

Spasticity is one of the most debilitating complications of neurologic conditions, such as stroke, brain injury, spinal cord injury, cerebral palsy, and multiple sclerosis. Although the exact pathophysiology is unknown, it is believed to result from an imbalance of ascending excitatory influences on and descending inhibitory components of the central nervous system. Clinically, spasticity manifests as abnormally increased muscle tone, associated with loss of range of motion, increased muscle stretch reflexes, clonus, weakness, and incoordination. If inadequately treated, spasticity leads to more disability and increase healthcare costs. Common complications of inadequately treated spasticity include joint and muscle contracture, pain, difficulty with performing activities of daily living and hygiene, and impaired transfers and ambulation.

Acquired brain injuries (ABI), including stroke, traumatic brain injury, and encephalopathy, often lead to long-term impairments, including spasticity. In severe cases, spasticity is difficult and frustrating to treat in this patient population, since the individuals may not tolerate the side effects of conventional therapies because of ABI-related deficits in arousal and cognition. Systemic medications, such as baclofen and tizanidine, are effective in controlling spasticity; however, they may also cause sleepiness and drowsiness, and impair memory and thinking processes—adverse effects that individuals with ABI may not tolerate.

Thus, "local" treatments, such as neurolysis and chemodenervation using botulinum toxin, have become superior treatment options in individuals with ABI, since they are devoid of the usual side effects of systemic medications. They are also effective in controlling spasticity, yet they do not impair arousal and cognition. The medical literature is replete with reports of the efficacy of botulinum toxin-A in the management of spasticity. Thus, the current challenge for clinicians and researchers at this time is to find ways to further enhance the efficacy of botulinum toxin. One way to achieve this is by exploiting certain properties of the toxin. Animal studies and clinical experience have shown that the effects of the drug is dose-dependent. One other property is the flexibility in preparing the volume of drug injected. Since botulinum toxin, as it is currently available (as BOTOX-A®) in the United States, requires reconstitution with preservative-free saline, there is flexibility for clinicians to manipulate the volume of solution that will be administered, without altering the dose.

Drug Treatments

Oral medications such as diazepam, baclofen, dantrolene sodium, and tizanidine are usually used as the first line of treatment to relax stiff, contracted, or overactive muscles. Some drugs have some risk side effects such as drowsiness, changes in blood pressure, and risk of liver damage that require continuous monitoring. Oral medications are most appropriate for children who need only mild reduction in muscle tone or who have widespread spasticity.

Botulinum toxin (BT-A), injected locally, has become a standard treatment for overactive muscles in children with spastic movement disorders such as CP. BT-A relaxes contracted muscles by keeping nerve cells from over-activating muscle. The relaxing effect of a BT-A injection lasts approximately 3 months. Undesirable side effects are mild and short-lived, consisting of pain upon injection and occasionally mild flu-like symptoms. BT-A injections are most effective when followed by a stretching program including physical therapy and splinting. BT-A injections work best for children who have some control over their motor movements and have a limited number of muscles to treat, none of which is fixed or rigid.

Intrathecal baclofen therapy uses an implantable pump to deliver baclofen, a muscle relaxant, into the fluid surrounding the spinal cord. Baclofen decreases the excitability of nerve cells in the spinal cord, which then reduces muscle spasticity throughout the body. The pump can be adjusted if muscle tone is worse at certain times of the day or night. The baclofen pump is most appropriate for individuals with chronic, severe stiffness or uncontrolled muscle movement throughout the body

Surgery

Orthopedic surgery is often recommended when spasticity and stiffness are severe enough to make walking and moving about difficult or painful. For many people with CP, improving the appearance of how they walk—their gait—is also important. Surgeons can lengthen muscles and tendons that are proportionately too short, which can improve mobility and lessen pain. Tendon surgery may help the symptoms for some children with CP but could also have negative long-term consequences. Orthopedic surgeries may be staggered at times appropriate to a child's age and level of motor development. Surgery can also correct or greatly improve spinal deformities in people with CP. Surgery may not be indicated for all gait abnormalities and the surgeon may request a quantitative gait analysis before surgery.

Surgery to cut nerves.

Selective dorsal rhizotomy (SDR) is a surgical procedure recommended for cases of severe spasticity when all of the more conservative treatments—physical therapy, oral medications, and intrathecal baclofen—have failed to reduce spasticity or chronic pain. A surgeon locates and selectively severs overactivated nerves at the base of the spinal column. SDR is most commonly used to relax muscles and decrease chronic pain in one or both of the lower or upper limbs. It is also sometimes used to correct an overactive bladder. Potential side effects include sensory loss, numbness, or uncomfortable sensations in limb areas once supplied by the severed nerve.

Complementary and Alternative Therapies

Many children and adolescents with CP use some form of complementary or alternative medicine. Controlled clinical trials involving some of the therapies have been inconclusive or showed no benefit and the therapies have not been accepted in mainstream clinical practice. Although there are anecdotal reports of some benefit in some children with CP, these therapies have not been approved by the U.S. Food and

Drug Administration for the treatment of CP. Such therapies include hyperbaric oxygen therapy, special clothing worn during resistance exercise training, certain forms of electrical stimulation, assisting children in completing certain motions several times a day, and specialized learning strategies. Also, dietary supplements, including herbal products, may interact with other products or medications a child with CP may be taking or have unwanted side effects on their own. Families of children with CP should discuss all therapies with their doctor.

Stem cell therapy is being investigated as a treatment for cerebral palsy, but research is in early stages and large-scale clinical trials are needed to learn if stem cell therapy is safe and effective in humans. Stem cells are capable of becoming other cell types in the body. Scientists are hopeful that stem cells may be able to repair damaged nerves and brain tissues. Studies in the United States are examining the safety and tolerability of umbilical cord blood stem cell infusion in children with CP.

Many children and adolescents with CP use some form of complementary or alternative medicine. Controlled clinical trials involving some of the therapies have been inconclusive or showed no benefit and the therapies have not been accepted in mainstream clinical practice. Although there are anecdotal reports of some benefit in some children with CP, these therapies have not been approved by the U.S. Food and Drug Administration for the treatment of CP. Such therapies include hyperbaric oxygen therapy, special clothing worn during resistance exercise training, certain forms of electrical stimulation, assisting children in completing certain motions several times a day, and specialized learning strategies. Also, dietary supplements, including herbal products, may interact with other products or medications a child with CP may be taking or have unwanted side effects on their own. Families of children with CP should discuss all therapies with their doctor.

Stem cell therapy is being investigated as a treatment for cerebral palsy, but research is in early stages and large-scale clinical trials are needed to learn if stem cell therapy is safe and effective in humans. Stem cells are capable of becoming other cell types in the body. Scientists are hopeful that stem cells may be able to repair damaged nerves and brain tissues. Studies in the United States are examining the safety and tolerability of umbilical cord blood stem cell infusion in children with CP.

Section 44.2

Assistive Technology for Managing Spasticity

This section contains text excerpted from the following sources: Text in this section begins with excerpts from "Orthotics for Pediatric Populations," U.S. Small Business Administration (SBA), July 31, 2013. Reviewed January 2018; Text under the heading "Types of Assistive Devices" is excerpted from "Cerebral Palsy: Hope Through Research," National Institute of Neurological Disorders and Stroke (NINDS), July 2013. Reviewed January 2018; Text beginning with the heading "Principles of Care" is excerpted from "Spasticity in Children and Young People with Non-Progressive Brain Disorders: Management of Spasticity and Co-Existing Motor Disorders and Their Early Musculoskeletal Complications," National Guideline Clearinghouse (NGC), Agency for Healthcare Research and Quality (AHRQ), July 2012. Reviewed January 2018.

Abnormalities in musculoskeletal development are common in children with disabilities, such as cerebral palsy and spina bifida, and represent a significant and growing proportion of the burden of disability in the United States. These abnormalities include impaired muscle tone and decreased voluntary muscle contraction, which can limit weight-bearing activities and contribute to the development of contractures and distortions of skeletal geometry, e.g., scoliosis. Orthotics are the most commonly prescribed medical device for children with a wide range of developmental, orthopedic, and neurological conditions (i.e., plagiocephaly, scoliosis, cerebral palsy, spina bifida, club foot, Down syndrome, muscular dystrophy, and others). They are used to correct bone alignment, reduce contracture/spasticity, restrict or assist movement, and reduce pain. Unfortunately, as many as 50 percent of prescribed medical devices are not used in this population because the child outgrows them, refuses to use them, or finds them unhelpful. This number may be partly reflective of the minimal innovation in the clinical orthotics field.

Orthotics prescribed today have changed little in the past forty years; they are, in general, esthetically unpleasing, rigid plastic and metal devices that restrict clothing and shoe choices. The clinical orthotics field has seen little of the innovative research that has revolutionized the prosthetics field in recent years. However, advances in material science, sensor technology, actuation, and rapid prototyping makes reinvigorating the orthotics field a possibility today. In parallel with these hardware technology developments, the last twenty years has brought advances in musculoskeletal modeling and computational power which allows for subject-specific models with individual variation in skeletal geometries to be created. This may be of particular importance given that orthotics are largely used in conjunction with other therapies, including botulinum toxin type A injections, physical and occupational therapy, and surgical interventions. These models may be used to inform the design of next generation orthotics to capitalize on the plasticity of the developing nervous and musculoskeletal systems while accounting for some of these other variables.

Types of Assistive Devices

Assistive devices such devices as computers, computer software, voice synthesizers, and picture books can greatly help some individuals with CP improve communications skills. Other devices around the home or workplace make it easier for people with CP to adapt to activities of daily living.

Orthotic devices help to compensate for muscle imbalance and increase independent mobility. Braces and splints use external force to correct muscle abnormalities and improve function such as sitting or walking. Other orthotics help stretch muscles or the positioning of a joint. Braces, wedges, special chairs, and other devices can help people sit more comfortably and make it easier to perform daily functions. Wheelchairs, rolling walkers, and powered scooters can help individuals who are not independently mobile.

Assistive devices such devices as computers, computer software, voice synthesizers, and picture books can greatly help some individuals with CP improve communications skills. Other devices around the home or workplace make it easier for people with CP to adapt to activities of daily living.

Orthotic devices help to compensate for muscle imbalance and increase independent mobility. Braces and splints use external force to correct muscle abnormalities and improve function such as sitting or walking. Other orthotics help stretch muscles or the positioning of a joint. Braces, wedges, special chairs, and other devices can help people sit more comfortably and make it easier to perform daily functions. Wheelchairs, rolling walkers, and powered scooters can help individuals who are not independently mobile.

Principles of Care

Children and young people with spasticity should have access to a network of care that uses agreed care pathways supported by effective communication and integrated team working. The network of care should provide access to a team of healthcare professionals experienced in the care of children and young people with spasticity. The network team should provide local expertise in paediatrics, nursing, physiotherapy, and occupational therapy. Access to other expertise, including orthotics, orthopaedic surgery, and/or neurosurgery and paediatric neurology, may be provided locally or regionally.

Orthotic Intervention for Spasticity

Orthoses are considered for children and young people with spasticity based on their individual needs and are aimed at specific goals, such as:

- Improving posture
- Improving upper limb function
- Improving walking efficiency
- Preventing or slowing development of contractures
- Preventing or slowing hip migration
- Relieving discomfort or pain
- Preventing or treating tissue injury, for example by relieving pressure points

When considering an orthosis, the network team discusses with the child or young person and their parents or carers the balance of possible benefits against risks. For example, they discuss its cosmetic appearance, the possibility of discomfort or pressure sores or of muscle wasting through lack of muscle use.

An assessment is made on whether an orthosis might:

- Cause difficulties with self-care or care by others
- Cause difficulties in relation to hygiene
- Be unacceptable to the child or young person because of its appearance

It is also important to ensure that orthoses are appropriately designed for the individual child or young person and are sized and fitted correctly. If necessary expert advice is sought from an orthotist within the network team.

A rigid orthosis may cause discomfort or pressure injuries in a child or young person with marked dyskinesia. They should be monitored closely to ensure that the orthosis is not causing such difficulties.

The network of care has a pathway that aims to minimize delay in:

- Supplying an orthosis once measurements for fit have been performed and

- Repairing a damaged orthosis

The network team informs children and young people who are about to start using an orthosis, and their parents or carers:

- How to apply and wear it

- When to wear it and for how long:

- An orthosis designed to maintain stretch to prevent contractures is more likely to be effective if worn for longer periods of time, for example at least 6 hours a day.

- An orthosis designed to support a specific function should be worn only when needed.

- When and where to seek advice

Children and young people and their parents or carers are also advised that they may remove an orthosis if it is causing pain that is not relieved despite their repositioning the limb in the orthosis or adjusting the strapping.

Specific Uses

Orthoses for children and young people with upper limb spasticity:

- Elbow gaiters to maintain extension and improve function

- Rigid wrist orthoses to prevent contractures and limit wrist and hand flexion deformity

- Dynamic orthoses to improve hand function (for example, a nonrigid thumb abduction splint allowing some movement for a child or young person with a 'thumb in palm' deformity)

For children and young people with equinus deformities that impair their gait:

- A solid ankle–foot orthosis if they have poor control of knee or hip extension

- A hinged ankle–foot orthosis if they have good control of knee or hip extension

Ankle–foot orthoses are considered for children and young people with serious functional limitations to improve foot position for sitting, transfers between sitting and standing, and assisted standing.

Ground reaction force ankle–foot orthoses are considered to assist with walking if the child or young person has a crouch gait and good passive range of movement at the hip and knee.

Body trunk orthoses are considered for children and young people with co-existing scoliosis or kyphosis if this will help with sitting.

Chapter 45

Treating Tremor

Tremors are unintentional trembling or shaking movements in one or more parts of your body. Most tremors occur in the hands. You can also have arm, head, face, vocal cord, trunk, and leg tremors. Tremors are most common in middle-aged and older people, but anyone can have them.

The cause of tremors is a problem in the parts of the brain that control muscles in the body or in specific parts of the body, such as the hands. They commonly occur in otherwise healthy people.

How Is Tremor Treated?

Although there is no cure for most forms of tremor, treatment options are available to help manage symptoms. In some cases, a person's symptoms may be mild enough that they do not require treatment.

Finding an appropriate treatment depends on an accurate diagnosis of the cause. Tremor caused by underlying health problems can sometimes be improved or eliminated entirely with treatment. For example, tremor due to thyroid hyperactivity will improve or even resolve (return to the normal state) with treatment of thyroid malfunction.

This chapter contains text excerpted from the following sources: Text in this chapter begins with excerpts from "Tremor," MedlinePlus, National Institutes of Health (NIH), September 9, 2016; Text beginning with the heading "How Is Tremor Treated?" is excerpted from "Tremor Fact Sheet," National Institute of Neurological Disorders and Stroke (NINDS), May 2017.

Also, if tremor is caused by medication, discontinuing the tremor caus-ing drug may reduce or eliminate this tremor.

If there is no underlying cause for tremor that can be modified, available treatment options include:

Medication

- Beta blocking drugs such as propranolol are normally used to treat high blood pressure but they also help treat essential tremor. Propranolol can also be used in some people with other types of action tremor. Other beta blockers that may be used include atenolol, metoprolol, nadolol, and sotalol.

- Antiseizure medications such as primidone can be effective in people with essential tremor who do not respond to beta block-ers. Other medications that may be prescribed include gabapen-tin and topiramate. However, it is important to note that some anti seizure medications can cause tremor.

- Tranquilizers (also known as benzodiazepines) such as alpra-zolam and clonazepam may temporarily help some people with tremor. However, their use is limited due to unwanted side effects that include sleepiness, poor concentration, and poor coordination. This can affect the ability of people to perform daily activities such as driving, school, and work. Also, when taken regularly, tranquilizers can cause physical dependence and when stopped abruptly can cause several withdrawal symptoms.

- Parkinson disease medications (levodopa, carbidopa) are used to treat tremor associated with Parkinson disease.

- Botulinum toxin injections can treat almost all types of tremor. It is especially useful for head tremor, which generally does not respond to medications. Botulinum toxin is widely used to con-trol dystonic tremor. Although botulinum toxin injections can improve tremor for roughly three months at a time, they can also cause muscle weakness. While this treatment is effective and usually well tolerated for head tremor, botulinum toxin treatment in the hands can cause weakness in the fingers. It can cause a hoarse voice and difficulty swallowing when used to treat voice tremor.

Focused Ultrasound

A new treatment for essential tremor uses magnetic resonance images (MRI) to deliver focused ultrasound to create a lesion in tiny areas of the brain's thalamus thought to be responsible for causing the tremors. The treatment is approved only for those individuals with essential tremor who do not respond well to anticonvulsant or beta blocking drugs.

Surgery

When people do not respond to drug therapies or have a severe tremor that significantly impacts their daily life, a doctor may recommend surgical interventions such as deep brain stimulation (DBS) or very rarely, thalamotomy. While DBS is usually well tolerated, the most common side effects of tremor surgery include dysarthria (trouble speaking) and balance problems.

- Deep brain stimulation (DBS) is the most common form of surgical treatment of tremor. This method is preferred because it is effective, has low risk, and treats a broader range of symptoms than thalamotomy. The treatment uses surgically implanted electrodes to send high frequency electrical signals to the thalamus, the deep structure of the brain that coordinates and controls some involuntary movements. A small pulse generating device placed under the skin in the upper chest (similar to a pacemaker) sends electrical stimuli to the brain and temporarily disables the tremor. DBS is currently used to treat parkinsonian tremor, essential tremor, and dystonia.

- Thalamotomy is a surgical procedure that involves the precise, permanent destruction of a tiny area in the thalamus. Currently, surgery is replaced by radiofrequency ablation to treat severe tremor when deep brain surgery is contraindicated—meaning it is unwise as a treatment option or has undesirable side effects. Radiofrequency ablation uses a radio wave to generate an electric current that heats up a nerve and disrupts its signaling ability for typically six or more months. It is usually performed on only one side of the brain to improve tremor on the opposite side of the body. Surgery on both sides is not recommended as it can cause problems with speech.

Lifestyle Changes

- Physical therapy may help to control tremor. A physical therapist can help people improve their muscle control, functioning, and strength through coordination, balancing, and other exercises. Some therapists recommend the use of weights, splints, other adaptive equipment, and special plates and utensils for eating.

- Eliminating or reducing tremor inducing substances such as caffeine and other medication (such as stimulants) can help improve tremor. Though small amounts of alcohol can improve tremor for some people, tremor can become worse once the effects of the alcohol wear off.

What Is the Prognosis?

Tremor is not considered a life-threatening condition. Although many cases of tremor are mild, tremor can be very disabling for other people. It can be difficult for individuals with tremor to perform normal daily activities such as working, bathing, dressing, and eating. Tremor can also cause "social disability." People may limit their physical activity, travel, and social engagements to avoid embarrassment or other consequences.

The symptoms of essential tremor usually worsen with age. Additionally, there is some evidence that people with essential tremor are more likely than average to develop other neurodegenerative conditions such as PD or Alzheimer disease (AD), especially in individuals whose tremor first appears after age 65.

Unlike essential tremor, the symptoms of physiologic and drug-induced tremor do not generally worsen over time and can often be improved or eliminated once the underlying causes are treated.

Chapter 46

Dystonia Treatments

The dystonias are a group of disorders characterized by excessive involuntary muscle contractions leading to abnormal postures and/or repetitive movements. There are many different clinical manifestations and many different causes. A careful assessment of the clinical manifestations is helpful for identifying syndromic patterns that focus diagnostic testing on potential causes. If a cause can be identified, specific etiology based treatments may be available. However, in the majority of cases, a specific cause cannot be identified, and treatments are based on symptoms.

Treatment options include counseling and education, oral medications, botulinum toxin injections, and several surgical procedures. A substantial reduction in symptoms and improved quality of life can be achieved in the majority of patients by combining these various options.

Treatment

There are many different treatment options that involve counseling and education, oral medications, intramuscular injection of botulinum neurotoxins (BoNT), physical and occupational therapy, and neurosurgical interventions. Subsequently, some suggestions are offered for how these individual ingredients can be combined for the best outcomes in different types of dystonia.

This chapter includes text excerpted from "Diagnosis and Treatment of Dystonia," U.S. Department of Health and Human Services (HHS), February 1, 2016.

Education and Counseling

Education and counseling are important for several reasons. Patients frequently are misdiagnosed for many years, and many are told they suffering from a psychiatric problem. Even for the most common and readily diagnosed subtypes of dystonia such as cervical dystonia, the mean time from onset of symptoms to diagnosis is 4–6 years. These delays in reaching a diagnosis often lead to frustration and mistrust of medical providers. Education and counseling are important for regaining trust so that patients are more likely to accept recommendations.

Education and counseling also are important because few therapies are curative. Achieving the best outcome often requires an empirical trial and error approach, which can sometimes amplify existing frustration and mistrust. A frank discussion of treatment options is essential to ensure that expectations are realistic. It is also worth bearing in mind that there is a high rate of psychiatric comorbidity in the dystonias including depression, anxiety, and social withdrawal. An open discussion of how these factors may influence overall quality of life is important.

Finally, many patients learn about their medical diagnoses and treatment options via the internet, which is not always a reliable source of information. Educating patients about the most reliable online sources of information can help to avoid misunderstandings. Most of these groups also provide informational brochures, newsletters and local patient support group meetings where patients can obtain new information.

Physical and Occupational Therapy

Patients frequently ask about the value of exercise and physical therapy, because they seem intuitively helpful for addressing abnormal muscle activity and pain. Although many patients seem to appreciate physical therapy, benefits often are temporary, and there are no large scale double blind studies that demonstrate objective benefits to justify regular application.

Several investigators have sought to demonstrate objective improvements using specific methods based on theories regarding the pathophysiology of dystonia. For example, the theory that dystonia results from maladaptive neuralplasticity has led to attempts to retrain normal patterns of activity via "constraint induced" movement training to limit abnormal movements while reinforcing normal ones, "sensorimotor retuning" with intensive exercises, "slow down" therapy, active exercise, and electromyography (EMG) biofeedback. Theories regarding maladaptive plasticity also have led to the opposing strategy of attempting to erase abnormal plasticity via lengthy periods of immobilization. Theories relating the pathophysiology of dystonia to defects in sensory processes or sensorimotor integration have led to attempts to alter sensory feedback as a treatment strategy. Various methods have been exploited including modification of sensory inputs, "kinesogenic taping," transcutaneous electrical nerve stimulation, and augmentation of somatosensory discrimination by Braille training.

Despite the enthusiasm for physical therapy in dystonia, systematic reviews have concluded that there is insufficient evidence to recommend any particular strategy. There are several reasons for the lack of clear guidelines. First, most of the studies have been quite small with outcomes that often were not reproducible, and the larger studies frequently demonstrated wide response variations among patients. Second, the reported benefits often have been quite small, transient, or subjective. The modest benefits of individual techniques have led to attempts to combine treatments using "multimodal" strategies, further obscuring the value of specific interventions. Third, there is a tradition in physical therapy to customize procedures according to the needs of individual patients. As a result, large studies using uniform protocols are scarce. Double blind and placebo controlled studies are rare also in part because of the difficulty in designing an appropriate control group to rule out nonspecific placebo effects. Finally, many of the methods are cumbersome and time consuming, limiting enthusiasm for clinical application.

Enthusiasm for specific strategies also is blunted by concerns that some well intentioned designs may be harmful. For example, significant improvements have been reported for patients with hand dystonia following 4–6 weeks of immobilization with a rigid splint. However, broad adoption has been limited by the long duration of splinting, side effects of hand clumsiness and weakness following splinting, and concerns that prolonged immobilization can trigger more severe fixed dystonia, sometimes as part of the complex regional pain syndrome. Similarly, transcutaneous electrical nerve stimulation has been reported to be helpful in some patients, yet detrimental to others. Despite these limitations, the available studies have provided some promising suggestions that deserve further exploration and development before more general recommendations can be formulated.

In the absence of solid evidence to guide more specific recommendations, it seems reasonable to incorporate general physical therapy methods according to patient preferences. These may include regular stretching exercises to mitigate against contractures, muscle relaxation methods to attenuate pulling and pain, and strengthening of antagonist muscles to balance abnormal postures. Various assistive devices also are available to allow more significantly disabled patients to function more independently.

Oral Medications

There are multiple articles summarizing oral medications for dystonia, including two systematic evidence based reviews. None of the commonly used drugs has been subject to large scale, double blinded, placebo controlled trials. None of them has been the U.S. Food and Drug Administration (FDA) approved for treatment of dystonia. Much of the evidence supporting the use of these drugs comes from small controlled trials, nonblinded trials, retrospective reviews, and anecdotal experience.

Acetylcholine Related Drugs

One of the most frequently prescribed classes of medications for the dystonias include anticholinergics such as trihexyphenidyl, benztropine, biperidin, ethopropazine, orphenadrine, and procyclidine. These drugs are thought to work by blocking muscarinic acetylcholine receptors in the basal ganglia. Their use is supported by multiple retrospective studies, and one prospective, double blind trial of trihexyphenidyl that showed clinically significant improvements in 71 percent of patients on an mean dose of 30 mg daily. However this study included only 31 patients with predominantly isolated dystonia, and a mean age of 19 years. Similar studies of children with dystonia associated with cerebral palsy showed that a significant proportion may worsen with anticholinergics. There are no prospective double blind, placebo controlled trials of anticholinergics for older adults, who are less likely to tolerate their many side effects.

Despite the limited and sometimes conflicting information, anticholinergics remain in broad use because they seem to be at least partly effective for many types of dystonia, regardless of the underlying etiology. Trihexyphenidyl must be started at a low dose, for example 2 mg twice daily. It can be increased by 2 mg every few days until benefits are observed or side effects emerge. Effective doses range from 6–40 mg daily, divided across 3–4 doses. Typical side effects include memory loss, confusion, restlessness, depression, dry mouth, constipation, urinary retention, blurry vision, or worsening of narrow angle glaucoma.

Dopamine Related Drugs

Medications that augment or suppress dopaminergic transmission in the basal ganglia may be extraordinarily helpful in select populations of patients with dystonia. Augmenting dopamine transmission with levodopa is dramatically effective in dopa responsive dystonia, which is most often caused by mutations in the *GCH1* gene encoding the enzyme Guanosine triphosphate (GTP) cyclohydrolase. Many patients respond to doses as low as half of a 25/100 mg tablet of carbidopa/levodopa twice daily, although others require larger doses. For an adequate trial of levodopa, the dose should be increased slowly to 1000 mg in an adult (or 20 mg/kg for children) divided across three daily doses for one month before concluding it will not be effective. In addition to levodopa, patients with classical dopa responsive dystonia respond to dopamine agonists and drugs that block dopamine metabolism such as monoamine oxidase inhibitors.

Levodopa is also at least partially effective in other disorders affecting dopamine synthesis that are caused by deficiency of tyrosine hydroxylase, sepiapterin reductase, and others. It may also be effective in some other rare disorders such as the dystonia in some cases of spinocerebellar ataxia type 375 or variant forms of ataxia telangiectasia, and for dystonia in Parkinson disease (PD). Aside from these specific populations, levodopa and dopamine agonists are not broadly useful for other types of dystonia, such as the more common adult onset isolated focal or segmental dystonias.

Medications that suppress dopaminergic transmission also may be useful for specific subgroups of patients. Although dopamine receptor antagonists have been used with variable success in small unblinded studies, their use is generally discouraged because the risk for development of acute dystonic reactions and tardive syndromes may lead to diagnostic confusion. However, depletion of dopamine with tetrabenazine does not carry these same risks, and it may be useful for some patients with dystonia, particularly those with tardive dystonia. It can be started at half of a 25 mg daily daily, and titrated up by a half tablet every 3–5 days, to a target of 25–100 mg daily. Dose limiting side effects include drowsiness, parkinsonism, depression, insomnia, nervousness, anxiety, and akathisia.

Gamma Aminobutyric Acid (GABA) Related Drugs

Another frequently prescribed group of medications is the benzodiazepines such as alprazolam, chlordiazepoxide, clonazepam, and diazepam. They are thought to work by amplifying transmission through gamma aminobutyric acid (GABA) receptors. There are no large double blind and controlled studies of the benzodiazepines in dystonia. Their use is supported by multiple small or retrospective studies. Anecdotal experience suggests they may be most useful for suppressing phasic aspects of dystonia, such as blinking in blepharospasm, or tremor dominant forms of dystonia. They also appear to be useful in the paroxysmal dyskinesias (PD), where dystonia can be a prominent feature. Common side effects include sedation, impaired mentation and coordination, and depression. There also is a risk for tachyphylaxis and dependency, so abrupt discontinuation or sudden large decreases in doses should be avoided.

Baclofen is a GABA receptor agonist that also is often used in dystonia. There are no controlled studies to guide recommendations for its use, but several retrospective studies and anecdotal reports suggest it is not often useful in childhood onset dystonias, especially those with coexisting spasticity of the lower limbs. Some adults also may benefit, but most do not. Effective oral doses range from 30–120 mg daily divided across 3–4 doses. Common side effects include sedation, nausea, impaired mentation, dizziness, and loss of muscle tone. Abrupt discontinuation or sudden large decreases in doses can be associated with withdrawal reactions that include delirium and seizures.

Baclofen also can be delivered intrathecally via chronically implanted minipumps, where it may be useful in a subpopulation of patients with dystonia. Here again, it has been most often employed in children where dystonia is combined with spasticity, especially in the lower limbs. The side effects are similar to those listed above for oral administration, with additional complications related to the implanted device. These complications include pump malfunction, catheter obstruction or leaks, or infection of the equipment.

Muscle Relaxants

Many patients request "muscle relaxants" because they seem intuitively useful for overactive and sore muscles. This is a broad category of medications with diverse mechanisms of action that include baclofen and benzodiazepines described above, along with carisoprodol, chlorzoxazone, cyclobenzeprine, metaxalone, methocarbamol, and orphenadrine. There are no formal studies to guide recommendations for the use of these drugs in dystonia, and responses vary widely. Nevertheless, many patients derive at least partial benefits, especially those with pain from uncontrolled muscle pulling.

Other Medications

A wide variety of other drugs have been advocated for specific forms of dystonia, generally based on small and nonblinded studies or anecdotal experiences. For example, carbamazepine and other anticonvulsants seem particularly useful for dystonic spasms in paroxysmal kinesigenic dyskinesia, and alcohol is useful in the myoclonus dystonia syndrome (MDS). Mexiletine and intravenous lidocaine may be helpful in some cases. Other options suggested for specific populations include amphetamines, cannabidiol, cyproheptidine, gabapentin, lithium, nabilone, riluzole, tizanidine, and zolpidem.

Botulinum Neurotoxins

Medical BoNTs are derived from a neurotoxic protein produced by the bacterium Clostridium botulinum (CB). The bacterial toxin causes a paralytic disorder known as botulism, but medical grade BoNT is purified and attenuated so that local intramuscular injections suppress overactive muscles in dystonia. There are seven distinct serotypes, A-G. Type A is marketed as onabotulinumtoxinA (Botox™), abobotulinumtoxinA (Dysport™), and incobotulinumtoxinA (Xeomin™). Type B is marketed as rimabotulinumtoxinB (Myobloc™). Their safety and efficacy have been the subject of multiple prior summaries, including several systematic evidence based reviews. They are very effective for many types of dystonia, significantly reducing abnormal movements and associated disability, and improving overall quality of life.

Many detailed resources are available for application of the BoNTs including target muscle selection, dosing, and the use of ancillary procedures for localization such as electromyography and ultrasound. The technical details associated with administration of BoNTs will not be reviewed here. Instead, the focus is on practical issues faced by physicians who may refer patients for BoNT treatments, and on some of the most common questions regarding their application. The first important issue involves the type of dystonia. The botulinum neurotoxins (BoNTs) are considered the treatment of first choice for most focal and segmental dystonias including blepharospasm, cervical dystonia, oromandibular and laryngeal dystonias, limb dystonias, and others. The benefits from injections usually emerge after 2–7 days, and they last for approximately 3–4 months. Most patients return for treatments 3–4 times yearly. BoNTs also can be valuable for patients with broader patterns of dystonia, where they are often under utilized. For these patients, the goal is to target the regions that cause the most discomfort. For example, patients with dyskinetic cerebral palsy

(DCP) often have generalized dystonia with prominent involvement of the neck, and treatment with BoNT can alleviate this discomfort ant reduce the risk of acquired myelopathy.

The BoNTs are dramatically effective for most focal dystonias, but it can be challenging to get good results with certain subtypes. Some patients with blepharospasm have coexisting apraxia of eyelid opening, which is more difficult to treat with BoNT. Injections into the pretarsal portion of the orbicularis oculi muscles may improve outcomes in these cases. Among patients with cervical dystonia (CD), those with prominent anterocollis can be more difficult to treat. Deep injections into prevertebral muscles have been advocated, although responses vary. For laryngeal dystonias, spasmodic adductor dysphonia responds more predictably than spasmodic abductor dysphonia. Oromandibular and lingual dystonias can sometimes be challenging to treat, although good outcomes can be achieved in experienced hands. Because there are so many small muscles that work together for coordinated activities, it can be difficult to achieve satisfactory outcomes for hand dystonias. Some patients enjoy dramatic benefits with very small doses, but achieving the right dose to avoid weakness or involvement of nearby muscles can be difficult to balance.

Another important issue involves side effects. There are no deleterious long-term side effects even after decades of treatment, apart from a small risk of developing resistance due to antibodies that neutralize the BoNT protein. However, the development of immunologically mediated resistance is rare with current preparations of BoNT. The short-term side effects depend mostly on local diffusion from the sites of injection. For blepharospasm the most common side effects are ptosis, local hematoma formation, tearing, and rarely blurry vision, or diplopia. For cervical dystonia the most common side effects are dysphagia, excessive neck muscle weakness, and occasionally dry mouth. For laryngeal dystonias the most common side effects are hoarsenss, or hypophonia, and rarely dysphagia and aspiration. For limb dystonias the most common side effects involve excessive weakening, or weakness of nearby muscles. Systemic side effects are unusual, but a few patients complain of a flu like syndrome for 3–5 days after their treatments.

A third issue involves the selection of a specific product. Many articles have summarized differences among the BoNTs regarding efficacy, side effects, and formulations. However, there are few scientifically rigorous comparisons, and the similarities are more striking than the differences. The choice of product depends largely on the experience and preferences of individual providers.

Surgical Interventions

Multiple surgical interventions are available for the treatment of the dystonias. Typically these more invasive approaches are reserved for patients who fail more conservative therapies. The most common intervention involves neuromodulation of brain activity via an implanted electrical impulse generator, although focal ablation of select brain areas and peripheral approaches that target nerves or muscles can be applied in some circumstances.

Neuromodulation

Neuromodulation is synonymous with deep brain stimulation (DBS). The term neuromodulation is increasingly preferred because some targets may not be "deep" and "stimulation" implies a mechanism that has not been established. Several extensive reviews on neuromodulation have been published recently, including a whole issue of the journal Movement Disorders. Here, the focus is on practical issues of relevance to any physician who may council patients regarding these options. The issues include patient selection for best outcomes, long-term expectations, and some ongoing debates.

Some patients with dystonia respond quite well to neuromodulation, while others derive no benefit. Many years of experience have provided some important insights into several factors that predict responses. Patients with isolated generalized dystonia syndromes (GDS) (previously "primary" dystonia) tend to respond most consistently, with the most objective blinded studies showing improvements in standardized dystonia rating scales of 40–60 percent. Among this patient population best outcomes appear to be associated with younger ages, shorter disease durations, and those who have the common *TOR1A* mutation for *DYT1* dystonia. There is insufficient evidence to predict outcomes in the more recently discovered genes including the *THAP1* gene for *DYT6*. Patients with fixed contractures or scoliosis do not do so well as those with more a more mobile syndrome.

Patients with isolated focal and segmental dystonias also appear to respond well to neuromodulation, although perhaps less predictably than those with isolated generalized dystonia. This group includes patients with relatively localized or segmental patterns involving the neck, face, trunk, or limbs. Patients with dystonic syndromes that are combined with other neurological features (previously "dystonia plus" or "secondary" dystonias) respond variably. Some subtypes consistently respond very well, for example myoclonus dystonia and tardive dystonia. Others have a consistently poor outcome (e.g., degenerative disorders) or are less predictable (e.g., cerebral palsy). One of the reasons for the poor outcomes in some populations is that it is difficult to detect a stable benefit for progressive degenerative disorders, or for disorders where dystonia is combined with other motor defects such as spasticity that are not expected to improve with neuromodulation. These populations should be considered for surgery only by very experienced centers after careful counseling, ideally as part of a methodical study aimed at elucidating risk/benefit profiles.

The long-term outcomes of neuromodulation are good, with benefits sustained for many years, and some studies reporting good outcomes even after 10 years. Ongoing access to an experienced center to adjust stimulator settings and address potential complications is essential. Benefits from surgery can be delayed for weeks or even months, requiring frequent visits to adjust stimulator settings for optimal outcomes. Return visits also should be anticipated every 2–4 years for battery replacement. In one study of 47 cases with *DYT1* dystonia followed by a very experienced multidisciplinary neuromodulation center for more than 10 years, 8.5 percent had delayed postoperative infection of equipment requiring antibiotics and/or equipment removal, 8.5 percent had malfunction of equipment such as impulse generator failure or lead defects, and 4.3 percent required revisions of lead location. These observations indicate that close follow-up by an experienced team is essential for long-term maintenance therapy. This requirement for return visits presents a barrier for some patients who may live far from experienced providers.

There are several unresolved questions that the counseling physician may be asked to address. One is the ideal surgical target. The internal segment of the globus pallidus (GPi) is the traditional target used by most centers. However, observations that patients with dystonia sometimes develop bradykinesia in unaffected body regions or gait failure have led to interest in other targets such as the subthalamic nucleus. On the other hand, neuromodulation of the subthalamic nucleus has been associated with dyskinesias, weight gain, and psychiatric changes. Others have targeted various regions of the thalamus, usually for focal hand dystonia (FHD) and those with prominent tremor. The "ideal" target remains unknown. Whether this target varies according to the subtype of dystonia also remains uncertain. As a result the selection of targets often is driven by the opinions of individual centers.

Another unresolved question involves the expected outcomes for patients with dystonias combined with other neurological features (previously "secondary" dystonias). Aside from tardive dystonia (TD) and myoclonus dystonia (MD), there is insufficient information to counsel interested patients regarding expectations. The lack of information should not be viewed as an absolute contraindication for surgery, but patients must be clearly informed about the chances for failure.

Ablative Approaches

Making controlled focal lesions in specific parts of the brain was the most common surgical procedure conducted for dystonia patients before neuromodulation became more popular. Lesions were made in a variety of locations, most notably the thalamus, globus pallidus, and cerebellum. Neuromodulation rapidly became more popular because it is more readily tunable, and because it is reversible in the event that intolerable side effects develop. However, neuromodulation has its own risk of complications related to the hardware, and it is expensive. Therefore, there is still a role for ablative procedures in some circumstances.

Ablative procedures may be useful in developing countries where the cost of equipment for neuromodulation and requirements for regular follow-up are prohibitive. Ablations are also useful for patients with a body habitus that presents a high risk for hardware related complications, such as those with severe dystonia and fixed contractions, or very young or otherwise small patients. They may be offered to patients who suffer repeated hardware infections, or merely do not wish to have chronically implanted hardware. They may also be appropriate as palliative procedures for patients with severe illness who cannot tolerate surgery to install and maintain the hardware, and for some progressive neurodegenerative disorders.

Peripheral Surgeries

Another category of surgeries often offered to patients with dystonia before BoNTs and neuromodulation became more popular involved directly sectioning or destroying overactive muscles or the nerves controlling them. These procedures are far less commonly used today, but they are still offered by some centers. They are covered briefly here for physicians encountering patients who may ask about them.

Selective peripheral denervation may be offered to patients with cervical dystonia who fail oral agents and botulinum toxins. The procedure involves extra spinal sectioning of nerves to specific muscles, so best outcomes are seen for patients with a limited number of muscles involved (e.g., pure torticollis or pure laterocollis). Success rates are reported from 60–90 percent. Side effects may include permanent somatosensory loss or dysesthesia in an isolated region of the neck, cosmetic changes associated with scaring or muscle atrophy, muscles weakness, and dysphagia. Abnormal movements may re-emerge after several weeks or years, a phenomenon that may reflect reinnervation or progression of the underlying disorder.

A variety of procedures are offered to patients with blepharospasm too. They include orbicularis myectomy, frontalis suspension, surgical shortening of the levator palpebrae, and removal of redundant eyelid skin. None of these procedures has been subject to rigorous trials, so they usually are offered only to patients who fail botulinum toxins. Included are patients who are resistant to the toxins, and those with coexisting apraxia of eyelid opening that may respond poorly to the toxins.

There also are several procedures in use for patients with laryngeal dystonia. Patients with spasmodic dysphonia may undergo thyroplasty to modify the cartilaginous structure of the larynx or thyroaretynoid myectomy (TAM). The most common approach involves sectioning the recurrent laryngeal nerve to the thyroarytenoid and annealing the stump to the ansa cervicalis. Complications can include transient or permanent voice impediment, dysphagia, and return of symptoms requiring re-operation.

Chapter 47

Plasmapheresis May Be Used to Treat Movement Disorders

Therapeutic apheresis is the process of transiently removing whole blood from the body, separating it into various components (e.g., cells, plasma, proteins, antibodies, antigen-antibody complexes, lipids, etc.), removing those components that contribute to disease, and then returning the remaining blood with possible addition of a blood component to the body. Several forms of therapeutic apheresis exist: therapeutic plasma exchange (plasma exchange; commonly known as TPE); white cell reduction (leukocytapheresis); platelet reduction (plateletapheresis); red cell exchange (erythrocytapheresis, or RBCX); low-density lipoprotein (LDL) apheresis; and extracorporeal photopheresis (ECP), which involves treating isolated leukocytes ex vivo with 8-methoxypsoralen and then exposing them to ultraviolet light before cells are returned to the patient.

This chapter contains text excerpted from the following sources: Text in this chapter begins with excerpts from "Therapeutic Apheresis," National Heart, Lung, and Blood Institute (NHLBI), November 29, 2012. Reviewed January 2018; Text under the heading "Procedure and Preparation for Apheresis" is excerpted from "Apheresis for Research," Clinical Center, National Institutes of Health (NIH), July 2013. Reviewed January 2018.

Apheresis medicine is that discipline of medicine, engineering, and science concerned with the care and management of patients and donors involved in extracorporeal blood separation interventions used in the treatment of disease or in the collection of various blood constituents. Apheresis has an undeserved reputation as an "old" science; one that in recent years has been overtaken at times by newer medical treatments. Yet it still is the only and often life-saving treatment for certain conditions. Apheresis remains the go-to procedure for treating many common and rare maladies alike and new treatment indications are being added. Although many specialists like hematologists, neurologists, and nephrologists see the evidence and benefits of therapeutic apheresis in their everyday work, the progress of Apheresis Medicine as a medical specialty has been generally slow. There is lack of good understanding pertaining to basic mechanisms of apheresis and optimal ways of applying apheresis to the improvement of underlying conditions as well as to the ability of apheresis to enhance other treatment modalities.

TPE in Neurological Diseases

Most neurological disorders treated with TPE are mediated by humoral immune responses, and the beneficial effect of TPE is believed to occur through removal of the offending inflammatory mediators (e.g., autoantibodies, cytokines, complement constituents). The efficacy of TPE in the treatment of neurologic diseases remains less clear. Although TPE is used in some neurologic diseases, confirmatory studies and trials are lacking. Many questions remain about the ability of TPE to affect central nervous systems and the ideal timing in accessing the blood-brain barrier.

Relapsing Remitting Multiple Sclerosis (RRMS). MS is the most common disease of the central nervous system in young adults. Although its pathogenesis is not fully understood, evidence suggests that MS is an autoimmune disease mediated by autoreactive T cells. Accordingly, MS treatments are based on immunomodulating or immunosuppressive drugs, which are more effective in the reduction of the relapse rate than in the reduction of the disability load accumulation. ECP promotes tolerance and down-regulation of inflammatory responses in patients with MS through the generation of tolerogenic dendritic cells and T regulatory cells.

Neuromelitis Optica (NMO). An inflammatory demyelinating disease of the central nervous system in which 85 percent of patients have associated antibody to aquaporin-4 and a relapsing course with poor prognosis. Growing evidence suggest patients with acute attacks may respond well to TPE. Prophylaxis to prevent further acute attacks includes immunosuppressive medications and immunomodulation such as rituximab, methotrexate, interferon, azathioprine, cyclophosphamide, prednisone, intravenous IgG, mitoxantrone, interferon, and mycophenolate mafetil. Some studies suggest that maintenance TPE may be beneficial in preventing further acute attacks. The primary purpose of using apheresis to study NMO would be to determine whether patients in an acute crisis improve to a greater degree when apheresis is initiated on day 1 of an attack in addition to steroid use versus steroid use alone.

Myasthenia Gravis (MG). Growing evidence suggest patients with muscle-specific kinase (MuSK) MG may respond differently to treatments than those with acetylcholine receptor-associated MG, thus treatment protocols were proposed to determine whether patients with anti-MuSK MG respond better to plasma exchange versus intravenous IgG administration during rapid deterioration.

Acute Disseminated Encephalomyelitis (ADEM). ADEM typically presents as fever, headache, and meningeal signs followed by acute encephalopathy, seizures, and multifocal neurological deficits. The pathogenesis of ADEM is not completely clear, but a significant association with certain HLA alleles has been reported. Patients with severe ADEM and who have contraindications to steroids or are not responsive to steroids are usually treated with either TPE or intravenous IgG. The dose and timing of intravenous IgG remains unclear. The mechanism of action of either TPE or IgG administration in this disease is yet to be elucidated. Both treatments have different requirements, availability, convenience, costs, and unique side effect profiles. Therefore, studies were proposed to assess whether TPE or intravenous IgG administration alone or as an adjunct to steroid therapy in severe ADEM would be beneficial in reducing hospital stays, ventilation days, complications, and the need for long-term rehabilitation.

Anti-NMDAR Encephalitis. Encephalitis associated with antibodies against the N-methyl-d-aspartate receptor (NMDAR) is characterized by a prodrome of headache, fever, nausea, vomiting, diarrhea, or symptoms of upper respiratory tract infection followed over a 2-week course by short-term memory deficits, psychiatric symptoms, decreased consciousness, seizures, and hypoventilation. A significant proportion of patients require hospitalization to manage seizures, receive mechanical ventilation, and treat hemodynamic instability. Because the disease is caused by an autoantibody, both intravenous IgG administration and TPE are predicted to have efficacy. Therefore, studies to determine the optimal treatment regimen via TPE or intravenous IgG alone or as an adjunct to steroid therapy is expected to help develop diagnostic criteria, define meaningful response criteria, improve patient outcomes, and be cost-effective.

Polymyositis is a rare disease that more commonly occurs with systemic autoimmune or connective tissue disease or known viral or bacterial infection, which often can make it difficult to diagnose. The fundamental immune process is mediated by CD8+ cytotoxic T cells, which invade non-necrotic muscle fibers that express the major histocompatibility class (MHC)-I antigen. Patients with polymyositis have overexpression of MHC-I on the surface of their muscle fibers. Treatment is predominately high-dose corticosteroids, with steroid-sparing therapy as second-line treatment. Intravenous IgG has also been shown to be an effective treatment. Further studies of the use of ECP in patients with polymyositis are expected to lead to a decrease in the dose of corticosteroids and faster patient improvement.

Procedure and Preparation for Apharesis

Various types of machines are used to do apheresis. These machines use sterile, disposable parts to prevent blood-borne infections. The needs of your protocol will usually determine the type of machine used for your apheresis.

During your procedure, you will receive a blood thinning medication (anticoagulant) so that your blood does not clot in the machine. Some people feel these minor side effects from this medication: tingling, numbness (around the lips, nose, and mouth), coolness all over, and slight nausea. These side effects usually come and go quickly, but if you have these symptoms or feel anything unusual, please tell your nurse immediately.

How Long Apheresis Takes

Depending on how much blood the apheresis machine needs to process, your apheresis could take between 1 and 5 hours.

After the Procedure

When the procedure is over, staff will remove the needles and put a bandage over each needle entry site. Please keep these bandages on for 3–4 hours.

Adjust your daily activity until the following day (about 24 hours):

- Avoid lifting heavy objects.

- Avoid strenuous exercise.

- Take the elevator, not the stairs.

- Drink lots of nonalcoholic/noncaffeinated beverages.

Chapter 48

Physical Strategies for Improving Movement Disorder Symptoms

Chapter Contents

Section 48.1

Why Exercise Helps People with Movement Disorders

This section contains text excerpted from the following sources: Text under the heading "Physical Activity for People with Disabilities" is excerpted from "2008 Physical Activity Guidelines for Americans," Office of Disease Prevention and Health Promotion (ODPHP), U.S. Department of Health and Human Services (HHS), October 2008. Reviewed January 2018; Text under the heading "Physical Activity May Reduce Age-Related Movement Problems" is excerpted from "Physical Activity May Reduce Age-Related Movement Problems," National Institutes of Health (NIH), March 23, 2015.

Physical Activity for People with Disabilities

The benefits of physical activity for people with disabilities have been studied in diverse groups. These groups include stroke victims, people with spinal cord injury, multiple sclerosis, Parkinson disease, muscular dystrophy, cerebral palsy, traumatic brain injury, limb amputations, mental illness, intellectual disability, and dementia.

Overall, the evidence shows that regular physical activity provides important health benefits for people with disabilities. The benefits include improved cardiovascular and muscle fitness, improved mental health, and better ability to do tasks of daily life. Sufficient evidence now exists to recommend that adults with disabilities should get regular physical activity.

Explaining the Guidelines

In consultation with their healthcare providers, people with disabilities should understand how their disabilities affect their ability to do physical activity. Some may be capable of doing medium to high amounts of physical activity, and they should essentially follow the Guidelines for adults.

Some people with disabilities are not able to follow the Guidelines for adults. These people should adapt their physical activity program to match their abilities, in consultation with their healthcare providers.

Studies show that physical activity can be done safely when the program is matched to an individual's abilities.

Key Guidelines for Adults with Disabilities

- Adults with disabilities, who are able to, should get at least 150 minutes per week (2 hours and 30 minutes) of moderate-intensity, or 75 minutes (1 hour and 15 minutes) per week of vigorous-intensity aerobic activity, or an equivalent combination of moderate and vigorous intensity aerobic activity. Aerobic activity should be performed in episodes of at least 10 minutes, and preferably, it should be spread throughout the week.

- Adults with disabilities, who are able to, should also do muscle-strengthening activities of moderate or high intensity that involve all major muscle groups on 2 or more days per week, as these activities provide additional health benefits.

- When adults with disabilities are not able to meet the above Guidelines, they should engage in regular physical activity according to their abilities and should avoid inactivity.

- Adults with disabilities should consult their healthcare providers about the amounts and types of physical activity that are appropriate for their abilities.

Meeting the Guidelines

People with disabilities are encouraged to get advice from professionals with experience in physical activity and disability because matching activity to abilities can require modifying physical activity in many different ways. Some people with disabilities also need help with their exercise program. For example, some people may need supervision when performing muscle strengthening activities, such as lifting weights.

Physical Activity May Reduce Age-Related Movement Problems

Age-related brain lesions known as white matter hyperintensities have been linked to movement problems and disabilities later in life. These lesions, which appear as bright spots on MRI images, can be used as a proxy measure of brain white matter disease. They are thought to reflect small blood vessel disease, and have also have been associated with dementia and other health issues in older people.

Previous research has found that seniors who are more physically active are at lower risk for walking difficulties and other movement problems. Researchers led by Dr. Debra A. Fleischman of Rush University Medical Center in Chicago examined whether physical activity can affect the link between age-related brain lesions and motor function in older adults. The study was partly funded by National Institutes of Health (NIH)'s National Institute on Aging (NIA), National Institute of Neurological Disorders and Stroke (NINDS), and National Institute of Minority Health and Health Disparities (NIMHD).

The researchers scanned the brains of 167 healthy older adults who were participating in a larger study of memory and aging. The participants' average age was 80. The investigators gave the participants various movement and strength tests. Participants also wore monitors on their wrists for up to 11 days to measure daily physical activity. The study appeared online in Neurology on March 11, 2015.

As expected, the researchers found that more physical activity was associated with better motor function. More age-related brain lesions were generally linked to poorer motor function. Physical activity levels were not related to the amount of lesions. However, among participants who were most active, the lesions weren't linked to poorer motor skills. Other factors like body mass index and vascular disease had no effect on the relationship between the brain lesions, daily activity, and motor function.

These results suggest that the level of physical activity later in life doesn't affect white matter hyperintensities but influences motor function via some other pathway. How physical activity might protect motor skills from the effects of these age-related brain lesions remains unknown. Previous studies suggest that physical activity may enhance brain health by increasing blood flow and other vascular functions in the brain.

"These results underscore the importance of efforts to encourage a more active lifestyle in older people to prevent movement problems, which is a major public health challenge," Fleischman says. "Physical activity may create a 'reserve' that protects motor abilities against the effects of age-related brain damage."

The associations found in this study suggest, but don't prove, that physical activity can protect against the loss of motor function caused by age-related brain lesions. The group is now monitoring brain scans over time to more closely examine the relationships between white matter hyperintensities, physical activity, and motor function.

Section 48.2

Battling Parkinson with Yoga

This section includes text excerpted from "Yoga: For Veterans
with Parkinson's Disease," U.S. Department of Veterans
Affairs (VA), April 28, 2017.

Yoga is very popular and is cited as a favorite complementary integrative health (CIH) therapy by many people living with Parkinson
disease (PD). People are often fearful of getting started in a yoga class
since there is often an incorrect portrayal of yoga in the media as being
only for flexible, skinny ballet dancers. Yoga, on the contrary, is a very
adaptable practice, with both functional and psychosocial benefits, that
can be suited to a wide variety of abilities.

Yoga has become synonymous with holding and moving between a
series of static postures (called asanas); however, this physical practice, called "hatha yoga," is only one part of the larger lifestyle of yoga
framework that includes branches such as philosophy, chanting and
selfless service. Hatha yoga combines physical postures to address
strength, flexibility, balance and mind-body-breath connection. Breathing practices (pranayama) and meditation are included to develop
greater self-awareness and can have tremendous benefit on the mental
state.

What Do We Know about Yoga in PD?

A review of the scientific literature shows a few studies that support
hatha yoga for people with PD. This is one area of research that is
just starting to build evidence. What studies do exist suggest modest
benefits for:

- **Mobility.** The issue of mobility has important implications for
  fall prevention in PD. Yoga participation can improve functional
  mobility and influences how a person with PD walks. Standing
  yoga poses target the hip extensor, knee extensor and ankle
  plantar flex or, which support center-of-gravity during walking
  and may improve overall stability.

- **Balance.** Balance training is an important component of PD therapy, because 40 percent of nursing home admissions are preceded by a fall. Research shows yoga-related improvements in balance (tandem, one-leg) and an associated decrease in a person's fear of falling; this can also help keep people with PD active in their communities.

- **Strength.** Gains in lower-body strength occur for PD patients following yoga practice and are associated with improved postural stability. Yoga requires isometric contraction (i.e., the joint angle and muscle length do not change) of specific muscle groups to stabilize the body as one performs the postures, and may mimic isokinetic contractions (i.e., variable resistance to a movement performed at constant speed) when performing controlled systemic movements from one pose to the next. These mechanisms may be the reason why yoga improves muscular strength.

- **Flexibility.** Improvements in flexibility and range of motion (ROM) are important since rigidity is a common clinical manifestation in PD. Research shows improvements in flexibility/ ROM of the shoulder, hip, and spine. Stooped posture is common in PD and can be related to short spinal flexors and weak spinal extensors; improved shoulder and spinal flexibility from yoga supports a more upright posture. Greater hip mobility from yoga may translate into improvements in shuffling gait which can be commonly seen in PD.

- **Mood and Sleep.** The psychosocial benefits associated with yoga are important for disease management, as they are not often addressed with classic medications used to replace the neurotransmitter dopamine in PD. Many classic medications used to treat anxiety are not safe in PD patients. The calming effect of yoga (by enhancing parasympathetic output) may lessen perceived stress, enhance relaxation, and benefit sleep in PD. Many patients with PD have apathy and fatigue which anecdotally are helped with yoga. Since the mind and the body are very connected in PD, any mental state benefits are tangibly translated into motor benefits. A yoga class can offer a support group, improved confidence, and self-efficacy. Caregivers can also participate and reap the rewards in the psychological realm as well.

Not everyone is lucky enough to live near a yoga instructor who has a deep understanding of PD—this makes it important to educate yourself, both about your specific PD needs and how yoga postures can help, so you can feel comfortable and confident with utilizing the yoga resources that are available in your own community.

Yoga Can Benefit People with Parkinson Both Physically and Cognitively!

Yoga is both physically and cognitively engaging by focusing on body-awareness during complex body positions. Yoga postures improve physical strength, flexibility, and balance. Yoga postures are also considered skill-acquisition exercises and can benefit our brains thinking patterns and processes to make our movements more efficient and effective.

Yoga helps to increase muscle mass that is useable in everyday life by focusing on functional movements. For example, one-leg balance poses such as the tree pose are helpful for climbing stairs; while the chair pose builds core and leg strength to help you get up out of bed and/or out of a seated position.

Yoga Is Actually a Form of Cueing/Attentional Training

The ability to move in Parkinson disease is not lost; rather the brain mechanisms that initiate movement are defective. Attentional training/cueing may provide a nonautomatic drive for movement, which may compensate for this faulty brain circuity and improve performance. Yoga breaks up complex sequences and/or postures into component parts, enabling a person to focus their attention on individual aspects of the posture and improve performance. Specific external cues given during a yoga class can also benefit performance in persons with Parkinson disease.

- Utilize visual cues (i.e., watch the yoga instructor or use a mirror) to help you coordinate your movement.

- Utilize props (i.e., blocks, straps, chairs) to get the experience of the full movement safely, and then take supports away as you progress.

- Talk to your yoga instructor about giving you hands-on adjustments while performing the poses. Subtle adjustments can help you with proper alignment and ensure you are not putting your body in a position that could be painful or result in injury.

- Focus on one aspect of the pose at a time to maintain your attention on your body in the present moment.

397

Know That Yoga Can Both Improve and Aggravate Your Parkinson Symptoms!

To avoid aggravating your symptoms, let your yoga instructor know that long holds may increase stiffness or muscle cramping. Instead of holding postures in stillness, try to move into the posture on an inhale breath, and relax out of the posture on an exhale breath. Yoga postures can be beneficial and improve rigidity, stiffness and slowness, especially in the chest muscles and spine. Focusing on yoga poses that safely extend the spine and/or deep diaphragmatic breathing exercises can create space in the chest and improve posture. Many of the floor poses in yoga allow you to practice getting up safely off the floor. This practice can increase confidence, reduce the fear of falling and increase the likelihood that you can get back up on your own if you do fall. Practice in the company of a caregiver first at least twice per day. You can use two stable supports one on either side at first if needed.

Use Yoga as an Opportunity to Focus on Posture

Stooped posture in Parkinson disease is common. It is attributed to shortened contracted spine flexors and weak extensors of the spine. Asymmetry of stiffness can lead to misalignment and can lead to misuse and disuse of muscles that can further worsen posture.

What Can Yoga Do?

- Strengthens your core, especially your transverse abdominal muscles.
- Lengthens your psoas muscle—a thick muscle that runs from under your armpits to your hips and connects your legs to your torso.
- Encourages gentle backbends to open upper spine.
- Creates self-awareness, and good habits, around how you hold your body in standing posture.

Chapter 49

Vocal Fold Paralysis and Its Treatment

What Is Vocal Fold Paralysis?

- Vocal fold paralysis (also known as vocal cord paralysis) is a voice disorder that occurs when one or both of the vocal folds don't open or close properly. Single vocal fold paralysis is a common disorder. Paralysis of both vocal folds is rare and can be life-threatening.

- The vocal folds are two elastic bands of muscle tissue located in the larynx (voice box) directly above the trachea (windpipe). When you breathe, your vocal folds remain apart and when you swallow, they are tightly closed. When you use your voice, however, air from the lungs causes your vocal folds to vibrate between open and closed positions.

- If you have vocal fold paralysis, the paralyzed fold or folds may remain open, leaving the air passages and lungs unprotected. You could have difficulty swallowing or food or liquids could accidentally enter the trachea and lungs, causing serious health problems.

This chapter includes text excerpted from "Vocal Fold Paralysis," National Institute on Deafness and Other Communication Disorders (NIDCD), March 6, 2017.

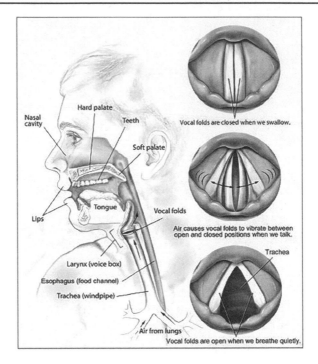

Figure 49.1. *Structures Involved in Speech and Voice Production*

What Causes Vocal Fold Paralysis?

Vocal fold paralysis may be caused by injury to the head, neck, or chest; lung or thyroid cancer; tumors of the skull base, neck, or chest; or infection (for example, Lyme disease). People with certain neurological conditions such as multiple sclerosis, or Parkinson disease, or who have sustained a stroke, may experience vocal fold paralysis. In many cases, however, the cause is unknown.

What Are the Symptoms?

Symptoms of vocal fold paralysis include changes in the voice, such as hoarseness or a breathy voice; difficulties with breathing, such as shortness of breath or noisy breathing; and swallowing problems, such as choking or coughing when you eat because food is accidentally entering the windpipe instead of the esophagus (the muscular tube that connects the throat to the stomach). Changes in voice quality, such as loss of volume or pitch, also may occur. Damage to both vocal folds, although rare, usually causes serious problems with breathing.

How Is Vocal Fold Paralysis Diagnosed?

Vocal fold paralysis is usually diagnosed by an otolaryngologist—a doctor who specializes in ear, nose, and throat disorders. He or she will ask you about your symptoms and when the problems began in order to help determine their cause. The otolaryngologist will also listen to your voice to identify breathiness or hoarseness. Using an endoscope—a tube with a light at the end—your doctor will look directly into the throat at the vocal folds. Some doctors also use a procedure called laryngeal electromyography (LEMG), which measures the electrical impulses of the nerves in the larynx, to better understand the areas of paralysis.

How Is Vocal Fold Paralysis Treated?

The most common treatments for vocal fold paralysis are voice therapy and surgery. Some people's voices will naturally recover sometime during the first year after diagnosis, which is why doctors often delay surgery for at least a year. During this time, your doctor will likely refer you to a speech language pathologist for voice therapy, which may involve exercises to strengthen the vocal folds or improve breath control while speaking. You might also learn how to use your voice differently, for example, by speaking more slowly or opening your mouth wider when you speak. Several surgical procedures are available, depending on whether one or both of your vocal folds are paralyzed. The most common procedures change the position of the vocal fold. These may involve inserting a structural implant or stitches to reposition the laryngeal cartilage and bring the vocal folds closer together. These procedures usually result in a stronger voice. Surgery is followed by additional voice therapy to help fine tune the voice.

When both vocal folds are paralyzed, a tracheotomy may be required to help breathing. In a tracheotomy, an incision is made in the front of the neck and a breathing tube is inserted through an opening, called a stoma, into the trachea. Rather than occurring through the nose and mouth, breathing now happens through the tube. Following surgery, therapy with a speech language pathologist helps you learn how to use the voice and how to properly care for the breathing tube.

Chapter 50

Stem Cell Research for Neurological and Movement Disorders

Stem cells possess the unique ability to differentiate into many distinct cell types in the body, including brain cells, but they also retain the ability to produce more stem cells, a process termed self-renewal. There are multiple types of stem cell, such as embryonic stem (ES) cells, induced pluripotent stem (iPS) cells, and adult or somatic stem cells. While various types of stem cells share similar properties there are differences as well. For example, ES cells and iPS cells are able to differentiate into any type of cell, whereas adult stem cells are more restricted in their potential. The promise of all stem cells for use in future therapies is exciting, but significant technical hurdles remain that will only be overcome through years of intensive research.

This chapter contains text excerpted from the following sources: Text in this chapter begins with excerpts from "Focus on Stem Cell Research," National Institute of Neurological Disorders and Stroke (NINDS), March 19, 2017; Text beginning with the heading "Parkinson Disease—a Major Target for Stem Cell Research" is excerpted from "Repairing the Nervous System with Stem Cells," National Institutes of Health (NIH), October 29, 2017.

Parkinson Disease—a Major Target for Stem Cell Research

The intensive research aiming at curing Parkinson disease with stem cells is a good example for the various strategies, successful results, and remaining challenges of stem cell-based brain repair. Parkinson disease is a progressive disorder of motor control that affects roughly 2 percent of persons 65 years and older. Triggered by the death of neurons in a brain region called the substantia nigra, Parkinson disease begins with minor tremors that progress to limb and bodily rigidity and difficulty initiating movement. These neurons connect via long axons to another region called the striatum, composed of subregions called the caudate nucleus and the putamen. These neurons that reach from the substantia nigra to the striatum release the chemical transmitter dopamine onto their target neurons in the striatum. One of dopamine's major roles is to regulate the nerves that control body movement. As these cells die, less dopamine is produced, leading to the movement difficulties characteristic of Parkinson disease. The causes of death of these neurons are not well understood.

For many years, doctors have treated Parkinson disease patients with the drug levodopa (L-dopa), which the brain converts into dopamine. Although the drug works well initially, levodopa eventually loses its effectiveness, and side-effects increase. Ultimately, many doctors and patients find themselves fighting a losing battle. For this reason, a huge effort is underway to develop new treatments, including growth factors that help the remaining dopamine neurons survive and transplantation procedures to replace those that have died.

Research on Fetal Tissue Transplants in Parkinson Disease

The strategy to use new cells to replace lost ones is not new. Surgeons first attempted to transplant dopamine-releasing cells from a patient's own adrenal glands in the 1980s. Although one of these studies reported a dramatic improvement in the patients' conditions, U.S. surgeons were only able to achieve modest and temporary improvement, insufficient to outweigh the risks of such a procedure. As a result, these human studies were not pursued further.

Another strategy was attempted in the 1970s, in which cells derived from fetal tissue from the mouse substantia nigra was transplanted into the adult rat eye and found to develop into mature dopamine neurons. In the 1980s, several groups showed that transplantation of this type of tissue could reverse Parkinson-like symptoms in rats and monkeys when placed in the damaged areas. The success of the animal studies led to several human trials beginning in the mid-1980s. In some cases, patients showed a lessening of their symptoms. Also, researchers could measure an increase in dopamine neuron function in the striatum of these patients by using a brain-imaging method called positron emission tomography (PET).

The National Institute of Health (NIH) has funded two large and well-controlled clinical trials in the past 15 years in which researchers transplanted tissue from aborted fetuses into the striatum of patients with Parkinson disease. These studies, performed in Colorado and New York, included controls where patients received quot; sham-quot; surgery (no tissue was implanted), and neither the patients nor the scientists who evaluated their progress knew which patients received the implants. The patients' progress was followed for up to eight years. Unfortunately, both studies showed that the transplants offered little benefit to the patients as a group. While some patients showed improvement, others began to suffer from dyskinesias, jerky involuntary movements that are often side effects of long-term L-dopa treatment. This effect occurred in 15 percent of the patients in the Colorado study and more than half of the patients in the New York study. Additionally, the New York study showed evidence that some patients' immune systems were attacking the grafts.

However, promising findings emerged from these studies as well. Younger and milder Parkinson patients responded relatively well to the grafts, and PET scans of patients showed that some of the transplanted dopamine neurons survived and matured. Additionally, autopsies on three patients who died of unrelated causes, years after the surgeries, indicated the presence of dopamine neurons from the graft. These cells appeared to have matured in the same way as normal dopamine neurons, which suggested that they were acting normally in the brain.

Researchers in Sweden followed the severity of dyskinesia in patients for eleven years after neural transplantation and found that the severity was typically mild or moderate. These results suggested that dyskinesias were due to effects that were distinct from the beneficial effects of the grafts. Dyskinesias may therefore be related to the ways that transplantation disturbs other cells in the brain and so may be minimized by future improvements in therapy. Another study that involved the grafting of cells both into the striatum (the target of dopamine neurons) and the substantia nigra (where dopamine neurons normally reside) of three patients showed no adverse effects and some modest improvement in patient movement. To determine the full extent of therapeutic benefits from such a procedure and confirm the reliability of these results, this study will need to be repeated with a larger patient population that includes the appropriate controls.

The limited success of these studies may reflect variations in the fetal tissue used for transplantation, which is of limited quantity and can not be standardized or well-characterized. The full complement of cells in these fetal tissue samples is not known at present. As a result, the tissue remains the greatest source of uncertainty in patient outcome following transplantation.

Stem Cells as a Source of Neurons for Transplantation in Parkinson Disease

The major goal for Parkinson investigators is to generate a source of cells that can be grown in large supply, maintained indefinitely in the laboratory, and differentiated efficiently into dopamine neurons that work when transplanted into the brain of a Parkinson patient. Scientists have investigated the behavior of stem cells in culture and the mechanisms that govern dopamine neuron production during development in their attempts to identify optimal culture conditions that allow stem cells to turn into dopamine-producing neurons.

Preliminary studies have been carried out using immature stem cell-like precursors from the rodent ventral midbrain, the region that normally gives rise to these dopamine neurons. In one study these precursors were turned into functional dopamine neurons, which were then grafted into rats previously treated with 6-hydroxy-dopamine (6-OHDA) to kill the dopamine neurons in their substantia nigra and induce Parkinson-like symptoms. Even though the percentage of surviving dopamine neurons was low following transplantation, it was sufficient to relieve the Parkinson-like symptoms. Unfortunately, these fetal cells cannot be maintained in culture for very long before they lose the ability to differentiate into dopamine neurons.

Cells with features of neural stem cells have been derived from ES-cells, fetal brain tissue, brain tissue from neurosurgery, and brain tissue that was obtained after a person's death. There is controversy about whether other organ stem cell populations, such as hematopoietic stem cells, either contain or give rise to neural stem cells

Many researchers believe that the more primitive ES cells may be an excellent source of dopamine neurons because ES-cells can be grown indefinitely in a laboratory dish and can differentiate into any cell type, even after long periods in culture. Mouse ES cells injected directly into

6-OHDA-treated rat brains led to relief of Parkinson-like symptoms. Further investigation showed that these ES cells had differentiated into both dopamine and serotonin neurons. This latter type of neuron is generated in an adjacent region of the brain and may complicate the response to transplantation. Since ES cells can generate all cell types in the body, unwanted cell types such as muscle or bone could theoretically also be introduced into the brain. As a result, a great deal of effort is being put into finding the right quot; recipequot; for turning ES cells into dopamine neurons—and only this cell type—to treat Parkinson disease. Researchers strive to learn more about normal brain development to help emulate the natural progression of ES cells toward dopamine neurons in the culture dish.

The availability of human ES cells has led to further studies to examine their potential for differentiation into dopamine neurons. Dopamine neurons from human embryonic stem cells have been generated. One research group used a special type of companion cell, along with specific growth factors, to promote the differentiation of the ES cells through several stages into dopamine neurons. These neurons showed many of the characteristic properties of normal dopamine neurons. Furthermore, evidence of more direct neuronal differentiation methods from mouse ES cells fuels hope that scientists can refine and streamline the production of transplantable human dopamine neurons.

One method with great therapeutic potential is nuclear transfer. This method fuses the genetic material from one individual donor with a recipient egg cell that has had its nucleus removed. The early embryo that develops from this fusion is a genetic match for the donor. This process is sometimes called quot; therapeutic cloning quote; and is regarded by some to be ethically questionable. However, mouse ES cells have been differentiated successfully in this way into dopamine neurons that corrected Parkinsonian symptoms when transplanted into 6-OHDA-treated rats. Similar results have been obtained using parthenogenetic primate stem cells, which are cells that are genetic matches from a female donor with no contribution from a male donor. These approaches may offer the possibility of treating patients with genetically-matched cells, thereby eliminating the possibility of graft rejection.

Activating the Brain's Own Stem Cells to Repair Parkinson Disease

Scientists are also studying the possibility that the brain may be able to repair itself with therapeutic support. This avenue of study is in its early stages but may involve administering drugs that stimulate the birth of new neurons from the brain's own stem cells. The concept is based on research showing that new nerve cells are born in the adult brains of humans. The phenomenon occurs in a brain region called the dentate gyrus of the hippocampus. While it is not yet clear how these new neurons contribute to normal brain function, their presence suggests that stem cells in the adult brain may have the potential to rewire dysfunctional neuronal circuitry.

The adult brain's capacity for self-repair has been studied by investigating how the adult rat brain responds to transforming growth factor alpha (TGFα), a protein important for early brain development that is expressed in limited quantities in adults. Injection of TGFα into a healthy rat brain causes stem cells to divide for several days before ceasing division. In 6-OHDAtreated (Parkinsonian) rats, however, the cells proliferated and migrated to the damaged areas. Surprisingly, the TGFα-treated rats showed few of the behavioral problems associated with untreated Parkinsonian rats.

These findings suggest that the brain can repair itself, as long as the repair process is triggered sufficiently. It is not clear, though, whether stem cells are responsible for this repair or if the TGF activates a different repair mechanism.

Part Six

Living with Movement Disorders

Chapter 51

Long-Term Care

In the year 2000, almost 10 million people needed some form of long-term care in the United States. Of this population, 3.6 million (37%) were under age 65 and 6 million (63%) were over age 65. Recent research suggests that most Americans turning age 65 will need long-term care at some point in their lives. This section of the website provides basic information so you can begin to think about how you will handle the need for long-term care. Your path will be unique to you, and based on your preferences and circumstances.

What is Long-Term Care?

Long-term care is a range of services and supports you may need to meet your personal care needs. Most long-term care is not medical care, but rather assistance with the basic personal tasks of everyday life, sometimes called Activities of Daily Living (ADLs), such as:

- Bathing
- Dressing
- Using the toilet
- Transferring (to or from bed or chair)
- Caring for incontinence
- Eating

This chapter includes text excerpted from "Find Your Path Forward," Administration for Community Living (ACL), October 10, 2017.

Other common long-term care services and supports are assistance with everyday tasks, sometimes called Instrumental Activities of Daily Living (IADLs) including:

- Housework

- Managing money

- Taking medication

- Preparing and cleaning up after meals

- Shopping for groceries or clothes

- Using the telephone or other communication devices

- Caring for pets

- Responding to emergency alerts such as fire alarms

Who Needs Care?

Recent research suggests that most Americans turning age 65 will need long-term care services at some point in their lives.

Age

- The older you are, the more likely you will need long-term care

Gender

- Women outlive men by about five years on average, so they are more likely to live at home alone when they are older

Disability

- Having an accident or chronic illness that causes a disability is another reason for needing long-term care

- Between ages 40 and 50, on average, eight percent of people have a disability that could require long-term care services

- 69 percent of people age 90 or more have a disability

Health Status

- Chronic conditions such as diabetes and high blood pressure make you more likely to need care

- Your family history such as whether your parents or grandparents had chronic conditions, may increase your likelihood

- Poor diet and exercise habits increase your chances of needing long-term care

Living Arrangements

- If you live alone, you're more likely to need paid care than if you're married, or single, and living with a partner

How Much Care Will You Need?

The duration and level of long-term care will vary from person to person and often change over time. Here are some statistics (all are "on average") you should consider:

- Someone turning age 65 today has almost a 70 percent chance of needing some type of long-term care services and supports in their remaining years

- **Women need care longer** (3.7 years) than men (2.2 years)

- **One-third of today's 65 year-olds** may never need long-term care support, but 20 percent will need it for longer than 5 years

Who Will Provide Your Care?

Long-term care services and support typically come from:

- An **unpaid caregiver** who may be a family member or friend

- A nurse, home health or home care aide, and/or therapist who comes to the home

- Adult day services in the area

- A **variety** of long-term care facilities

A caregiver can be your family member, partner, friend or neighbor who helps care for you while you live at home. About 80 percent of care at home is provided by unpaid caregivers and may include an array of emotional, financial, nursing, social, homemaking, and other services. On average, caregivers spend 20 hours a week giving care. More than half (58 percent) have intensive caregiving responsibilities that may include assisting with a personal care activity, such as bathing or feeding.

Information on caregivers show that:

- About 65.7 million people in the United States (one in four adults) were unpaid family caregivers to an adult or child in 2009

- About two-thirds are women

- Fourteen percent who care for older adults are themselves age 65 or more

- Most people can live at home for many years with help from unpaid family and friends, and from other paid community support

Where Can You Receive Care?

Most long-term care is provided at home. Other kinds of long-term care services and supports are provided by community service organizations and in long-term care facilities.

Examples of **home care services** include:

- An unpaid caregiver who may be a family member or friend

- A nurse, home health or home care aide, and/or therapist who comes to the home

Community support services include:

- Adult day care service centers

- Transportation services

- Home care agencies that provide services on a daily basis or as needed

Often these services supplement the care you receive at home or provide time off for your family caregivers.

Outside the home, a variety of facility-based programs offer more options:

- **Nursing homes** provide the most comprehensive range of services, including nursing care and 24-hour supervision

- Other facility-based choices include **assisted living, board and care homes, and continuing care retirement communities**. With these providers, the level of choice over who delivers your care varies by the type of facility. You may not get to choose who will deliver services, and you may have limited say in when they arrive.

Participant Directed Services are a way to provide services that lets you control what services you receive, who provides them, and how and when those services are delivered. They provide you with information and assistance to choose and plan for the services and supports that work best for you including:

- Who you want to provide your services (can include family and friends
- Whether you want to use a home care service agency

In **facility-based services** you generally don't have the option to hire someone independently, but you should have choices about:

- Which staff members provide your care
- The schedule you keep
- The meals you eat

In **home and community-based settings**, you should have the ability to participate or **direct the development** of a service plan, provide feedback on services and activities, and request changes as needed.

Who Pays for Long-Term Care?

Consumer surveys reveal common misunderstandings about which public programs pay for long-term care services. It is important to clearly understand what is and isn't covered.

Medicare:

Only pays for long-term care if you require skilled services or rehabilitative care:

- In a nursing home for a maximum of 100 days, however, the average Medicare covered stay is much shorter (22 days).
- At home if you are also receiving skilled home health or other skilled in-home services. Generally, long-term care services are provided only for a short period of time.
- Does not pay for nonskilled assistance with Activities of Daily Living (ADL), which make up the majority of long-term care services
- You will have to pay for long-term care services that are not covered by a public or private insurance program

Medicaid:

- Does pay for the largest share of long-term care services, but to qualify, your income must be below a certain level and you must meet minimum state eligibility requirements

- Such requirements are based on the amount of assistance you need with ADL

- Other federal programs such as the Older Americans Act and the Department of Veterans Affairs pay for long-term care services, but only for specific populations and in certain circumstances

Health Insurance:

Most employer-sponsored or private health insurance, including health insurance plans, cover only the same kinds of limited services as Medicare

If they do cover long-term care, it is typically only for skilled, short-term, medically necessary care

There are an increasing number of private payment options including:

- Long-term care insurance

- Reverse mortgages

- Life insurance options

- Annuities

Chapter 52

Prevention of Falls

A simple thing can change your life—like tripping on a rug, or slipping on a wet floor. If you fall, you could break a bone, like thousands of older men and women do each year. For older people, a break can be the start of more serious problems, such as a trip to the hospital, injury, or even disability.

If you or an older person you know has fallen, you're not alone. More than one in three people age 65 years or older falls each year. The risk of falling—and fall related problems—rises with age.

Many Older Adults Fear Falling

The fear of falling becomes more common as people age, even among those who haven't fallen. It may lead older people to avoid activities such as walking, shopping, or taking part in social activities.

But don't let a fear of falling keep you from being active. Overcoming this fear can help you stay active, maintain your physical health, and prevent future falls. Doing things like getting together with friends, gardening, walking, or going to the local senior center helps you stay healthy. The good news is, there are simple ways to prevent most falls.

This chapter includes text excerpted from "Prevent Falls and Fractures," National Institute on Aging (NIA), National Institutes of Health (NIH), March 15, 2017.

Causes and Risk Factors for Falls

Many things can cause a fall. Your eyesight, hearing, and reflexes might not be as sharp as they were when you were younger. Diabetes, heart disease, or problems with your thyroid, nerves, feet, or blood vessels can affect your balance. Some medicines can cause you to feel dizzy or sleepy, making you more likely to fall. Other causes include safety hazards in the home or community environment.

Scientists have linked several personal risk factors to falling, including muscle weakness, problems with balance and gait, and blood pressure that drops too much when you get up from lying down or sitting (called postural hypotension). Foot problems that cause pain and unsafe footwear, like backless shoes or high heels, can also increase your risk of falling.

Confusion can sometimes lead to falls. For example, if you wake up in an unfamiliar environment, you might feel unsure of where you are. If you feel confused, wait for your mind to clear or until someone comes to help you before trying to get up and walk around.

Some medications can increase a person's risk of falling because they cause side effects like dizziness or confusion. The more medications you take, the more likely you are to fall.

Take the Right Steps to Prevent Falls

If you take care of your overall health, you may be able to lower your chances of falling. Most of the time, falls and accidents don't "just happen." Here are a few tips to help you avoid falls and broken bones:

- **Stay physically active.** Plan an exercise program that is right for you. Regular exercise improves muscles and makes you stronger. It also helps keep your joints, tendons, and ligaments flexible. Mild weight bearing activities, such as walking or climbing stairs, may slow bone loss from osteoporosis.

- **Have your eyes and hearing tested.** Even small changes in sight and hearing may cause you to fall. When you get new eyeglasses or contact lenses, take time to get used to them. Always wear your glasses or contacts when you need them If you have a hearing aid, be sure it fits well and wear it.

- **Find out about the side effects of any medicine you take.** If a drug makes you sleepy or dizzy, tell your doctor or pharmacist.

- **Get enough sleep.** If you are sleepy, you are more likely to fall.

- **Limit the amount of alcohol you drink.** Even a small amount of alcohol can affect your balance and reflexes. Studies show that the rate of hip fractures in older adults increases with alcohol use.

- **Stand up slowly.** Getting up too quickly can cause your blood pressure to drop. That can make you feel wobbly. Get your blood pressure checked when lying and standing.

- **Use an assistive device if you need help feeling steady when you walk.** Appropriate use of canes and walkers can prevent falls. If your doctor tells you to use a cane or walker, make sure it is the right size for you and the wheels roll smoothly. This is important when you're walking in areas you don't know well or where the walkways are uneven. A physical or occupational therapist can help you decide which devices might be helpful and teach you how to use them safely.

- **Be very careful when walking on wet or icy surfaces.** They can be very slippery! Try to have sand or salt spread on icy areas by your front or back door.

- **Wear nonskid, rubber soled, low heeled shoes, or lace up shoes with nonskid soles that fully support your feet.** It is important that the soles are not too thin or too thick. Don't walk on stairs or floors in socks or in shoes and slippers with smooth soles.

- **Always tell your doctor if you have fallen since your last checkup, even if you aren't hurt when you fall.** A fall can alert your doctor to a new medical problem or problems with your medications or eyesight that can be corrected. Your doctor may suggest physical therapy, a walking aid, or other steps to help prevent future falls.

What to Do If You Fall

Whether you are at home or somewhere else, a sudden fall can be startling and upsetting. If you do fall, stay as calm as possible.

Take several deep breaths to try to relax. Remain still on the floor or ground for a few moments. This will help you get over the shock of falling.

Decide if you are hurt before getting up. Getting up too quickly or in the wrong way could make an injury worse.

If you think you can get up safely without help, roll over onto your side. Rest again while your body and blood pressure adjust. Slowly get up on your hands and knees, and crawl to a sturdy chair.

Put your hands on the chair seat and slide one foot forward so that it is flat on the floor. Keep the other leg bent so the knee is on the floor. From this kneeling position, slowly rise and turn your body to sit in the chair.

If you are hurt or cannot get up on your own, ask someone for help or call 911. If you are alone, try to get into a comfortable position and wait for help to arrive.

Carrying a mobile or portable phone with you as you move about your house could make it easier to call someone if you need assistance. An emergency response system, which lets you push a button on a special necklace or bracelet to call for help, is another option.

Keep Your Bones Strong to Prevent Falls

Falls are a common reason for trips to the emergency room and for hospital stays among older adults. Many of these hospital visits are for fall-related fractures. You can help prevent fractures by keeping your bones strong.

Having healthy bones won't prevent a fall, but if you fall, it might prevent breaking a hip or other bone, which may lead to a hospital or nursing home stay, disability, or even death. Getting enough calcium and vitamin D can help keep your bones strong. So can physical activity. Try to get at least 150 minutes per week of physical activity.

Other ways to maintain bone health include quitting smoking and limiting alcohol use, which can decrease bone mass and increase the chance of fractures. Also, try to maintain a healthy weight. Being underweight increases the risk of bone loss and broken bones.

Osteoporosis is a disease that makes bones weak and more likely to break. For people with osteoporosis, even a minor fall may be dangerous. Talk to your doctor about osteoporosis.

Chapter 53

Dressing with Ease,
Style, and Comfort

People with movement disorders can suffer from isolation and emotional issues that affect their health and quality of life. Their self-esteem can decrease because there is a constant dependence on someone for simple daily tasks and a perceived social stigma that they are different from others. However, a person with a movement disability need not go through a dejected life. There are many ways to cope through those hard feelings. Some of them include working on self-acceptance, focusing on the person's strengths rather than weaknesses or inability, fighting social stigma, or getting help from professionals.

Dressing can boost a person's self-confidence. However, a major challenge faced by people with movement disorders is dressing and undressing. When people with movement disorders are able to dress well with ease, style, and comfort, it helps build confidence in the person.

How Can People with Movement Disorders Dress Well?

There are several clothing options available for people with limited mobility. A person with a movement disability can make their own dressing decisions with the support of guardians or caregivers. Clothing that is easier to put on and take off is helpful for a disabled person.

Some options include open-back shirts and jackets, high-back jeans for seated users, zippers replaced with Velcro, large toggles, custom prosthetics, and many others.

Available Dressing Options

Lightweight and stretch-knit fabrics allow easy movement for a person with disability. Garments with openings in the front and wide armholes eliminate the need for hand movements and are easier to be worn and taken off. Some people have problems with hand/finger coordination; however, large buttons that are easily removable are useful—they can be hidden in shirts, dresses, blouses, and pants.

Fabric loops can be fitted on to pants and underwear to make them easier to be put on and pulled off. Also for toileting purposes, trousers with elastic waistbands and French-cut underpants with wide-leg openings are helpful. For women, wraparound skirts with openings in the back or drop seat pants help while traveling and in accommodating weight changes. Culottes give women the look of a skirt and the usefulness of pants. People who have a weaker side should dress the weaker side first as this helps them wear the dress more confidently and reduce any crease in the dress. Few people find it more comfortable to wear clothes while lying down while few others prefer sitting while wearing their pants or inner garments.

When the disorder makes a person sit for a long time, he or she should choose comfortable clothing such as loose tops, short jackets, capes, or ponchos. The type of clothing could be cotton or polyester blend, or a flexible fabric that moves with the body. The comfort of the fabric is based on its heat retention, moisture absorption, and feel. Another option is fleece, which is both fashionable and functional. Soft and slippery fabric like nylon pajamas, dresses, gowns, and nylon lingerie allow the body to slide easily. People who have a breathing problem can use wider necklines and should avoid hairy fabrics like mohair. Clothing choices should depend on comfort, texture, color, and accessibility that suits and helps the person who has a movement disorder.

Dressing aids such as a dressing stick with a hook, buttoners, zipper pulls, stocking aid, and long-handled shoehorn are helpful and easily available for a person with a movement disability. The buttoners help in pulling the buttons through the button holes, zipper pulls help to open and close zips, and the shoehorn assists in getting the shoes on.

Footwear choices depend on the condition of movement disorder. People with weak ankles are checked by a physical therapist and are recommended for the right kind of footwear Some healthcare providers advise patients to wear leg braces for support; wearing knee-high fashion boots is a good way of covering leg braces. Rubber soles in shoes may cause slipping; hence, moccasins are advised. Light and supportive shoes are best for walking along with brace support. Some shoes also have Velcro fasteners that help the person to easily put on the shoes; and laced shoes, if replaced with elastic laces, offer more support.

References

1. "Dressing with Ease, Style and Comfort," ALS Association, n.d.

2. "Dressing in Style for Persons with Disabilities," Serving People with Disability, n.d.

3. Hansen, Tom. "Dressing with Disabilities," Accessible Systems, June 27, 2017.

Chapter 54

Assistive Technology Can Help People with Movement Disorders Live More Independently

Mobility aids help you walk or move from place to place if you are disabled or have an injury. They include:

- Crutches
- Canes
- Walkers
- Wheelchairs
- Motorized scooters

This chapter contains text excerpted from the following sources: Text in this chapter begins with excerpts from "Mobility Aids," MedlinePlus, National Institutes of Health (NIH), September 16, 2016; Text under the heading "Mobility Options for People with Disabilities" is excerpted from "ADA Requirements—Wheelchairs, Mobility Aids, and Other Power-Driven Mobility Devices," ADA.gov, U.S. Department of Justice (DOJ), January 31, 2014. Reviewed January 2018; Text under the heading "What Are Some Types of Assistive Devices and How Are They Used?" is excerpted from "What Are Some Types of Assistive Devices and How Are They Used?" *Eunice Kennedy Shriver* National Institute of Child Health and Human Development (NICHD), December 1, 2016.

You may need a walker or cane if you are at risk of falling. If you need to keep your body weight off your foot, ankle or knee, you may need crutches. You may need a wheelchair or a scooter if an injury or disease has left you unable to walk.

Choosing these devices takes time and research. You should be fitted for crutches, canes and walkers. If they fit, these devices give you support, but if they don't fit, they can be uncomfortable and unsafe.

Mobility Options for People with Disabilities

Wheelchairs

Most people are familiar with the manual and power wheelchairs and electric scooters used by people with mobility disabilities. The term "wheelchair" is defined in the new rules as "a manually-operated or power-driven device designed primarily for use by an individual with a mobility disability for the main purpose of indoor or of both indoor and outdoor locomotion."

Other Power-Driven Mobility Devices

In recent years, some people with mobility disabilities have begun using less traditional mobility devices such as golf cars or Segways®. These devices are called "other power-driven mobility device" (OPDMD) in the rule. OPDMD is defined in the new rules as "any mobility device powered by batteries, fuel, or other engines— that is used by individuals with mobility disabilities for the purpose of locomotion, including golf cars, electronic personal assistance mobility devices—such as the Segway® PT, or any mobility device designed to operate in areas without defined pedestrian routes, but that is not a wheelchair." When an OPDMD is being used by a person with a mobility disability, different rules apply under the Americans with Disabilities Act (ADA) than when it is being used by a person without a disability.

What Are Some Types of Assistive Devices and How Are They Used?

Some examples of assistive technologies are:

- People with physical disabilities that affect movement can use mobility aids, such as wheelchairs, scooters, walkers, canes, crutches, prosthetic devices, and orthotic devices, to enhance their mobility.

- Hearing aids can improve hearing ability in persons with hearing problems.

- Cognitive assistance, including computer or electrical assistive devices, can help people function following brain injury.

- Computer software and hardware, such as voice recognition programs, screen readers, and screen enlargement applications, help people with mobility and sensory impairments use computer technology.

- In the classroom and elsewhere, assistive devices, such as automatic page-turners, book holders, and adapted pencil grips, allow learners with disabilities to participate in educational activities.

- Closed captioning allows people with hearing impairments to enjoy movies and television programs.

- Barriers in community buildings, businesses, and workplaces can be removed or modified to improve accessibility. Such modifications include ramps, automatic door openers, grab bars, and wider doorways.

- Lightweight, high-performance wheelchairs have been designed for organized sports, such as basketball, tennis, and racing.

- Adaptive switches make it possible for a child with limited motor skills to play with toys and games.

- Many types of devices help people with disabilities perform such tasks as cooking, dressing, and grooming. Kitchen implements are available with large, cushioned grips to help people with weakness or arthritis in their hands. Medication dispensers with alarms can help people remember to take their medicine on time. People who use wheelchairs for mobility can use extendable reaching devices to reach items on shelves.

Chapter 55

Rehabilitation Engineering for Physical Functions

What Is Rehabilitation Engineering?

Rehabilitation engineering is the use of engineering principles to:

- develop technological solutions and devices to assist individuals with disabilities, and

- aid the recovery of physical and cognitive functions lost because of disease or injury.

Rehabilitation engineers design and build devices and systems to meet a wide range of needs that can assist individuals with mobility, communication, hearing, vision, and cognition. These tools help people with day-to-day activities related to employment, independent living, and education.

Rehabilitation engineering may involve relatively simple observations of how individuals perform tasks, and making accommodations to eliminate further injuries and discomfort. On the other end of the spectrum, rehabilitation engineering includes sophisticated brain computer interfaces that allow a severely disabled individual to operate

This chapter includes text excerpted from "Rehabilitation Engineering," National Institute of Biomedical Imaging and Bioengineering (NIBIB), November 2016.

computers and other devices simply by thinking about the task they want to perform.

Rehabilitation engineers also improve upon standard rehabilitation methods to regain functions lost due to congenital disorders, disease (such as stroke or joint replacement) or injury (such as limb loss) to restore mobility.

How Can Future Rehabilitation Engineering Research Improve the Quality of Life for Individuals?

Ongoing research in rehabilitation engineering involves the design and development of innovative technologies and techniques that can help people regain physical or cognitive functions. For example:

- **Rehabilitation robotics**, to use robots as therapy aids instead of solely as assistive devices. Smart rehabilitation robotics aid mobility training in individuals suffering from impaired movement, such as following a stroke.

- **Virtual rehabilitation**, which uses virtual reality simulation exercises for physical and cognitive rehabilitation. These tools are entertaining, motivate patients to exercise, and provide objective measures such as range of motion. The exercises can be performed at home by a patient and monitored by a therapist over the Internet (known as telerehabilitation), which offers convenience as well as reduced costs.

- **Physical prosthetics**, such as smarter artificial legs with powered ankles, exoskeletons, dextrous upper limbs and hands. This is an area where researchers continue to make advances in design and function to better mimic natural limb movement and user intent.

- **Advanced kinematics**, to analyze human motion, muscle electrophysiology and brain activity to more accurately monitor human functions and prevent secondary injuries.

- **Sensory prosthetics**, such as retinal and cochlear implants to restore some lost function to provide navigation and communication, increasing independence and integration into the community.

- **Brain computer interfaces**, to enable severely impaired individuals to communicate and access information. These technologies use the brain's electrical impulses to allow individuals to move a computer cursor or a robotic arm that can reach and grab items, or send text messages.

- **Modulation of organ function**, as interventions for urinary and fecal incontinence and sexual disorders. Recent developments in neuromodulation of the peripheral nervous system offer the promise to treat organ function in the case of a spinal cord injury (SCI).

- **Secondary disorder treatment**, such as pain management.

What Are National Institute of Biomedical Imaging and Bioengineering (NIBIB)-Funded Researchers Developing in the Area of Rehabilitation Engineering?

Promising research currently supported by NIBIB includes a wide range of approaches and technological development. Several examples are described below.

Restoring muscle control. People with spinal cord injuries have limited or no ability to control muscle groups below the site of the injury. This often requires assistive mobility devices (crutches, wheelchairs, or powered wheelchairs) and part- or full-time caregiver support. One research team is investigating a technological approach to bypass the injury. They have built a fully-implantable system that uses a sensor to measure voluntary muscle contractions above the injury; the sensor in turn sends electrical signals to trigger muscle activity below the injury. The technology has enabled restoration of standing, stepping, cycling, and hand grasp. Another research team is using electrical stimulus in conjunction with physical therapy to more effectively train the central nervous system (CNS) to enhance the function of the few remaining neurons at the site of the injury. The team uses a completely noninvasive system to train the nervous system below the injury how to walk. This approach has improved walking speed long after the therapy has ended. Another approach uses implantable spinal cord stimulators, originally designed to reduce pain, to alter the neural activity in the spine to restore control of standing and stepping in patients. All of these teams are planning to attain FDA approval for Phase I safety trials.

Prosthesis control. Standard-of-care prostheses for amputees, while increasing in sophistication, lack the ability to reliably detect a user's fine motor commands. Several teams are developing technologies to more accurately record and transmit the user's intent to use their hands to grasp, grip or pinch by recording the electrical signals sent by the user. By implanting electrodes in the residual arm muscles, peripheral nerves, spinal cord, and brain, it is possible to detect these electrical signals, convert them into digital commands, and drive the motors in a hand prosthesis to significantly improve function. Researchers are fine-tuning the system for each limb as well as the different needs of each amputee. By exploring all of these approaches simultaneously, it should be possible to advance the state of the art faster. Several studies have FDA approval for clinical trials, and the others are still undergoing preclinical research prior to advancing to trial.

Closed-loop braces for limbs, spine. Traditional orthoses, or braces, were purely mechanical, passive devices to provide structural, postural, and functional characteristics of the musculoskeletal system. By incorporating electronic sensors, controllers, and motors, it is possible to greatly increase functional performance for users. One approach is to build an ankle-foot brace with a hydraulically adjustable stiffness to mimic the muscles and tendons in a healthy individual. This team is developing a child-size version of the device, which adjusts to maintain a proper fit as the child grows. Another approach is to develop a hydraulic system to use forces from a user's un-impaired or less-impaired limb to support motion by the impaired limb. And yet a third approach is to build an electromechanical control system capable of supporting a complete range of motion for individuals with thoracic/lumbar vertebrae that are compressed or crushed.

Chapter 56

Coping with Chronic Illness and Depression

Depression is a real illness. Treatment can help you live to the fullest extent possible, even when you have another illness.

It is common to feel sad or discouraged after a heart attack, a cancer diagnosis, or if you are trying to manage a chronic condition like pain. You may be facing new limits on what you can do and feel anxious about treatment outcomes and the future. It may be hard to adapt to a new reality and to cope with the changes and ongoing treatment that come with the diagnosis. Your favorite activities, like hiking or gardening, may be harder to do.

Temporary feelings of sadness are expected, but if these and other symptoms last longer than a couple of weeks, you may have depression. Depression affects your ability to carry on with daily life and to enjoy work, leisure, friends, and family. The health effects of depression go beyond mood—depression is a serious medical illness with many symptoms, including physical ones. Some symptoms of depression are:

- Feeling sad, irritable, or anxious.

- Feeling empty, hopeless, guilty, or worthless.

- Loss of pleasure in usually-enjoyed hobbies or activities, including sex.

This chapter includes text excerpted from "Chronic Illness and Mental Health," National Institute of Mental Health (NIMH), December 18, 2015.

- Fatigue and decreased energy, feeling listless.

- Trouble concentrating, remembering details, and making decisions.

- Not being able to sleep, or sleeping too much. Waking too early.

- Eating too much or not wanting to eat at all, possibly with unplanned weight gain or loss.

- Thoughts of death, suicide or suicide attempts.

- Aches or pains, headaches, cramps, or digestive problems without a clear physical cause and/or that do not ease even with treatment.

People with Other Chronic Medical Conditions Have a Higher Risk of Depression

The same factors that increase risk of depression in otherwise healthy people also raise the risk in people with other medical illnesses. These risk factors include a personal or family history of depression or loss of family members to suicide.

However, there are some risk factors directly related to having another illness. For example, conditions such as Parkinson disease and stroke cause changes in the brain. In some cases, these changes may have a direct role in depression. Illness-related anxiety and stress can also trigger symptoms of depression.

Depression is common among people who have chronic illnesses such as the following:

- Cancer

- Coronary heart disease (CHD)

- Diabetes

- Epilepsy

- Multiple sclerosis (MS)

- Stroke

- Alzheimer disease (AD)

- Human immunodeficiency virus infection and acquired immune deficiency syndrome (HIV/AIDS)

- Parkinson disease (PD)

- Systemic lupus erythematosus (SLE)

- Rheumatoid arthritis (RA)

Sometimes, symptoms of depression may follow a recent medical diagnosis but lift as you adjust or as the other condition is treated. In other cases, certain medications used to treat the illness may trigger depression. Depression may persist, even as physical health improves.

Research suggests that people who have depression and another medical illness tend to have more severe symptoms of both illnesses. They may have more difficulty adapting to their co-occurring illness and more medical costs than those who do not also have depression.

It is not yet clear whether treatment of depression when another illness is present can improve physical health. However, it is still important to seek treatment. It can make a difference in day-to-day life if you are coping with a chronic or long-term illness.

People with Depression Are at Higher Risk for Other Medical Conditions

It may have come as no surprise that people with a medical illness or condition are more likely to suffer from depression. The reverse is also true: the risk of developing some physical illnesses is higher in people with depression.

People with depression have an increased risk of CVD, diabetes, stroke, and AD, for example. Research also suggests that people with depression are at higher risk for osteoporosis relative to others. The reasons are not yet clear. One factor with some of these illnesses is that many people with depression may have less access to good medical care. They may have a harder time caring for their health, for example, seeking care, taking prescribed medication, eating well, and exercising.

Ongoing research is also exploring whether physiological changes seen in depression may play a role in increasing the risk of physical illness. In people with depression, scientists have found changes in the way several different systems in the body function, all of which can have an impact on physical health:

- Signs of increased inflammation

- Changes in the control of heart rate and blood circulation

- Abnormalities in stress hormones

- Metabolic changes typical of those seen in people at risk for diabetes

It is not yet clear whether these changes, seen in depression, raise the risk of other medical illness. However, the negative impact of depression on mental health and everyday life is clear.

Depression Is Treatable Even When Other Illness Is Present

Do not dismiss depression as a normal part of having a chronic illness. Effective treatment for depression is available and can help even if you have another medical illness or condition. If you or a loved one think you have depression, it is important to tell your healthcare provider and explore treatment options.

You should also inform the healthcare provider about all treatments or medications you are already receiving, including treatment for depression (prescribed medications and dietary supplements). Sharing information can help avoid problems with multiple medications interfering with each other. It also helps the provider stay informed about your overall health and treatment issues.

Recovery from depression takes time, but treatment can improve the quality of life even if you have a medical illness. Treatments for depression include:

- Cognitive behavioral therapy (CBT), or talk therapy, that helps people change negative thinking styles and behaviors that may contribute to their depression. Interpersonal and other types of time-limited psychotherapy have also been proven effective, in some cases combined with antidepressant medication.

- Antidepressant medications, including, but not limited to, selective serotonin reuptake inhibitors (SSRIs) and serotonin and norepinephrine reuptake inhibitors (SNRIs).

- While electroconvulsive therapy (ECT) is generally reserved for the most severe cases of depression, newer brain stimulation approaches, including transcranial magnetic stimulation (TMS), can help some people with depression without the need for general anesthesia and with few side effects.

Chapter 57

Parenting a Child with a Movement Disorder: Special Concerns

Chapter Contents

Section 57.1

Caring for a Child with Special Needs

This section contains text excerpted from the following sources: Text in this section begins with excerpts from "Responsible Fatherhood Toolkit: Resources from the Field," National Responsible Fatherhood Clearinghouse, U.S. Department of Health and Human Services (HHS), January 6, 2015; Text under the heading "Parenting Strategies for your Child with Special Needs" is excerpted from "Parenting Your Child with Developmental Delays and Disabilities," Child Welfare Information Gateway, U.S. Department of Health and Human Services (HHS), February 7, 2017.

Many families face the challenges associated with raising a child with special needs, a term that covers a broad range of conditions or chronic illnesses such as cerebral palsy, developmental delay, attention deficit hyperactivity disorder (ADHD), dyslexia, autism, Down syndrome, depression, asthma, sickle cell anemia, and cystic fibrosis. According to the 2009–10 National Survey of Children with Special Health Care Needs (NS-CSHCN) approximately 15 percent of children in the United States are estimated to have special health needs and 23 percent of households with children include a child with special health needs. Special health needs exist across a wide spectrum and may involve medical, behavioral, developmental, learning, or mental health issues. But all involve worries and concerns that often lead to feelings of isolation and helplessness for parents.

Experts note that parents of children with special needs often experience grief as they struggle to adapt to their situation. Different kinds of grief exist, and parents should understand there is not a "typical" grief process. In her poem "Welcome to Holland,"Emily Perl Kingsley compares the experience to planning a fabulous vacation in one place, but then having to get accustomed to being somewhere very different. She pointed out that "the pain of that will never, ever, ever, ever, go away because the loss of that dream is a very significant loss," but if you spend your life mourning you may never be free to enjoy the special things about your new destination. Practitioners can help both fathers and mothers navigate what can ultimately be a rewarding journey of resilience.

From a Father's Perspective

Practitioners with personal experience with children with special needs and who work with fathers of children with special health needs describe the feelings fathers may experience:

- Loneliness and isolation
  - James May, a pioneer in the area of fathers of children with special needs, pointed out that feelings of embarrassment about their child's lack of developmental appropriateness and the tendency to have fewer social supports than women lead to high feelings of isolation for many men.
  - At a Fathers Network meeting in Columbia, South Carolina, one father remarked: "All the other dads at the lunch table talked about how successful their kids were in their little league football games the over last weekend ... I'm just thrilled my son is out of pull-up diapers.
- "Hunter-provider" anxiety
  - Many men in fatherhood programs feel ineffective as they struggle to find steady employment and balance their roles as fathers, husbands, and providers. These feelings may amplify when they face the demands and costs of medical or therapeutic care for their children.
  - Greg Schell of the Washington State Fathers Network reported that approximately 86 percent of children with special healthcare needs require prescription medications, 52 percent need specialty medical care, 33 percent need vision care, 25 percent require mental healthcare, 23 percent need specialized therapies, and 11 percent need special medical equipment.
- Strained marital relationships
  - Although divorce rates for couples who have children with special needs are nearly identical to divorce rates of other families, practitioners note that parents in these families often report low rates of marriage satisfaction.
  - Ray Morris noted, "Having a child with special needs can put a strain on even the most solid marriage."
- Feelings of inadequacy
  - According to W.C. Hoecke, some fathers say their partners have become "super saints" or "super educators." They

perceive their partners as "having all the information and answers" and feel their own perspective often is overlooked or ignored in dealing with their child's issues. These feelings can increase if mothers are the "primary receivers of information" and fathers have to rely on "second-hand information" from mothers.

- A father in the Family Connection of South Carolina program said: "I feel I can't compete with her level of informational knowledge about my child's disability, treatments, or knowledgeable care for my child."

Based on their experiences working with fathers who have children with special needs that span a broad spectrum, practitioners in the field also maintain that:

- Responsive fathering is a strong predictor of better developmental outcomes for children, including improved emotional regulation, communication skills, and cognitive and language development.

- Increased father involvement in early intervention services can ease the overall workload for mothers, reduce maternal stress, and strengthen family cohesion. However, fathers' needs often are overlooked.

- Fathers and mothers of children with special needs have many of the same issues and concerns, but there might be differences in how they respond to their child's condition, what they do to cope, and what they find helpful.

- If professionals are not involving fathers with father-specific services, they are missing important opportunities to maximize critical gains and supports for the children.

- Fathers want information about their child's condition and development, what can be done to help, and what services are available to help their child and the family as a whole.

- Fathers want someone outside the family to talk to about their worries and concerns; however, they might not be very good at seeking this type of help. Also, most fathers prefer male support groups because they feel more comfortable sharing their concerns with other men.

- Working is a common coping strategy for fathers and important for their identity and self-esteem. Fathers want flexibility from employers and service providers so they can respond to their children's needs, attend appointments, and be involved in decisions and care for their child.

Parenting Strategies for your Child with Special Needs

- If your child is diagnosed with a disability, remember that you are not alone. Meet and interact with other families of children with special needs, including those with your child's identified disability. You may have many questions about how your child's diagnosis affects your whole family.

- Seek information. Learn the specifics about your child's special needs. When your child is diagnosed with a disability, you should begin interventions as early as possible so your child can make the best possible progress.

- Find resources for your child. Seek referrals from your physician or other advisors to find professionals and agencies that will help your child. Keep in mind that some services that assist your child may also provide programs to benefit your entire family.

- Locate or start a support group. You may appreciate the opportunity to give and receive assistance or encouragement from others who can truly identify with your experience.

- Take a break and give yourself the gift of time to regroup, reestablish your relationships with family members, or reconnect with friends. You will be a better champion for your child when you take the time to care of yourself as well.

- Don't let your child's delay or disability label become the entire focus. Your child has special challenges but is also a member of your family. Seeing your child grow and develop as an individual and part of the family is one of the great pleasures of being a parent.

Section 57.2

Bullying and Disability

This section includes text excerpted from "Bullying and Children
and Youth with Disabilities and Special Health Needs,"
StopBullying.gov, U.S. Department of Health and
Human Services (HHS), October 1, 2017.

What Is Bullying?

Bullying is unwanted, aggressive behavior among school aged children. It involves a real or perceived power imbalance and the behavior is repeated, or has the potential to be repeated, over time.

Both kids who are bullied and kids who bully others may have serious, lasting problems.

Children with physical, developmental, intellectual, emotional, and sensory disabilities are more likely to be bullied than their peers. Any number of factors—physical vulnerability, social skill challenges, or intolerant environments—may increase their risk. Research suggests that some children with disabilities may bully others as well.

Kids with special health needs, such as epilepsy or food allergies, may also be at higher risk of being bullied. For kids with special health needs, bullying can include making fun of kids because of their allergies or exposing them to the things they are allergic to. In these cases, bullying is not just serious; it can mean life or death.

A small but growing amount of research shows that:

- Children with attention deficit hyperactivity disorder (ADHD) are more likely than other children to be bullied. They also are somewhat more likely than others to bully their peers.

- Children with autism spectrum disorder (ASD) are at increased risk of being bullied and left out by peers. In a study of 8–17-year-olds, researchers found that children with ASD were more than three times as likely to be bullied as their peers.

- Children with epilepsy are more likely to be bullied by peers, as are children with medical conditions that affect their appearance, such as cerebral palsy, muscular dystrophy, and spina bifida. These children frequently report being called names related to their disability.

- Children with hemiplagia (paralysis of one side of their body) are more likely than other children their age to be bullied and have fewer friends.

- Children who have diabetes and are dependent on insulin may be especially vulnerable to peer bullying.

- Children who stutter may be more likely to be bullied. In one study, 83 percent of adults who stammered as children said that they were teased or bullied; 71 percent of those who had been bullied said it happened at least once a week.

- Children with learning disabilities (LD) are at a greater risk of being bullied. At least one study also has found that children with LD may also be more likely than other children to bullying their peers.

Effects of Bullying

Kids who are bullied are more likely to have:

- Depression and anxiety. Signs of these include increased feelings of sadness and loneliness, changes in sleep and eating patterns, and loss of interest in activities they used to enjoy. These issues may persist into adulthood.

- Health complaints.

- Decreased academic achievement—grade point average (GPA) and standardized test scores—and school participation. They are more likely to miss, skip, or drop out of school.

Bullying, Disability Harassment, and the Law

Bullying behavior can become "disability harassment," which is prohibited under Section 504 of the Rehabilitation Act of 1973 and Title II of the *Americans with Disabilities Act (ADA) of 1990*. According to the U.S. Department of Education (ED), disability harassment is "intimidation or abusive behavior toward a student based on disability that creates a hostile environment by interfering with or denying a student's participation in or receipt of benefits, services, or opportunities in the institution's program."

Disability harassment can take different forms including verbal harassment, physical threats, or threatening written statements. When a school learns that disability harassment may have occurred, the school must investigate the incident(s) promptly and respond appropriately. Disability harassment can occur in any location that is connected with school—classrooms, the cafeteria, hallways, the playground, athletic fields, or school buses. It also can occur during school-sponsored events.

What Parents Can Do

If you believe a child with special needs is being bullied:

- Be supportive of the child and encourage him or her to describe who was involved and how and where the bullying happened. Be sure to tell the child that it is not his or her fault and that nobody deserves to be bullied or harassed. Do not encourage the child to fight back. This may make the problem worse.

- Ask the child specific questions about his or her friendships. Be aware of signs of bullying, even if the child doesn't call it that. Children with disabilities do not always realize they are being bullied. They may, for example, believe that they have a new friend although this "friend" is making fun of them.

- Talk with the child's teacher immediately to see whether he or she can help to resolve the problem.

- Put your concerns in writing and contact the principal if the bullying or harassment is severe or the teacher doesn't fix the problem. Explain what happened in detail and ask for a prompt response. Keep a written record of all conversations and communications with the school.

- Ask the school district to convene a meeting of the Individualized Education Program (IEP) or the Section 504 teams. These groups ensure that the school district is meeting the needs of its students with disabilities. This meeting will allow parents to explain what has been happening and will let the team review the child's IEP or 504 plans and make sure that the school is taking steps to stop the harassment. Parents, if your child needs counseling or other supportive services because of the harassment, discuss this with the team. Work with the school to help establish a system-wide bullying prevention program that includes support systems for bullied children. As the ED recognizes, "creating a supportive school climate is the most important step in preventing harassment."

- Explore whether the child may also be bullying other younger, weaker students at school. If so, his or her IEP may need to be modified to include help to change the aggressive behavior.

- Be persistent. Talk regularly with the child and with school staff to see whether the behavior has stopped.

Chapter 58

Caring for Someone with Disabilities

If you are a family member who cares for someone with a disability, whether a child or an adult, combining personal, caregiving, and everyday needs can be challenging.

Caregiving Tips for Families of People with Disabilities

These general caregiving tips provide families with information on how to stay healthy and positive. Keep in mind that these tips can be used to address many family issues. Information, support, advocacy, empowerment, care, and balance can be the foundation for a healthy family and are appropriate no matter what the challenge.

Be Informed

- Gather information about your family member's condition, and discuss issues with others involved in the care of your family member. Being informed will help you make more knowledgeable health decisions and improve your understanding about any challenges your family might face.

- Notice how others care for the person with special needs. Be aware of signs of mental or physical abuse.

This chapter includes text excerpted from "Disability and Health—Family Caregivers," Centers for Disease Control and Prevention (CDC), August 3, 2017.

Get Support

- Family members and friends can provide support in a variety of ways and oftentimes want to help. Determine if there are big or small things they can do to assist you and your family.

- Join a local or online support group. A support group can give you the chance to share information and connect with people who are going through similar experiences. A support group may help combat the isolation and fear you may experience as a caregiver.

- Don't limit your involvement to support groups and associations that focus on a particular need or disability. There are also local and national groups that provide services, recreation, and information for people with disabilities.

- Friends, family, healthcare providers, support groups, community services, and counselors are just a few of the people available to help you and your family.

Be an Advocate

- Be an advocate for your family member with a disability. Caregivers who are effective advocates may be more successful at getting better service.

- Ask questions. For example, if your family member with a disability uses a wheelchair and you want to plan a beach vacation, find out if the beaches are accessible via a car, ramp, portable walkway mat, or other equipment.

- Inform other caregivers of any special conditions or circumstances. For example, if your family member with a disability has a latex allergy, remind dental or medical staff each time you visit them.

- Document the medical history of your family member with a disability, and keep this information current.

- Make sure your employer understands your circumstances and limitations. Discuss your ability to travel or to work weekends or evenings. Arrange for flexible scheduling when needed.

- Become familiar with the Americans with Disabilities Act (ADA), the Family Medical Leave Act (FMLA), and other state and national provisions. Know how and when to apply them to your situation.

Be Empowering

- Focus on what you and your family member with a disability can do.

- Find appropriate milestones and celebrate them.

- If someone asks you questions about the family member with a disability, let him or her answer when possible. Doing so may help empower the individual to engage with others.

- When appropriate, teach your family member with a disability to be as independent and self-assured as possible. Always keep health and safety issues in mind.

- Man on elliptical machine

Take Care of Yourself

- Take care of yourself. Caring for a family member with a disability can wear out even the strongest caregiver. Stay healthy for yourself and those you care for.

- Work hard to maintain your personal interests, hobbies, and friendships. Don't let caregiving consume your entire life. This is not healthy for you or those you care for. Balance is key.

- Allow yourself not to be the perfect caregiver. Set reasonable expectations to lower stress and make you a more effective caregiver.

- Delegate some caregiving tasks to other reliable people.

- Take a break. Short breaks, like an evening walk or relaxing bath, are essential. Long breaks are nurturing. Arrange a retreat with friends or get away with a significant other when appropriate.

- Don't ignore signs of illness: if you get sick, see a healthcare provider. Pay attention to your mental and emotional health as well. Remember, taking good care of yourself can help the person you care for as well. Exercising and eating healthy also are important.

Keep Balance in the Family

- Family members with a disability may require extra care and attention. Take time for all family members, taking into account the needs of each individual. For example, it's important for parents of a child with a disability to also spend time with each other and with any other children they might have.

• Consider respite care. "Respite" refers to short-term, temporary care provided to people with disabilities so that their families can take a break from the daily routine of caregiving.

Emergency and Disaster Preparedness

It is important that people with disabilities and their caregivers make plans to protect themselves in the event of an emergency or disaster. Emergencies and disasters can strike quickly and without warning and can force people to leave their home or be confined in their home. For the millions of Americans who have disabilities, emergencies such as acts of terrorism, and disasters such as fires and floods, present a real challenge.

Chapter 59

Social Security Benefits for People with Disabilities

Disability is something most people don't like to think about. But the chances that you'll become disabled probably are greater than you realize. Studies show that a 20-year-old worker has a 1-in-4 chance of becoming disabled before reaching full retirement age.

Social Security pay disability benefits through two programs: the Social Security disability insurance (SSDI) program and the Supplemental Security Income (SSI) program.

Who Can Get Social Security Disability Benefits?

Social Security pays benefits to people who can't work because they have a medical condition that's expected to last at least one year or result in death. Federal law requires this very strict definition of disability. While some programs give money to people with partial disability or short-term disability, Social Security does not. Certain family members of disabled workers can also receive money from Social Security.

This chapter includes text excerpted from "Disability Benefits," U.S. Social Security Administration (SSA), January 15, 2017.

How Do I Meet the Earnings Requirement for Disability Benefits?

In general, to get disability benefits, you must meet two different earnings tests:

1. A recent work test, based on your age at the time you became disabled; and

2. A duration of work test to show that you worked long enough under Social Security. Certain blind workers have to meet only the duration of work test.

How Do I Apply for Disability Benefits?

There are two ways that you can apply for disability benefits. You can:

1. Apply online at www.socialsecurity.gov; or

2. Call their toll-free number, 800-772-1213, to make an appointment to file a disability claim at your local Social Security office or to set up an appointment for someone to take your claim over the telephone. The disability claims interview lasts about one hour. If you're deaf or hard of hearing, you may call their toll-free TTY number, 800-325-0778, between 7 a.m. and 7 p.m. on business days.

If you schedule an appointment, you'll receive a Disability Starter Kit to help you get ready for your disability claims interview.

You have the right to representation by an attorney or other qualified person of your choice when you do business with Social Security.

When Should I Apply and What Information Do I Need?

You should apply for disability benefits as soon as you become disabled. Processing an application for disability benefits can take three to five months. To apply for disability benefits, you'll need to complete an application for Social Security benefits. You can apply online at www.socialsecurity.gov.

The information required includes:

- Your Social Security number (SSN);

- Your birth or baptismal certificate;

- Names, addresses, and phone numbers of the doctors, caseworkers, hospitals, and clinics that took care of you, and dates of your visits;

- Names and dosage of all the medicine you take;

- Medical records from your doctors, therapists, hospitals, clinics, and caseworkers that you already have in your possession;

- Laboratory and test results;

- A summary of where you worked and the kind of work you did; and

- A copy of your most recent W-2 Form (Wage and Tax Statement) or, if you're self-employed, your federal tax returns for the past year.

In addition to the basic application for disability benefits, you'll also need to fill out other forms. One form collects information about your medical condition and how it affects your ability to work. Other forms give doctors, hospitals, and other healthcare professionals who have treated you, permission to send us information about your medical condition.

Don't delay applying for benefits if you can't get all of this information together quickly. The U.S. Social Security Administration (SSA) will help you get it.

Who Decides If I Am Disabled?

The Social Security Administration (SSA) reviews the application to make sure you meet some basic requirements for disability benefits. They will check whether you worked enough years to qualify. Also, they will evaluate any current work activities. If you meet these requirements, they will process your application and forward your case to the Disability Determination Services (DDS) office in your state.

This state agency completes the initial disability determination decision for the SSA. Doctors and disability specialists in the state agency ask your doctors for information about your condition. They'll consider all the facts in your case. They'll use the medical evidence from your doctors, hospitals, clinics, or institutions where you've been treated and all other information. They'll ask your doctors about:

- Your medical condition(s);

- When your medical condition(s) began;

- How your medical condition(s) limit your activities;
- Medical tests results; and
- What treatment you've received.

They'll also ask the doctors for information about your ability to do work-related activities, such as walking, sitting, lifting, carrying, and remembering instructions. Your doctors don't decide if you're disabled.

The state agency staff may need more medical information before they can decide if you're disabled. If your medical sources can't provide needed information, the state agency may ask you to go for a special examination. It is preferable to ask your own doctor, but sometimes the exam may have to be done by someone else. Social Security will pay for the exam and for some of the related travel costs.

How SSA Make the Decision

The SSA use a five-step process to decide if you're disabled.

1. **Are you working?** If you're working and your earnings average more than a certain amount each month, you generally won't be considered to be disabled. The amount changes each year. If you're not working, or your monthly earnings average to the current amount or less, the state agency then looks at your medical condition.

2. **Is your medical condition "severe"?** For you to be considered to have a disability by Social Security's definition, your medical condition must significantly limit your ability to do basic work activities—such as lifting, standing, walking, sitting, and remembering—for at least 12 months. If your medical condition isn't severe SSA won't consider you to be disabled. If your condition is severe, they will proceed to step three.

3. **Does your impairment(s) meet or medically equal a listing?** The SSA list of impairments (the listings) describes medical conditions that they consider severe enough to prevent a person from completing substantial gainful activity, regardless of age, education, or work experience. If your medical condition (or combination of medical conditions) isn't on this list, the state agency looks to see if your condition is as severe as a condition on the list. If the severity of your medical condition meets or equals the severity of a listed impairment, the state

agency will decide that you have a qualifying disability. If the severity of your condition doesn't meet or equal the severity level of a listed impairment, the state agency goes on to step four.

4. **Can you do the work you did before?** At this step, SSA will decide if your medical impairment(s) prevents you from performing any of your past work. If it doesn't, they will decide you don't have a qualifying disability. If it does, they will proceed to step five.

5. **Can you do any other type of work?** If you can't do the work you did in the past, they look to see if there's other work you can do despite your impairment(s). They consider your age, education, past work experience, and any skills you may have that could be used to do other work. If you can't do other work, they will decide that you're disabled. If you can do other work, they will decide that you don't have a qualifying disability.

How Will SSA Tell Me Their Decision?

SSA Will Tell You Their Decision

When the state agency makes a determination on your case, they will send a letter to you. If your application is approved, the letter will show the amount of your benefit, and when your payments start. If your application isn't approved, the letter will explain why and tell you how to appeal the determination if you don't agree with it.

What If I Disagree?

If you disagree with a decision made on your claim, you can appeal it. The steps you can take are explained in The Appeals Process, which is available from Social Security.

Chapter 60

Legal Issues in Planning for Incapacity

Advance Care Planning (ACP) is not just about old age. At any age, a medical crisis could leave someone too ill to make his or her own healthcare decisions. Even if you are not sick now, making healthcare plans for the future is an important step toward making sure you get the medical care you would want, even when doctors and family members are making the decisions for you.

What Is Advance Care Planning?

Advance care planning involves learning about the types of decisions that might need to be made, considering those decisions ahead of time, and then letting others know about your preferences. These preferences are often put into an advance directive, a legal document that goes into effect only if you are incapacitated and unable to speak for yourself. This could be the result of disease or severe injury—no matter how old you are. It helps others know what type of medical care you want. It also allows you to express your values and desires related to end-of-life care. You might think of an advance directive as a living document—one that you can adjust as your situation changes because of new information or a change in your health.

This chapter includes text excerpted from "Advance Care Planning: Healthcare Directives," National Institute on Aging (NIA), National Institutes of Health (NIH), May 17, 2017.

Medical Research and Advance Care Planning

Research shows that advance directives can make a difference and that people who document their preferences in this way are more likely to get the care they prefer at the end of life than people who do not.

Decisions That Could Come up near Death

Sometimes when doctors believe a cure is no longer possible and you are dying, decisions must be made about the use of emergency treatments to keep you alive. Doctors can use several artificial or mechanical ways to try to do this. Decisions that might come up at this time include:

Cardiopulmonary resuscitation (CPR). CPR might restore your heartbeat if your heart stops or is in a life-threatening abnormal rhythm. The heart of a young, otherwise healthy person might resume beating normally after CPR. An otherwise healthy older person, whose heart is beating erratically or not beating at all, might also be helped by CPR. CPR is less likely to work for an older person who is ill, can't be successfully treated, and is already close to death. It involves repeatedly pushing on the chest with force, while putting air into the lungs. This force has to be quite strong, and sometimes ribs are broken or a lung collapses. Electric shocks known as defibrillation and medicines might also be used as part of the process.

Ventilator use. Ventilators are machines that help you breathe. A tube connected to the ventilator is put through the throat into the trachea (windpipe) so the machine can force air into the lungs. Putting the tube down the throat is called intubation. Because the tube is uncomfortable, medicines are used to keep you sedated (unconscious) while on a ventilator. If you can't breathe on your own after a few days, a doctor may perform a tracheotomy or "trach" (rhymes with "make"). During this bedside surgery, the tube is inserted directly into the trachea through a hole in the neck. For long-term help with breathing, a trach is more comfortable, and sedation is not needed. People using such a breathing tube aren't able to speak without special help because exhaled air goes out of the trach rather than past their vocal cords.

Artificial nutrition or artificial hydration. A feeding tube and/or intravenous (IV) liquids are sometimes used to provide nutrition when a person is not able to eat or drink. These measures can be helpful if you are recovering from an illness. However, if you are near death, these could actually make you more uncomfortable. For example, IV liquids, which are given through a plastic tube put into a vein, can increase the burden on failing kidneys. Or if the body is shutting down near death, it is not able to digest food properly, even when provided through a feeding tube. At first, the feeding tube is threaded through the nose down to the stomach. In time, if tube feeding is still needed, the tube is surgically inserted into the stomach.

Comfort care. Comfort care is anything that can be done to soothe you and relieve suffering while staying in line with your wishes. Comfort care includes managing shortness of breath; offering ice chips for dry mouth; limiting medical testing; providing spiritual and emotional counseling; and giving medication for pain, anxiety, nausea, or constipation. Often this is done through hospice, which may be offered in the home, in a hospice facility, in a skilled nursing facility, or in a hospital.

Getting Started

Start by thinking about what kind of treatment you do or do not want in a medical emergency. It might help to talk with your doctor about how your present health conditions might influence your health in the future. For example, what decisions would you or your family face if your high blood pressure leads to a stroke? Medicare or private health insurance may cover these discussions with your doctor.

If you don't have any medical issues now, your family medical history might be a clue to thinking about the future. Talk with your doctor about decisions that might come up if you develop health problems similar to those of other family members.

In considering treatment decisions, your personal values are key. Is your main desire to have the most days of life, or to have the most life in your days? What if an illness leaves you paralyzed or in a permanent coma and you need to be on a ventilator? Would you want that?

What makes life meaningful to you? If your heart stops or you have trouble breathing, would you want to undergo life-saving measures if it meant that, in the future, you could be well enough to spend time with your family? Even if the emergency leaves you simply able to spend your days listening to books on tape or gazing out the window watching the birds and squirrels compete for seeds in the bird feeder, you might be content with that.

But, there are many other scenarios. Here are a few. What would you decide?

- If a stroke leaves you paralyzed and then your heart stops, would you want CPR? What if you were also mentally impaired by a stroke—does your decision change?

- What if you become unable to feed yourself near the end of life? Would you want a feeding tube used to give you nutrition?

- What if you are permanently unconscious and then develop pneumonia? Would you want antibiotics and a ventilator used?

For some people, staying alive as long as medically possible is the most important thing. An advance directive can help make sure that happens.

Your decisions about how to handle any of these situations could be different at age 40 than at age 85. Or they could be different if you have an incurable condition as opposed to being generally healthy. An advance directive allows you to provide instructions for these types of situations and then to change the instructions as you get older or if your viewpoint changes.

Do You or a Family Member Have Alzheimer Disease (AD)?

Many people are unprepared to deal with the legal and financial consequences of a serious illness such as Alzheimer disease (AD). Advance planning can help people with AD and their families clarify their wishes and make well-informed decisions about healthcare and financial arrangements.

Making Your Wishes Known

There are two main elements in an advance directive—a living will and a durable power of attorney for healthcare. There are also other documents that can supplement your advance directive. You can choose which documents to create, depending on how you want decisions to be made. These documents include:

Living will. A living will is a written document that helps you tell doctors how you want to be treated if you are dying or permanently unconscious and cannot make decisions about emergency treatment. In a living will, you can say which of the procedures you would want, which ones you wouldn't want, and under which conditions each of your choices applies.

Durable power of attorney for healthcare. A durable power of attorney for healthcare is a legal document naming a healthcare proxy, someone to make medical decisions for you when you are unable to do so. Your proxy, also known as a representative, surrogate, or agent, should be familiar with your values and wishes. This means that he or she will be able to decide as you would when treatment decisions need to be made. A proxy can be chosen in addition to or instead of a living will. Having a healthcare proxy helps you plan for situations that cannot be foreseen, like a serious auto accident.

Some people are reluctant to put specific health decisions in writing. For them, naming a healthcare agent might be a good approach, especially if there is someone they feel comfortable talking with about their values and preferences. In this case, the proxy can evaluate each situation or treatment option independently.

Other advance care planning documents. You might also want to prepare documents to express your wishes about a single medical issue or something not covered in your advance directive. A living will usually covers only the specific life-sustaining treatments discussed earlier. You might want to give your healthcare proxy specific instructions about other issues, such as blood transfusion or kidney dialysis. This is especially important if your doctor suggests that, given your health condition, such treatments might be needed in the future.

Two medical issues that might arise at the end of life are do-not-resuscitate (DNR) orders and organ and tissue donation.

A **DNR order** tells medical staff in a hospital or nursing facility that you do not want them to try to return your heart to a normal rhythm if it stops or is beating unevenly. Even though a living will might say CPR is not wanted, it is helpful to have a DNR order as part of your medical file if you go to a hospital. Posting a DNR next to your bed might avoid confusion in an emergency situation. Without a DNR order, medical staff will make every effort to restore the normal rhythm of your heart. A nonhospital DNR will alert emergency medical personnel to your wishes regarding CPR and other measures to restore your heartbeat if you are not in the hospital. A similar document that is less familiar is called a DNI (do not intubate) order. A DNI tells medical staff in a hospital or nursing facility that you do not want to be put on a breathing machine.

Organ and tissue donation allows organs or body parts from a generally healthy person who has died to be transplanted into people who need them. Commonly, the heart, lungs, pancreas, kidneys, corneas, liver, and skin are donated. There is no age limit for organ and tissue donation.

At the time of death, family members may be asked about organ donation. If those close to you, especially your proxy, know how you feel about organ donation, they will be ready to respond. There is no cost to the donor's family for this gift of life. If the person has requested a DNR order but wants to donate organs, he or she might have to indicate that the desire to donate supersedes the DNR. That is because it might be necessary to use machines to keep the heart beating until the medical staff is ready to remove the donated organs.

What Are Physician Orders for Life-Sustaining Treatment (POLST) and Medical Orders for Life-Sustaining Treatment (MOLST)?

A number of States use an advance care planning form known as POLST (Physician Orders for Life-Sustaining Treatment) or MOLST (Medical Orders for Life-Sustaining Treatment). This form provides more detailed guidance about your medical care preferences.

The form is filled out by your doctor, or sometimes a nurse practitioner or physician's assistant, after discussing your wishes with you and your family. Once signed by your doctor, this form has the same authority as any other medical order. Check with your State department of health to find out if this form is available where you live.

What about Pacemakers and ICDs?

Some people have pacemakers to help their hearts beat regularly. If you have one and are near death, it may not necessarily keep you alive. But, you might have an ICD (implantable cardioverter-defibrillator) placed under your skin to shock your heart back into regular beatings if the rhythm becomes irregular. If other life-sustaining measures are not used, the ICD may also be turned off. You need to state in your advance directive what you want done if the doctor suggests it is time to turn it off.

Selecting Your Healthcare Proxy

If you decide to choose a proxy, think about people you know who share your views and values about life and medical decisions. Your proxy might be a family member, a friend, your lawyer, or someone with whom you worship. It's a good idea to also name an alternate proxy. It is especially important to have a detailed living will if you choose not to name a proxy.

You can decide how much authority your proxy has over your medical care—whether he or she is entitled to make a wide range of decisions or only a few specific ones. Try not to include guidelines that make it impossible for the proxy to fulfill his or her duties. For example, it's probably not unusual for someone to say in conversation, "I don't want to go to a nursing home," but think carefully about whether you want a restriction like that in your advance directive. Sometimes, for financial or medical reasons, that may be the best choice for you.

Of course, check with those you choose as your healthcare proxy and alternate before you name them officially. Make sure they are comfortable with this responsibility.

Making It Official

Once you have talked with your doctor and have an idea of the types of decisions that could come up in the future and whom you would like as a proxy, if you want one at all, the next step is to fill out the legal forms detailing your wishes. A lawyer can help but is not required. If you decide to use a lawyer, don't depend on him or her to help you understand different medical treatments. That's why you should start the planning process by talking with your doctor.

Many states have their own advance directive forms. The American Bar Association (ABA) has a list of advance care planning forms by state. Your local Area Agency on Aging can help you locate the right forms. You can find your area agency phone number by calling the Eldercare Locator toll-free at 800-677-1116 or by visiting www.eldercare.gov.

Some states want your advance directive to be witnessed; some want your signature notarized. A notary is a person licensed by the state to witness signatures. You might find a notary at your bank, post office, or local library, or call your insurance agent. Some notaries charge a fee.

Some people spend a lot of time in more than one state—for example, visiting children and grandchildren. If that's your situation also, you might consider preparing an advance directive using forms for each state—and keep a copy in each place, too.

After You Set Up Your Advance Directive

Give copies of your advance directive to your healthcare proxy and alternate proxy. Give your doctor a copy for your medical records. Tell key family members and friends where you keep a copy. If you have to go to the hospital, give staff there a copy to include in your records. Because you might change your advance directive in the future, it's a good idea to keep track of who receives a copy.

Review your advance care planning decisions from time to time—for example, every 10 years, if not more often. You might want to revise your preferences for care if your situation or your health changes. Or, you might want to make adjustments if you receive a serious diagnosis; if you get married, separated, or divorced; if your spouse dies; or if something happens to your proxy or alternate. If your preferences change, make sure your doctor, proxy, and family know about them.

What happens if you have no advance directive or have made no plans and you become unable to speak for yourself? In such cases, the state where you live will assign someone to make medical decisions on your behalf. This will probably be your spouse, your parents if they are available, or your children if they are adults. If you have no family members, the state will choose someone to represent your best interests.

Always remember, an advance directive is only used if you are in danger of dying and need certain emergency or special measures to keep you alive but are not able to make those decisions on your own. An advance directive allows you to continue to make your wishes about medical treatment known.

Nobody can predict the future. You may never face a medical situation where you are unable to speak for yourself and make your wishes known. But having an advance directive may give you and those close to you some peace of mind.

Advance Directive Wallet Card

You might want to make a card to carry in your wallet indicating that you have an advance directive and where it is kept. Here is a slightly revised example of the wallet card offered by the Office of the Attorney General in Maryland. It uses the phrase "healthcare agent" instead of "healthcare proxy." You might want to print this to fill out and carry with you.

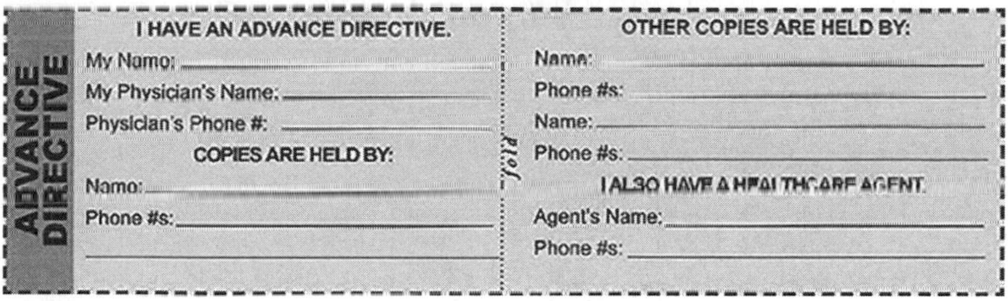

ADVANCE DIRECTIVE

I HAVE AN ADVANCE DIRECTIVE.

My Name: ______

My Physician's Name: ______

Physician's Phone #: ______

COPIES ARE HELD BY:

Name: ______

Phone #s: ______

______

fold

OTHER COPIES ARE HELD BY:

Name: ______

Phone #s: ______

Name: ______

Phone #s: ______

I ALSO HAVE A HEALTHCARE AGENT.

Agent's Name: ______

Phone #s: ______

Figure 60.1. *Wallet Card*

Part Seven

Clinical Trials and Research on Movement Disorders

Chapter 61

Introduction to Clinical Research

What Is Clinical Research?

Clinical research is research conducted with human subjects, or material of human origin, in which the researcher directly interacts with human subjects. Clinical research helps doctors and researchers to find new and better ways to understand, detect, control, and treat illness. A clinical research study is a way to find answers to difficult scientific or health questions. For example, the study might explore the best ways to treat people with colon cancer. By studying cancer cells from patients, researchers may be able to determine the specific genetic mutations (changes in gene sequence) that caused the normal, healthy cells to become cancerous, and may help doctors decide on the best drugs to prescribe or surgeries to perform. Clinical research today may help other doctors in the future screen their healthy patients before they ever develop cancer.

What Is a Protocol?

All clinical studies are based on a set of rules or directions called a protocol. A protocol describes what types of people are eligible to

This chapter includes text excerpted from "FAQ about Clinical Research," National Human Genome Research Institute (NHGRI), August 11, 2017.

participate in the study; determines the schedule of tests, procedures, medications, and dosages; and sets the length of the study.

What Is a Clinical Trial?

A clinical trial is a research study in which one or more human subjects are prospectively assigned to one or more interventions (which may include placebo or other control) to evaluate the effects of those interventions on health-related biomedical or behavioral outcomes.

What Are Clinical Trial "Phases?"

Clinical trials of experimental drugs proceed through four phases:

- In Phase I clinical trials, researchers test a new drug or treatment for the first time in a small group of normal, healthy volunteers (about 20–80) to evaluate its safety, determine a safe dosage range, and identify side effects.

- In Phase II clinical trials, the study drug or treatment is given to a larger group of people (about 100–300), including patients with the particular disease, to see if the drug or treatment is effective, and to further evaluate its safety.

- In Phase III clinical trials, the study drug or treatment is given to large groups of people (from 1,000–3,000), including patients, to confirm its effectiveness, monitor side effects, compare it to other commonly used treatments, and collect information that will allow the drug or treatment to be used safely.

- Phase IV clinical trials are done after the drug or treatment has been approved by the U.S. Food and Drug Administration (FDA) and marketed for public use. These studies continue testing the drug or treatment to collect information about its effect in various populations and gather data on any side effects associated with long-term use.

What Are "Blind" or "Masked" Studies?

In many clinical trials, one group of patients will be given an experimental drug or treatment, while a control group is given either a standard treatment for the illness, or a placebo (a harmless "fake" drug), or no treatment at all.

In a "blinded" or "masked" study, participants do not know whether they are getting the drug being tested, or whether they are in the control group. The goal is to prevent the so-called "placebo effect" from influencing the results of the experiment. The placebo effect is the phenomenon of patients feeling better simply because they think they are receiving a helpful drug or treatment.

Sometimes, clinical trials are "double-blind" or "double-masked." That means that neither the participants, nor the study staff members, know who is receiving the experimental drug and who is in the control group. Studies are performed in this way so that neither the patients' nor the doctors' expectations about the experimental drug can influence the observations and results.

Should I Volunteer for Clinical Research?

Clinical research is a vital part of finding new treatments and cures for diseases. Carefully conducted clinical studies are the fastest way to find treatments that are safe and effective. By volunteering for a clinical study, you would be participating in research that may result in a new treatment for a deadly or debilitating disease.

Before you agree to participate in a study, you must be given complete information about the study, known as "informed consent." Informed consent involves two essential components: a document and a process. The informed consent document gives a summary of the research project (including the study's purpose, research procedures, potential benefits and risks, etc.) and explains the individual's rights as a research participant. This document is part of an informed consent process, which consists of conversations between the research team and the participant, and may include other supporting material such as study brochures. The informed consent process provides research participants with ongoing explanations that will help them make informed decisions about whether to begin or continue participating in the research project.

Chapter 62

Clinical Trials on Parkinson Disease

Chapter Contents

Section 62.1

Neural Correlates of Cognition in Parkinson Disease

This section includes text excerpted from "Neural Correlates of Cognition in Parkinson Disease," ClinicalTrials.gov, National Institutes of Health (NIH), December 2017.

Brief Summary

Cognitive impairment in Parkinson disease (PD) has far-reaching effects on both motor outcomes and quality of life in PD patients. Furthermore, deep brain stimulation (DBS), now an evidence-based treatment for certain cases of PD, has the risk of causing deficits in multiple areas of cognition.

As such, the purpose of this study is to understand the neuroanatomical and neurophysiologic basis for impaired cognition in PD. The aim is to identify neural correlates of cognition by measuring brain signal activity while PD patients are engaged in cognition on a computer.

Detailed Description

Study Participants: For this study, the investigators will recruit approximately 100 healthy control participants and 100 Parkinson disease (PD) patients that are undergoing deep brain stimulation (DBS) as routine standard of care.

Screening: For healthy control participants, investigators will approach adults, aged 18–90, for possible involvement in the study. Potential participants will be asked if they have ever been diagnosed with a movement disorder, psychiatric disorder, or dementia. For PD patients undergoing evaluation for DBS, investigators will first consult with their neurologist and neurosurgeon. Next, investigators will approach the participant and explain the study.

Healthy Controls: Healthy controls will complete standardized questionnaires and play a computer game to assess cognition, taking no longer than 30 minutes.

PD Participants: As part of the usual DBS process in the treatment of side effects of PD at University of Florida (UF), PD participants will asked to participate in this trial. There are three evaluation time points: before surgery, during surgery, and possibly after surgery. Before surgery, the PD patients will complete standardized questionnaires and be trained on a computer game to assess cognition. During surgery, the participants will play the same computer game while brain signals are recorded. When the patients return to University of Florida for DBS programming visits within 12 months after surgery, they will repeat the standardized questionnaires and computer game once again.

Outcome Measures

Primary Outcome Measures:

1. Change in behavioral performance (Time Frame: Baseline, before surgery, during surgery, and up to 1 year after surgery)

   - Behavioral performance will be assessed by the computer game that assess cognition. All computer games used in this study will have a similar form. The computer will record responses to each trial during the computer game.

Secondary Outcome Measures:

1. Change in Score on Questionnaire for Impulsive-Compulsive Disorders in Parkinson Disease-Rating Scale (QUIP-RS) (Time Frame: Baseline, before surgery, during surgery, and up to 1 year after surgery)

   - Assess the scores from a standard clinical questionnaire called QUIP-RS. Scores range from 0–112.

2. Change in Score on Montreal Cognitive Assessment (MoCA) (Time Frame: Baseline, before surgery, during surgery, and up to 1 year after surgery)

   - Assess the scores from standard clinical questionnaire called MoCA. Scores range from 0–30.

3. Local field potential brain signal (Time Frame: At time of surgery)

   - Measuring Brain signal while Parkinson disease patients play a computer game during surgery. Local field potential is measured in Hertz (Hz)

Eligibility Criteria

Ages Eligible for Study: 18–90 Years (Adult, Senior)
Sexes Eligible for Study: All
Accepts Healthy Volunteers: Yes
Criteria

Controls:

- Inclusion Criteria: Healthy adults between the ages of 18–90.

- Exclusion Criteria: Participants that have known movement disorders, psychiatric disorders, or any type of dementia.

PD-DBS Participants:

- Inclusion Criteria: Persons undergoing DBS surgery for the implantation of electrodes for the treatment of motor disorders

- Exclusion Criteria: Failure of the DBS surgical candidacy screening process

Section 62.2

Motivational Interviewing and Physical Activity Change in Parkinson Disease

This section includes text excerpted from "Motivational Interviewing and Physical Activity Change in Parkinson Disease," ClinicalTrials. gov, National Institutes of Health (NIH), November 22, 2017.

Brief Summary

The purpose of this study is to test the efficacy of a 6-month telephone-based motivational interviewing intervention and a web-based application intervention to improve physical activity in participants with Parkinson disease.

Detailed Description

Participants will be randomized into one of four groups to examine two separate interventions. The groups are: motivational interviewing (a counseling/coaching style), a web-based application for participants to keep track of their physical activity, a combination of the motivational interviewing and the web-based application, and an educational program on various issues related to Parkinson disease. The intervention will last 6 months with a follow-up appointment at 9 months. Participants will be asked to come to Galter Pavilion at Northwestern Memorial Hospital or Shirley Ryan AbilityLab a total of five times over the course of the nine months.

Outcome Measures

Primary Outcome Measures:

1. Test the efficacy of the Motivational Interviewing (MI) Intervention and the Web-Based Self-Monitoring Application Intervention by monitoring the change in physical activity using data collected from an Actigraph activity monitor. (Time Frame: Assessment will occur at baseline, 3 months, 6 months, and 9 months.)

   • Participants will wear an Actigraph activity monitor for one week every quarter to collect data about physical activity throughout the duration of the study. Time spent doing physical activity will be compared at each assessment for this outcome.

2. Test the efficacy of the MI Intervention and the Web-Based Self-Monitoring Application Intervention by monitoring the change in physical activity using the Physical Activity Scale for Individuals with Physical Disabilities (PASIPD). (Time Frame: Assessment will occur at baseline, 3 months, 6 months, and 9 months.)

   • PASIPD is a 13-item 7-day physical activity recall questionnaire designed to evaluate physical activity levels in people with physical disabilities by soliciting information about leisure time activities, household activities, and work-related activities.

Secondary Outcome Measures:

1. Test the efficacy of the Motivational Interviewing (MI) intervention and the Web-Based Self-Monitoring Application Intervention for improving balance using the Berg Balance Scale (BBS). (Time Frame: Assessment will occur at baseline, 3 months, 6 months, and 9 months.)

- The Berg Balance Scale is a 14-item performance measure to assess static balance and fall risk.

2. Test the efficacy of the Motivational Interviewing (MI) intervention and the Web-Based Self-Monitoring Application Intervention for improving balance using the

    - Activities-Specific Balance Confidence Scale (ABC). (Time Frame: Assessment will occur at baseline, 3 months, 6 months, and 9 months.)

    - Activities-Specific Balance Confidence Scale is a 16-item self-report measure of confidence in performing various activities of daily living without falling.

3. Test the efficacy of the Motivational Interviewing (MI) intervention and the Web-Based Self-Monitoring Application Intervention for improving balance using the Unified Parkinson Disease Rating Scale (UPDRS). (Time Frame: Assessment will occur at baseline, 3 months, 6 months, and 9 months.)

    - The UPDRS is an assessment that monitors the progression of Parkinson disease. For this outcome, the "postural stability" portion of the assessment will be used to determine balance improvements.

4. Test the efficacy of the Motivational Interviewing (MI) intervention and the Web-Based Self-Monitoring Application Intervention for improving quality of life using the assessment measure Neuro-QOL. (Time Frame: Assessment will occur at baseline, 3 months, 6 months, and 9 months.)

    - The Neuro-QOL is a set of self-report measures that assess the health-related quality of life of adults and children with neurological disorders.

5. Test the efficacy of the Motivational Interviewing (MI) intervention and the Web-Based Self-Monitoring Application Intervention for improving quality of life using the assessment measure Patient-Reported Outcomes Measurement Information System (PROMIS). (Time Frame: Assessment will occur at baseline, 3 months, 6 months, and 9 months.)

    - PROMIS Global Health is a 10-item scale rating physical and mental health and overall quality of life.

Eligibility Criteria

Ages Eligible for Study: 18 Years and older (Adult, Senior)
Sexes Eligible for Study: All
Accepts Healthy Volunteers: No
Criteria

Inclusion Criteria:

- Community dwelling
- Age 18 or older
- Physician confirmed diagnosis of PD with Hoehn and Yahr stage ≤3
- Ability to ambulate independently (walker is allowed) for distance of 50 feet or 10 minutes at a time
- Does not meet current CDC physical activity guidelines of 150 minutes of moderate to vigorous physical activity per week
- and plans to have a smartphone, tablet, or computer and access to the Internet for the next 9 months
- Willing to monitor activity on their smartphone, tablet, or computer via a web-based application during the 9-month program
- Currently uses the Internet in a basic capacity

Exclusion Criteria:

- Inability to speak and understand English
- Has a cardiovascular disorder or other health condition that would make exercise unsafe according to their physician
- Patients who are currently receiving physical therapy or received physical therapy one month prior to study enrollment
- Cognitive impairment as defined by inability to provide informed consent and to self-report feelings and behaviors
- Montreal Cognition Scale (MOCA): rating of less than 24, indicative of cognitive dysfunction
- Patients who indicate it is not recommended they participate in increased physical activity as indicated by the Physical Activity Restriction Questionnaire (PAR-Q)
- Patients who are in other studies that monitor fitness or physical activity

479

Section 62.3

Effect on Parkinson Disease after Therapeutic Induction of Craniosacral Integrated Therapy

This section includes text excerpted from "Effect on Parkinson Disease after Therapeutic Induction of Craniosacral Integrated Therapy," ClinicalTrials.gov, National Institutes of Health (NIH), July 13, 2016.

Brief Summary

NIH is studying and researching the effect of CranioSacral Integrative therapy on Parkinson-diseased patients for 3 months. With a therapeutic induction via manual CranioSacral integrative therapy for 90 minutes per session with a total of 2 session divided equally in a month (biweekly intervention). At the end of 3 months each patient will have total of 9 hours of CranioSacral Integrative therapy induced, NIH will document the symptoms and shortcomings of the patients at evaluation, before and after therapeutic treatment on a measured scale ranging from 1–10. Finally graphically and statistically measure the quality of change in the symptoms at the end of 3 months and provide executive summary of the research finding, which the investigators expect to be a positive one.

Outcome Measures

Primary Outcome Measures:

1. reduction in tremors due to Parkinson disease in the patient (Time Frame: 3 months)

    *   Measurement of the tremors and quality of the coordination of the medial leminiscus system on 1–10 (1 being zero tremors and 10 being out of control tremors) scale at the evaluation and at beginning and at the end of each treatment session and in the end will provide a graphical and statistical display in the change in the tremors relative to the therapeutic induction

Secondary Outcome Measures:

1. Quality of Proprioception (Time Frame: 3 months)

   - will evaluate the patients ability to move within space and time with certain precision and measure it on a scale of 1–10 (1 being very precise with fine motor movement and 10 being out of control fine motor movements)at the time of evaluation and at the beginning and end of each therapeutic treatment and finally document it graphically and statistically, the change in the overall motor movements like walking and quality of gait.

Other Outcome Measures:

1. Overall emotional State and sleep quality (Time Frame: 3 months)

   - will evaluate the overall emotional and sleeping habits on the measurement scale of 1–10 where 1 being emotionally stable and positive with 8 hours of quality sleep and 10 being emotionally unstable and have less than 4 hours of sleep at night and at the end of research will graphically and statistically provide the outcome of the above mentioned measure.

Eligibility Criteria

Ages Eligible for Study: 18 Years and older (Adult, Senior)
Sexes Eligible for Study: All
Accepts Healthy Volunteers: Yes
Criteria

Inclusion Criteria:

- Must be diagnosed with Parkinson disease

Exclusion Criteria:

- Anyone without Parkinson disease

Chapter 63

Daily and Weekly Rehabilitation Delivery for Young Children with Cerebral Palsy (DRIVE)

Brief Summary

The purpose of this study is to determine the optimal frequency and intensity of physical therapy for children with cerebral palsy aged 6–24 months of age. Participants will be randomly assigned to one of three groups: daily, intermediate, or weekly physical therapy. Short and long term effects will be evaluated to determine the best 'dose' of rehabilitation for children with cerebral palsy, including frequency (number of sessions per week and the number of weeks), intensity (how hard the patient works), and time (how many total hours) of rehabilitation treatment.

Detailed Description

Determining optimal frequency of treatment for young children with cerebral palsy (CP) has implications for shaping the future of pediatric

This chapter includes text excerpted from "Daily and Weekly Rehabilitation Delivery for Young Children with Cerebral Palsy (DRIVE)," ClinicalTrials.gov, National Institutes of Health (NIH), August 5, 2016.

rehabilitation. There are wide variations in the number of hours per week of treatment in current outpatient rehabilitation programs for children with CP, suggesting clinical uncertainty. Usual weekly therapy at 1–2 hours per week for 6 months or longer is the most commonly implemented frequency of dose for children with CP 6–24 months of age. However, this decision about frequency is often made based on clinical reasoning and scheduling, not on principles of rehabilitation, child development, or evidence from strongly designed randomized controlled trials. The proposed study will fill this gap by directly comparing the effects of 3 frequency levels of therapy—concentrated daily, intermediate, and usual weekly in children with CP 6–24 months of age at the initiation of treatment and following these patients for 2 years.

In this prospective longitudinal study, children with Cerebral Palsy (n=75), 6–24 months of age, will be randomly assigned to one of three groups: daily, intermediate, or weekly physical therapy. The treatment phase of this study design is 5 months for a total of 40 hours of one-on-one therapy for both groups. Level 1 daily therapy is 2 hours of therapy per day for 20 straight weekdays. Level 2 intermediate therapy is 2 hours of therapy per day 3 days per week for 6.6 weeks. Level 3 usual weekly therapy is 2 hours of therapy one day per week for 20 weeks. Researchers will directly compare the effects of 3 these frequency levels of therapy at the initiation of treatment and following these patients for 2 years. Results will provide quantitative evidence of frequency-response, which is critical for informing clinical decision-making, health policy, and guidelines for reimbursement.

Outcome Measures

Primary Outcome Measures:

1. Change in Gross Motor Function Measure (GMFM)-88 (Time Frame: Baseline (pre-treatment) and 3 months, 6 months, 12 months, 18 months, and 24 months after initiation of treatment)

   - GMFM evaluates change in gross motor function over time or with intervention in children with CP from 5 months to 16 years. It has been used widely in the field to determine functional motor change following intervention.

Secondary Outcome Measures:

1. Change in Goal Attainment Scaling (GAS) (Time Frame: Baseline (pre-treatment) and 3 months, 6 months, 12 months, 18 months, and 24 months after initiation of treatment)

- GAS creates patient, family, and clinical anchors as the external criterion for improvement by establishing activity or participation goals that reflect what an individual, family, and clinician consider meaningful or relevant. The GAS method allows for goals to be defined at different levels of mastery and assigned numerical values for score calculation, similar to a Likert scale. The scale will have 5 points representing different levels of mastery of the individual patient's goal. A score of -2 represents baseline, -1 less change than expected, 0 for the expected level of change, and +1 and +2 for achievement of more change than expected. To attempt to ensure ordinality, each level on the scale will be described and will reflect a single dimension of change that is measurable, achievable, and relevant

2. Change in Bayley Scales of Infant Development III (Time Frame: Baseline (pre-treatment) and 3 months, 6 months, 12 months, 18 months, and 24 months after initiation of treatment)

   - *The Bayley Scales of Infant and Toddler Development-Third Edition* is an individually administered test designed to assess developmental functioning of infants and toddlers. The Bayley-III assesses development in five areas: cognitive, language, motor, social-emotional, and adaptive behavior.

3. Change in Pediatric Evaluation and Disability Inventory (PEDI) (Time Frame: Baseline (pre-treatment) and 3 months, 6 months, 12 months, 18 months, and 24 months after initiation of treatment)

   - Administered as a parent survey. The PEDI is a descriptive measure of a child's current functional performance and can track changes over time. The PEDI measures both capability and performance of functional activities in three content domains: self-care, mobility, and social function. It can be used as a comprehensive clinical assessment of key functional capabilities and performance in children between the ages of six months and seven years.

Eligibility Criteria

Ages Eligible for Study: 6 Months to 24 Months (Child)
Sexes Eligible for Study: All

Accepts Healthy Volunteers: No
Criteria

Inclusion Criteria:

- an age of 6 months—24 months at the initiation of treatment. The age will be corrected for any eligible children born preterm until they are 2 years of age, as is standard clinical and research practice

- a diagnosis or risk for CP in GMFCS levels III, IV and V or motor delay

- ability to tolerate a 2 hour therapy session based on parent report and evaluating therapists, the same criteria the investigators used for the pilot study.

Exclusion Criteria:

- uncontrollable seizures or any comorbid condition that prevents full participation during treatment sessions

- participation in another daily treatment program in the last 6 months

- auditory, or visual conditions that prevent full participation during treatment sessions

- the family is unable to commit to the prescribed dose or follow up evaluations

Chapter 64

Growth and Development of the Striatum in Huntington Disease (Kids-HD)

Brief Summary

Huntington disease (HD) is an autosomal dominant disease manifested in a triad of cognitive, psychiatric, and motor signs and symptoms. HD is caused by a triplet repeat (CAG) expansion in the gene *Huntingtin (HTT)*. This disease has classically been conceptualized as a neurodegenerative disease. However, recent evidence suggests that abnormal brain development may play an important role in the etiology of HD. HTT is expressed during development and through life. In animal studies, the *HTT* gene has been shown to be vital for brain development. This suggests that a mutant form of *HTT* (gene-expanded or CAG repeats of 40 and above) would affect normal brain development. In addition, studies in adults who are gene-expanded for HD, but have not yet manifested the illness, (preHD subjects) have significant changes in the structure of their brain, even up to 20 years before onset of clinical diagnosis. How far back these changes are evident is unknown. One possibility is that these brain changes

This chapter includes text excerpted from "Growth and Development of the Striatum in Huntington Disease (Kids-HD)," ClinicalTrials.gov, National Institutes of Health (NIH), June 1, 2017.

are present throughout life, due to changes in brain development, though initially associated with only subtle functional abnormalities.

In an effort to better understand the developmental aspects of this brain disease, the current study proposes to evaluate brain structure and function in children, adolescents, and young adults (ages 6–18) who are at risk for developing HD—those who have a parent or grandparent with HD. Brain structure will be evaluating using magnetic resonance imaging (MRI) with quantitative measures of the entire brain, cerebral cortex, as well as white matter integrity via diffusion tensor imaging (DTI). Brain function will be assessed by cognitive tests, physical and neurologic evaluation, behavioral assessment, and quantitative craniofacial structure assessment. Subjects that are gene-expanded (GE) will be compared to subjects who are gene nonexpanded (GNE) and as well to matched healthy controls. Changes in brain structure and/or function in the GE group, compared to both GNE and control groups, would lend support to the notion that this disease has an important developmental component.

Outcome Measures

Primary Outcome Measures:

1   Volume of brain structures as measured by MRI [Time Frame: 6–7 hour testing day]

- MRI and DTI data will be analyzed to assess brain structure based upon variables including global volume, total cerebral spinal fluid, subregion volumes, cortical surface anatomy including cortical depth, surface area and gyral shape, and symmetry between brain hemispheres, all in consideration of age, gender, and height. Results will be evaluated for comparative differences between the GE group, the GNE group, and the healthy control group. In addition, these measures of brain structure will be paired with corresponding measures of brain function to evaluate brain development based upon growth and performance.

Secondary Outcome Measures:

1. Quantitative assessment of cognitive skills and motor skills [Time Frame: 6–7 hour testing day]

- Participants undergo a cognitive battery which will quantify skills such as attention, learning, memory. In addition, motor skill (both fine and gross) will be assessed and quantified.

Results will be analyzed for comparative differences between the GE group, the GNE group, and the healthy control group. In addition, these measures of brain function will be paired with appropriate measures of brain structure to evaluate brain development based upon growth and performance.

Biospecimen Retention: Samples with DNA

Biospecimens are collected and retained for both case and control participants for genetic testing purposes. Specimens are either a single sample of 1–2 teaspoons of blood drawn from the arm or 1 teaspoon of saliva via collection device.

Biospecimens will be tested for the number of CAG repeats in the Huntington gene. Each sample obtained will be coded with a randomly assigned number and never linked with personal identifiers. The results from the genetic analysis will be sent directly to the data manager on the project, who is the ONLY research member with access to this data. This person has no direct contact with study participants.

Eligibility Criteria

Ages Eligible for Study: 6–18 Years (Child, Adult)
Sexes Eligible for Study: All
Accepts Healthy Volunteers: Yes
Sampling Method: Non-Probability Sample

Study Population

Young people ages 6–18 years old who have a parent or grandparent that has been diagnosed with HD.

Criteria

Inclusion Criteria:

- Family history of HD.

- Age 6–18 years.

- Age-appropriate knowledge of HD and personal risk.

Exclusion Criteria:

- Metal in body, including braces.

- History of head trauma, brain tumor, seizures, and epilepsy.

- History of major surgery and/or significant ongoing medical issue(s).

Chapter 65

Physical Telerehabilitation in Multiple Sclerosis

Brief Summary

The study aims to evaluate the efficacy of the MS HAT (Multiple Sclerosis Home Automated Telemanagement) System as an adjunct to the current standard of medical care for patients with MS (PwMS). The individual patient with MS will be the unit of analysis. For each participant, the investigators will assess the effect of Home Automated Telemanagement (HAT) on functional outcomes, levels of disablement including impairment, activity and participation, socio-behavioral parameters, and satisfaction with medical care as described below.

Detailed Description

People with multiple sclerosis may develop severe disability over the time. Physical therapy including regular exercise helps patients with severe disability to maintain muscle strength, reduce disease symptoms and improve quality of life. However physical therapy programs at clinical settings require constant travel which may limit access of patients with mobility disability to these services on continuous basis. Technology can allow patients with mobility disability

---

This chapter includes text excerpted from "Physical Telerehabilitation in Multiple Sclerosis," ClinicalTrials.gov, National Institutes of Health (NIH), July 27, 2017.

exercise at home under supervision of their rehabilitation team. Currently it is unclear how effective this approach is. The study aims to demonstrate that the patients who were helped by the new technology to exercise at home will have better fitness, less symptoms and better quality of life. If so, other patients with significant mobility disability will be able to take advantage of this technology. This approach can be extended to people with different diseases causing mobility impairment and it can be used not only for physical but also for cognitive and occupational rehabilitation.

Outcome Measures

Primary Outcome Measures:

1. Cardiorespiratory fitness (Time Frame: Baseline up to 6 months)

    • Cardiorespiratory fitness will be measured by oxygen consumption

Secondary Outcome Measures:

1. MS Self-efficacy scale (Time Frame: Baseline up to 6 months)

    • MS Self-efficacy scale is a 14-point questionnaire designed to assess the psychological adjustment and quality-of-life of individuals with MS.

2. Exercise adherence (Time Frame: Baseline up to 6 months)

    • Exercise adherence will be measured by the number of sessions completed by the participant out of the number of exercise sessions prescribed.

3. Center for Epidemiologic Studies Depression Scale (CES-D) (Time Frame: Baseline up to 6 months)

    • The CES-D is a 20 point questionnaire based on self-reported frequency of symptoms related to depression during the past week.

4. Berg Balance Scale (BBS) (Time Frame: Baseline up to 6 month)

    • BBS is a clinical 14-item scale designed to measure balance

5. 2-Minute Walk Test (2MWT) (Time Frame: Baseline up to 6 months)

    • Total distance walked in meters will be recorded.

Eligibility Criteria

Ages Eligible for Study: 22 Years and older (Adult, Senior)
Sexes Eligible for Study: All
Accepts Healthy Volunteers: No
Criteria

Inclusion Criteria:

- Age >21

- Confirmed diagnosis of Multiple Sclerosis based on McDonald criteria

- EDSS range 5.0-8.0

- Mini-Mental State Examination (MMSE) > 22 or presence of a caregiver to assist in daily exercise regimen

Exclusion Criteria:

- Coronary artery disease

- Congestive heart failure

- Uncontrolled hypertension

- Epilepsy

- Pacemaker or implanted defibrillator

- Unstable fractures or other musculoskeletal diagnoses

Chapter 66

The Study of Skeletal Muscle Blood Flow in Becker Muscular Dystrophy

Brief Summary

This pilot study tests the hypothesis that the medication nitric oxide extract from beetroot juice improves blood flow to the skeletal muscle during exercise. The investigators will use cutting edge technology with contrast enhanced ultrasound to visualize the microvascular blood supply to the forearm. Animal studies have shown reversal of muscle damage with improved delivery of blood to the exercising muscle. This research aims to understand the mechanism of action of this medication in a way it has never been studied before. The results may help benefit individuals with muscular dystrophy in the future.

Detailed Description

The subjects are asked to perform a graded hand-grip exercise while blood flow to the skeletal muscle is visualized by contrast enhanced ultrasound.

This is done at baseline and after taking the study agent.

This chapter includes text excerpted from "The Study of Skeletal Muscle Blood Flow in Becker Muscular Dystrophy," ClinicalTrials.gov, National Institutes of Health (NIH), March 6, 2017.

Outcome Measures

Primary Outcome Measures:

1. Change in Skeletal Muscle Blood Flow (Time Frame: At baseline and within one hours after taking beetroot juice or Tadalafil)

    - Exercise induced skeletal muscle perfusion is measured by contrast-enhanced ultrasound (CEU) during graded voluntary contraction on a hand grip dynamometer.

Secondary Outcome Measures:

1. Change in Measured Functional Sympatholysis (Time Frame: At baseline, and within an hour after taking beetroot juice or Tadalafil)

    - Functional sympatholysis (attenuation of exercise induced skeletal muscle vasoconstriction) is assessed using a lower body negative pressure chamber.

2. Change in Measured Flow Mediated Dilation (FMD) (Time Frame: At baseline, and within an hour after taking beetroot juice or Tadalafil)

    - Endothelial function is assessed by measuring flow-mediated dilation (FMD) by Doppler ultrasound.

Eligibility Criteria

Ages Eligible for Study: 18 Years to 45 Years (Adult)
Sexes Eligible for Study: Male
Accepts Healthy Volunteers: Yes
Criteria

Inclusion Criteria:

- Healthy man, aged 18–45 years, currently taking no medication. OR
- Clinical diagnosis of Becker Muscular Dystrophy (BMD), aged 18–45 years, and currently taking no medication.

Exclusion Criteria:

- Hypertension, diabetes, heart failure, liver disease
- ECG evidence of prolonged QT interval (measure of the time between the start of the Q wave and the end of the T wave in the heart's electrical cycle)

Chapter 67

Exploring the Brain's Relationship to Habits

Research may impact development of treatments for movement disorders such as Parkinson and Huntington diseases, as well as conditions such as autism.

The basal ganglia, structures deep in the forebrain already known to control voluntary movements, also may play a critical role in how people form habits, both bad and good, and in influencing mood and feelings.

"This system is not just a motor system," says Ann Graybiel."We think it also strongly affects the emotional part of the brain."

Graybiel, an investigator at the McGovern Institute of the Massachusetts Institute of Technology (MIT) and a professor in MIT's Department of Brain and Cognitive Sciences, believes that a core function of the basal ganglia is to help humans develop habits that eventually become automatic, including habits of thought and emotion.

"Many everyday movements become habitual through repetition, but we also develop habits of thought and emotion," she says."If cognitive and emotional habits are also controlled by the basal ganglia, this may explain why damage to these structures can lead not only to movement disorders, but also to repetitive and intrusive thoughts, emotions and desires."

This chapter includes text excerpted from "Exploring the Brain's Relationship to Habits," National Science Foundation (NSF), January 4, 2013. Reviewed January 2018.

497

Graybiel's research focuses on the brain's relationship to habits—how we make or break them—and the neurobiology of the habit system. She and her team have identified and traced neural loops that run from the outer layer of the brain—"the thinking cap," as she calls it—to a region called the striatum, which is part of the basal ganglia, and back again. These loops, in fact, connect sensory signals to habitual behaviors.

Graybiel's work ultimately could have an impact not just on such classic movement disorders as Parkinson and Huntington diseases, but in other conditions where repetitive movements commonly occur, such as Tourette syndrome, autism, or obsessive-compulsive disorder (OCD), the latter when sufferers experience unwanted and repeated thoughts, feelings, ideas, sensations or behaviors that make them feel driven to do something, for example, repeatedly washing their hands.

Moreover, the research could have an immediate value for trying to understand "what happens in the brain as addiction occurs, as bad habits form, not just good habits," she says. "There are many psychiatric and neurologic conditions in which these same brain regions are disordered.

"These conditions may in part be influenced by the very system we are working on. We are working with models of anxiety and depression, stress and some of these movement disorders."

It turns out that the emotional circuits of the brain have strong ties to the striatum, she says. Graybiel's research suggests that activity in the striatum strongly affects the emotional decisions that people make: whether to accept a good outcome or a potentially bad one, for example, and that there are circuits favoring good outcomes, and, surprisingly, other circuits that favor bad ones.

"This work ties into new research suggesting that there are brain systems for 'good' and brain systems for 'bad,'" she says. "What is intriguing is that we may have identified the circuits that decide between the two."

Recently, Graybiel, an early National Science Foundation grantee, won the prestigious Kavli Prize in neuroscience (along with Cornelia Isabella Bargmann of Rockefeller University and Winfried Denk of the Max Planck Institute for Medical Research) for their groundbreaking research "elucidating basic neuronal mechanisms underlying perception and decision."

These prizes recognize scientists for their seminal advances in astrophysics, nanoscience and neuroscience, and include a cash award of $1 million in each field.

Graybiel's lab was the first to discover more than three decades ago, that neurotransmitters in the striatum had a precise and unique organization—compartments similar to layers—a finding that surprised most scientists at the time.

"We couldn't see this organization in regular old anatomy, but we found this with chemical markers, by using stains," she says. "Imagine if you look at a desert and everything looks plain and uniform, just all sand. Then you put on special glasses, and all of a sudden, you could see the chemical composition of the sands. The whole landscape looks totally different, and that's what happened when we did this stain.

"We now know that all over the brain, these molecules are highly ordered," she adds. "They are communication lines, and connections from a to b and b to c, and these connections all work because of these chemical communication molecules. We happened to find that the deep brain, which looked so primitive, wasn't as primitive as people thought. We found that if we looked at the chemicals and then at the inputs and the outputs, everything was organized with respect to these chemical compartments."

Graybiel and her team also determined that communication molecules known to be related to human disorders, such as dopamine, a key neurotransmitter, were prominently organized in this way. Dopamine dysfunction is associated with the development of Parkinson disease.

"As we looked more and more, we found that we could trace connections from the neocortex to the striatum," she says. "They were all organized in compartments either in the compartments we called striosomes or in the compartments that surrounded them."

The striosomes are one of two complementary chemical compartments within the striatum. The second compartment is known as the matrix.

Following upon this, "the next thing we found was that the whole thing looked like a learning machine because of the way it all was organized," she says. "We decided to study learning. In order to do that, we had to learn to record the neural activity. It turns out that the system is tremendously active as we learn habits. That's how we began."

Graybiel uses electrical recordings, behavioral tests and gene-based approaches to study these issues, and has seen remarkable changes in neural activity within the striatum as animals learned new habits.

"The activity in this part of the brain changed as the animals learned, and they were highly correlated with the learning," she says. "We take the animals to 'school' every day, and give them practice. They do learn habits—to run to the right, or do something when a click occurs, until it's habitual. As they learn, there are all these changes in the neural activity."

She and her lab also found that these changes are coordinated with activity patterns in the hippocampus, a brain structure involved with memory of facts and events. Currently, she and her lab are studying new methods to influence the activity in the striatum, and genes found in the brain region thought to be involved in the brain's response to abusive drugs, as well as to therapeutic drugs, such as those to treat Parkinson.

Their work suggests a new view of how the core brain structures involved in Parkinson disease are affected by dopamine depletion, and how this key neurotransmitter might influence the ability to maintain movement and thought.

"Hopefully, our basic science work can lead to new therapeutic approaches to these disorders, not only in drug treatments but also other novel treatments that affect the on-going activity of neurons in the basal ganglia," she says. "There is nothing I would rather do than to help in the search for new therapies to treat the range of disorders related to the system we study, from Parkinson disease to OCD to addiction, and maybe, just maybe, to help the rest of us unlearn bad habits."

Chapter 68

Space Technologies in the Rehabilitation of Movement Disorders

More than 50 years have passed since the first human spaceflight. As the duration of the flights has increased considerably, and amount of in-orbit activities has become greater, the need to maintain healthy bones and muscles in space has become more critical. Bones and muscles rely on performing daily activities in the presence of Earth's gravity to stay healthy. In space, traditional Earth-based methods to maintain bones and muscles, such as physical exercise, are challenging due to constraints that include such factors as crew time and vehicle size.

To meet these challenges, specialists from the Institute of Biomedical Problems in Russia and their commercial partner, Zvezda, developed the Penguin suit to provide loading along the length of the body (axial loading) in a way that compensates for the lack of daily loading that the body usually experiences under the Earth's gravity. The first testing of the suit in space was performed in 1971 aboard the Salyut-1 station. Now the Penguin suit is actively used on the International Space Station as a regular component of the Russian countermeasure system of health maintenance.

This chapter includes text excerpted from "Space Technologies in the Rehabilitation of Movement Disorders," National Aeronautics and Space Administration (NASA), November 19, 2015.

Since the early 1990s, Professor Inessa Kozlovskaya and her team at the Institute of Biomedical Problems in Russia have implemented the use of this axial loading suit in clinical rehabilitation practice. The clinical version of the Penguin suit, the Adeli, was developed at the Institute of Pediatrics Russian Academy of Science under the leadership of Professor Ksenia Semyonova and is used for the comprehensive treatment of cerebral palsy in children. The treatment method is focused on restoring functional links of the body through a corrective flow of sensory information to the muscles, thereby improving the health of the tissues being loaded. This results in the correction of walking patterns and stabilization of balance in a relatively short period of time, including for those cerebral palsy children with deep motor disturbances. The Adeli suit was licensed in 1992 and has been continuously developed since. These methods have become one of the most popular and widely used in Russian médical clinics for rehabilitation of children with infantile cerebral paralysis.

New methods were also developed for patients undergoing motor rehabilitation after stroke and brain trauma. Paralytic and paretic alterations of motor functions that are the most frequent after-effects of these diseases typically lead to significant limitations in motor and social activity of these patients, decrease their functional abilities and obstruct their rehabilitation. Given all of the complexities and importance of the rehabilitation of these patients, another clinical modification of the Penguin suit was developed called the "Regent suit." The complex effect of the Regent suit on the body is based on an increase of the axial loading on skeletal structures and an increase in resistive loads on muscles during movement, which results in an increase of sensory information to the nervous system that is important for counteracting the development of pathological posture and for normalization of vertical stance and walking control. The Regent suit is effectively used at the early stage of rehabilitation for patients having movement disorders after cerebrovascular accident and cranium-brain traumas.

The clinical studies of the efficacy of the Regent suit in the rehabilitation of motor disorders in patients with limited lesions of the central nervous system were performed in acute and chronic studies with the participation of hundreds of stroke and brain trauma patients in the hospital No 83 Federal Medical-Biological Agency of Russia under leadership of professor Sergey Shvarkov, and in the Center of Speech Pathology and Neurorehabilitation under leadership of professor Vicktor Shklovsky. The efficacy of the suit in patients with post stroke hcmiparcsis was assessed at the Scientific Center of Neurology under leadership of professor Ludmila Chernikova. These studies have shown that use of the suit results in a significant decrease in paresis and spasticity in the lower leg muscle groups, as well as an improvement of sensitivity in distal parts of lower limbs, and an overall improvement of locomotor functions. The positive effect on high mental functions was noticed at the same time, namely, an improvement of speech characteristics, an increase of active vocabulary, and an improvement in the patient's ability to recognize objects.

The use of the Regent suit is a complex, drug-free approach to the treatment of motor disorders. The method is closely related to the natural function of walking, activates all of the muscles involved in posture and spatial orientation and is very safe. It allows for shorter treatment time, can be used both under hospital and outpatient conditions and allows for a wide range of adjustments that allow individualized rehabilitation programs based on uniqueness of the neurological deficit and functional abilities of each patient. Today the Regent suit is applied in 43 medical institutions in Russia and abroad, and the results related to using both the Adeli and Regent suits are based on numerous observations and clinical studies.

Part Eight

Additional Help and Information

Chapter 69

Glossary of Terms Related to Movement Disorders

agonist: A drug capable of combining with a receptor and initiating action.

antagonist: A drug that opposes the effects of another by physiological or chemical action or by a competitive mechanism.

anticholinergic drugs: Drugs that interfere with production or uptake of the neurotransmitter acetylcholine.

apoptosis: Also called programmed cell death. A form of cell death in which a programmed sequence of events leads to the elimination of old, unnecessary, and unhealthy cells.

arrhythmia: An abnormal heart rhythm. The heartbeats may be too slow, too rapid, too irregular, or too early.

ataxia (ataxic): The loss of muscle control.

ataxia-telangiectasia: A rare, childhood neurological disorder that causes degeneration in the part of the brain that controls motor movements and speech.

athetoid: Making slow, sinuous, involuntary, writhing movements, especially with the hands.

This glossary contains terms excerpted from documents produced by several sources deemed reliable.

atrophy: A decrease in size or wasting away of a body part or tissue.

autonomic dysreflexia: A potentially dangerous complication of spinal cord injury in which blood pressure rises to dangerous levels. If not treated, autonomic dysreflexia can lead to stroke and possibly death.

axial traction: The application of a mechanical force to stretch the spine; used to relieve pressure by separating vertebral surfaces and stretching soft tissues.

axon: The long, thin extension of a nerve cell that conducts impulses away from the cell body.

basal ganglia: A region located at the base of the brain composed of four clusters of neurons, or nerve cells. This area is responsible for body movement and coordination.

biopsy: A procedure in which tissue or other material is removed from the body and studied for signs of disease.

botulinum toxin: A drug commonly used to relax spastic muscles; it blocks the release of acetylcholine, a neurotransmitter that energizes muscle tissue.

bradykinesia: A gradual loss of spontaneous movement.

cardiomyopathy: Heart muscle weakness that interferes with the heart's ability to pump blood.

cerebral palsy: A functional disorder caused by damage to the brain during pregnancy, delivery, or shortly after birth. It is characterized by movement disorders, including spasticity (tight limb muscles), purposeless movements, rigidity (severe spasticity), lack of balance, or a combination of these disorders.

cervical: The part of the spine in the neck region.

chemodenervation: A treatment that relaxes spastic muscles by interrupting nerve impulse pathways via a drug, such as botulinum toxin, which prevents communication between neurons and muscle tissue.

chorea: An abnormal voluntary movement disorder, one of a group of neurological disorders called dyskinesias, which are caused by overactivity of the neurotransmitter dopamine in the areas of the brain that control movement.

choreoathetoid: A condition characterized by aimless muscle movements and involuntary motions.

chromosomes: Genetic structures that contain deoxyribonucleic acid.

computed tomography (CT): A technique used for diagnosing brain disorders. CT uses a computer to produce a high-quality image of brain structures.

contracture: Chronic shortening of a muscle or tendon that limits movement of a bony joint, such as the elbow.

cortex: Part of the brain responsible for thought, perception, and memory. Huntington disease affects the basal ganglia and cortex.

corticobasal degeneration: A progressive neurological disorder characterized by nerve cell loss and atrophy (shrinkage) of multiple areas of the brain including the cerebral cortex and the basal ganglia.

cytokine: A small protein released by immune cells that has a specific effect on the interactions between cells, or communications between cells, or on the behavior of cells.

deep brain stimulation: A treatment that uses an electrode implanted into part of the brain to stimulate it in a way that temporarily inactivates some of the signals it produces.

dementia: Loss of intellectual abilities.

dendrite: A short arm-like protuberance from a neuron. Dendrite is from the Greek for "branched like a tree."

deoxyribonucleic acid (DNA): The substance of heredity containing the genetic information necessary for cells to divide and produce proteins. DNA carries the code for every inherited characteristic of an organism.

developmental delay: Behind schedule in reaching the milestones of early childhood development.

disk: Shortened terminology for an intervertebral disk, a disk-shaped piece of specialized tissue that separates the bones of the spinal column.

dopamine: A chemical messenger, deficient in the brains of Parkinson disease patients, that transmits impulses from one nerve cell to another.

dyskinesias: Abnormal involuntary twisting and writhing movements that can result from long-term use of high doses of levodopa.

dysphagia: Difficulty in swallowing.

dystonias: Movement disorders in which sustained muscle contractions cause twisting and repetitive movements or abnormal postures.

dystrophin: A protein that helps maintain the shape and structure of muscle fibers.

electroencephalogram: A technique for recording the pattern of electrical currents inside the brain.

electromyography: A special recording technique that detects muscle activity.

embryonic stem cells: Undifferentiated cells from the embryo that have the potential to become a wide variety of specialized cell types.

Friedreich ataxia: An inherited disease that causes progressive damage to the nervous system resulting in symptoms ranging from muscle weakness and speech problems to heart disease.

gait analysis: A technique that uses cameras, force plates, electromyography, and computer analysis to objectively measure an individual's pattern of walking.

gastrostomy: A surgical procedure that creates an artificial opening in the stomach for the insertion of a feeding tube.

gene: The basic unit of heredity, composed of a segment of DNA containing the code for a specific trait.

hemiparesis: Paralysis affecting only one side of the body.

Huntington disease: A progressively disabling movement disorder that affects the individual's judgment, memory, and other cognitive functions.

hypotonia: Decreased muscle tone.

intrathecal baclofen: Baclofen that is injected into the cerebrospinal fluid of the spinal cord to reduce spasticity.

intubation: The process of putting a tube into a hollow organ or passageway, often into the airway.

levodopa: A drug used in the treatment of Parkinson disease.

ligament: A tough band of connective tissue that connects various structures such as two bones.

lumbar: The part of the spine in the middle back, below the thoracic vertebrae and above the sacral vertebrae.

magnetic resonance imaging (MRI): An imaging technique that uses radio waves, magnetic fields, and computer analysis to create a picture of body tissues and structures.

merosin: A protein found in the connective tissue that surrounds muscle fibers.

mitochondria: Microscopic, energy-producing bodies within cells that are the cells' "power plants."

mutation: In genetics, any defect in a gene.

myasthenia gravis: A chronic autoimmune neuromuscular disease characterized by varying degrees of weakness of the skeletal (voluntary) muscles of the body.

myelin: A structure of cell membranes that forms a sheath around axons, insulating them and speeding conduction of nerve impulses.

myoclonus: A condition in which muscles or portions of muscles contract involuntarily in a jerky fashion.

myopathy: Any disorder of muscle tissue or muscles.

neural prostheses: Prosthetic devices that can respond to signals from the brain.

neuroacanthocytosis: A rare movement disorder marked by progressive muscle weakness and atrophy, progressive cognitive loss, chorea, and acanthocytosis.

neurogenic pain: Generalized pain that results from nervous system malfunction.

neuromodulation: A series of techniques employing electrical stimulation or the administration of medication by means of devices implanted in the body. These techniques allow the treatment of a range of disorders including certain forms of pain, spasticity, tremor, and urinary problems.

neuron: Also known as a nerve cell; the structural and functional unit of the nervous system. A neuron consists of a cell body and its processes: an axon and one or more dendrites.

neuroprotective: Describes substances that protect nervous system cells from damage or death.

neurotransmitter: A chemical released from neurons that transmits an impulse to another neuron, muscle, organ, or other tissue.

orthostatic hypotension: A sudden drop in blood pressure when a person stands up from a lying-down position. It may cause dizziness, lightheadedness, and, in extreme cases, loss of balance or fainting.

orthotic devices: Special devices, such as splints or braces, used to treat posture problems involving the muscles, ligaments, or bones.

pallidotomy: A surgical procedure in which a part of the brain called the globus pallidus is lesioned in order to improve symptoms of tremor, rigidity, and bradykinesia.

palsy: Paralysis, or the lack of control over voluntary movement.

paralysis: The inability to control movement of a part of the body.

paraplegia: A condition involving complete paralysis of the legs.

parkinsonian gait: A characteristic way of walking that includes a tendency to lean forward; small, quick steps as if hurrying forward (called festination); and reduced swinging of the arms.

parkinsonism: A term referring to a group of conditions that are characterized by four typical symptoms: tremor, rigidity, postural instability, and bradykinesia.

periodic limb movement disorder: A disorder characterized by repetitive stereotyped movements of the limbs, primarily the legs, during sleep.

positron emission tomography (PET): A tool used to diagnose brain functions and disorders. PET produces three-dimensional, colored images of chemicals or substances functioning within the body.

postural instability: Impaired balance that causes a tendency to lean forward or backward and to fall easily.

pressure sore: A reddened area or open sore caused by unrelieved pressure on the skin over bony areas such as the hip-bone or tailbone.

prevalence: The number of cases of a disease that are present in a particular population at a given time.

ptosis: An abnormal drooping of the eyelids.

quadriplegia: Paralysis of both the arms and legs.

receptor: A structure on the surface or interior of a cell that selectively receives and binds to a specific substance.

recessive: A trait that is apparent only when the gene or genes for it are inherited from both parents.

regeneration: Repair, regrowth, or restoration of tissues; opposite of degeneration.

respite care: Rest or relief from caretaking obligations.

restless legs syndrome (RLS): A neurological disorder characterized by unpleasant sensations in the legs and an uncontrollable urge to move them for relief.

Rett syndrome: A childhood neurodevelopmental disorder that affects females almost exclusively. Loss of muscle tone is usually the first symptom.

rhizotomy: An operation to disconnect specific nerve roots in order to stop severe spasticity.

rigidity: A symptom of the disease in which muscles feel stiff and display resistance to movement even when another person tries to move the affected part of the body, such as an arm.

selective dorsal rhizotomy: A surgical procedure in which selected nerves are severed to reduce spasticity in the legs.

selective dorsal rhizotomy (SDR): Describes stiff muscles and awkward movements.

spastic diplegia (or diparesis): A form of cerebral palsy in which spasticity affects both legs, but the arms are relatively or completely spared.

spastic hemiplegia (or hemiparesis): A form of cerebral palsy in which spasticity affects an arm and leg on one side of the body.

spastic quadriplegia (or quadriparesis): A form of cerebral palsy in which all four limbs are paralyzed or weakened equally.

spina bifida: A neural tube defect (a disorder involving incomplete development of the brain, spinal cord, and/or their protective coverings) caused by the failure of the fetus's spine to close properly during the first month of pregnancy.

spinal muscular atrophy (SMA): A group of hereditary diseases that cause weakness and wasting of the voluntary muscles in the arms and legs of infants and children.

spinal shock: A temporary physiological state that can occur after a spinal cord injury in which all sensory, motor, and sympathetic functions of the nervous system are lost below the level of injury.

stem cell: Special cells that have the ability to grow into any one of the body's more than 200 cell types.

striatum: Part of the basal ganglia of the brain. The striatum is composed of the caudate nucleus, putamen, and ventral striatum.

substantia nigra: Movement-control center in the brain where loss of dopamine-producing nerve cells triggers the symptoms of Parkinson disease; substantia nigra means "black substance," so called because the cells in this area are dark.

synapse: A specialized junction between two nerve cells. At the synapse, a neuron releases neurotransmitters that diffuse across the gap and activate receptors situated on the target cell.

T-cell: An immune system cell that produces substances called cytokines, which stimulate the immune response.

tardive dyskinesia: A neurological syndrome caused by the long-term use of neuroleptic drugs. It is characterized by repetitive, involuntary, purposeless movements.

thalamotomy: A procedure in which a portion of the brain's thalamus is surgically destroyed, usually reducing tremors.

thoracic: The part of the spine at the upper-back to mid-back level.

Tourette syndrome: A neurological disorder characterized by repetitive, stereotyped, involuntary movements, and vocalizations called tics.

trait: Any genetically determined characteristic.

tremor: An involuntary trembling or quivering.

ultrasound: A technique that bounces sound waves off tissue and bone and uses the pattern of echoes to form an image, called a sonogram.

ventricles: Cavities within the brain that are filled with cerebrospinal fluid.

vertebrae: The 33 hollow bones that make up the spine.

Wilson disease: A rare inherited disorder in which excessive amounts of copper accumulate in the body.

Chapter 70

Directory of Agencies That Provide Information about Movement Disorders

Government Agencies That Provide Information about Movement Disorders

Administration for Community Living (ACL)
330 C St. S.W.
Washington, DC 20201
Toll-Free: 800-677-1116
Phone: 202-401-4634
Website: www.acl.gov

Agency for Healthcare Research and Quality (AHRQ)
Office of Communications and Knowledge Transfer
5600 Fishers Ln.
Seventh Fl.
Rockville, MD 20857
Phone: 301-427-1104
Website: www.ahrq.gov

Resources in this chapter were compiled from several sources deemed reliable; all contact information was verified and updated in January 2018.

Centers for Disease Control and Prevention (CDC)
1600 Clifton Rd.
Atlanta, GA 30329-4027
Toll-Free: 800-232-4636
Toll-Free TTY: 888-232-6348
Website: www.cdc.gov
E-mail: cdcinfo@cdc.gov

Clearinghouse on Disability Information
Office of Special Education
and Rehabilitative Services
(OSERS), U.S. Department of
Education (ED)
400 Maryland Ave. S.W.
Washington, DC 20202
Toll-Free: 800-872-5327
Toll-Free TTY: 888-320-6942
Website: www.ed.gov/about/
offices/list/osers/index.htm

Eunice Kennedy Shriver National Institute of Child Health and Human Development (NICHD)
P.O. Box 3006
Rockville, MD 20847
Toll-Free: 800-370-2943
Toll-Free Fax: 866-760-5947
Website: www.nichd.nih.gov
E-mail: NICHDInformation
ResourceCenter@mail.nih.gov

Healthfinder®
National Health Information
Center (NHIC)
1101 Wootton Pkwy
Rockville, MD 20852
Website: www.healthfinder.gov
E-mail: healthfinder@hhs.gov

National Cancer Institute (NCI)
BG 9609 MSC 9760
9609 Medical Center Dr.
Bethesda, MD 20892-9760
Toll-Free: 800-4-CANCER
(800-422-6237)
Website: www.cancer.gov

National Eye Institute (NEI)
Information Office
31 Center Dr. MSC 2510
Bethesda, MD 20892-2510
Phone: 301-496-5248
Website: www.nei.nih.gov
E-mail: 2020@nei.nih.gov

National Human Genome Research Institute (NHGRI)
Communications and Public
Liaison Branch
Bldg. 31 Rm. 4B09
9000 Rockville Pike
Bethesda, MD 20892-2152
Phone: 301-402-0911
Fax: 301-402-2218
Website: www.genome.gov

National Institute of Arthritis and Musculoskeletal and Skin Diseases (NIAMS)
NIAMS Information
Clearinghouse
Bethesda, MD 20892-3675
Toll-Free: 877-22-NIAMS
(877-226-4267)
Phone: 301-495-4484
TTY: 301-565-2966
Fax: 301-718-6366
Website: www.niams.nih.gov
E-mail: NIAMSinfo@mail.nih.gov

National Institute of Diabetes and Digestive and Kidney Diseases (NIDDK)
Health Information Center
Toll-Free: 800-860-8747
Toll-Free TTY: 866-569-1162
Website: www.niddk.nih.gov

National Institute of Mental Health (NIMH)
6001 Executive Blvd.
Rm. 6200 MSC 9663
Bethesda, MD 20892-9663
Toll-Free: 866-615-6464
Toll-Free TTY: 866-415-8051
TTY: 301-443-8431
Fax: 301-443-4279
Website: www.nimh.nih.gov
E-mail: nimhinfo@nih.gov

National Institute of Neurological Disorders and Stroke (NINDS)
NIH Neurological Institute
P.O. Box 5801
Bethesda, MD 20824
Phone: 301-496-5751
Website: www.ninds.nih.gov
E-mail: braininfo@ninds.nih.gov

National Institute on Aging (NIA)
31 Center Dr. MSC 2292
Bldg. 31 Rm. 5C27
Bethesda, MD 20892
Toll-Free: 800-222-2225
Toll-Free TTY: 800-222-4225
Website: www.nia.nih.gov
E-mail: niaic@nia.nih.gov

National Institute on Deafness and Communication Disorders (NIDCD)
31 Center Dr. MSC 2320
Bethesda, MD 20892-2320
Toll-Free: 800-241-1044
Toll-Free TTY: 800-241-1055
Website: www.nidcd.nih.gov
E-mail: nidcdinfo@nidcd.nih.gov

National Institute on Disability, Independent Living, and Rehabilitation Research (NIDILRR)
330 C St. S.W.
Rm. 1304
Washington, DC 20201
TTY: 202-245-7316
Fax: 202-205-0392
Website: www.acl.gov/about-acl/about-national-institute-disability-independent-living-and-rehabilitation-research
E-mail: nidilrr-mailbox@acl.hhs.gov

National Institute on Drug Abuse (NIDA)
6001 Executive Bdwy.
Rm. 5213
Bethesda, MD 20892-9561
Phone: 301-443-1124
Website: www.nida.nih.gov

National Institutes of Health (NIH)
9000 Rockville Pike
Bethesda, MD 20892
Phone: 301-496-4000
TTY: 301-402-9612
Website: www.nih.gov
E-mail: NIHinfo@od.nih.gov

National Women's Health Information Center (NWHIC)
200 Independence Ave. S.W.
Washington, DC 20201
Toll-Free: 800-994-9662
Website: www.womenshealth.gov

U.S. Department of Health and Human Services (HHS)
200 Independent Ave. S.W.
Washington, DC 20201
Toll-Free: 877-696-6775
Website: www.hhs.gov

U.S. Food and Drug Administration (FDA)
10903 New Hampshire Ave.
Silver Spring, MD 20993
Toll-Free: 888-463-6332
Website: www.fda.gov

U.S. National Library of Medicine (NLM)
8600 Rockville Pike
Bethesda, MD 20894
Toll-Free: 888-346-3656
Phone: 301-594-5983
Website: www.nlm.nih.gov/research/umls
E-mail: custserv@nlm.nih.gov

U.S. Social Security Administration (SSA)
1100 W. High Rise
6401 Security Blvd.
Baltimore, MD 21235
Toll-Free: 800-772-1213
Toll-Free TTY: 800-325-0778
Website: www.ssa.gov

Private Agencies That Provide Information about Movement Disorders

The ALS Association
1275 K St. N.W., Ste. 250
Washington, DC 20005
Toll-Free: 800-782-4747
Phone: 202-407-8580
Fax: 202-464-8869
Website: www.alsa.org
E-mail: alsinfo@alsa-national.org

ALS Therapy Development Institute
300 Technology Sq.
Ste. 400
Cambridge, MA 02139
Phone: 617-441-7200
Website: www.als.net
E-mail: info@als.net

American Academy of Neurology (AAN)
201 Chicago Ave.
Minneapolis, MN 55415
Toll-Free: 800-879-1960
Phone: 612-928-6000
Fax: 612-454-2746
Website: www.aan.com

American Academy of Pediatrics (AAP)
345 Park Blvd.
Itasca, IL 60143
Toll-Free: 800-433-9016
Fax: 847-434-8000
Website: www.aap.org
E-mail: kidsdocs@aap.org

American Association of Neurological Surgeons (AANS)
American Association of Neurological Surgeons Executive Office
5550 Meadowbrook Dr.
Rolling Meadows, IL 60008-3852
Toll-Free: 888-566-AANS
(888-566-2267)
Phone: 847-378-0500
Fax: 847-378-0600
Website: www.aans.org
E-mail: info@aans.org

American Heart Association (AHA)
National Center
7272 Greenville Ave.
Dallas, TX 75231
Toll-Free: 800-AHA-USA-1
(800-242-8721)
Website: www.heart.org

American Liver Foundation (ALF)
39 Bdwy.
Ste. 2700
New York, NY 10006
Toll-Free: 800-GO LIVER
(800-465-4837)
Phone: 212-668-1000
Website: www.liverfoundation.org
E-mail: info@liverfoundation.org

American Parkinson Disease Association (APDA)
135 Parkinson Ave.
Staten Island, NY 10305
Toll-Free: 800-223-2732
Fax: 718-981-4399
Website: www.apdaparkinson.org
E-mail: apda@apdaparkinson.org

American Psychological Association (APA)
750 First St. N.E.
Washington, DC 20002-4242
Toll-Free: 800-374-2721
Phone: 202-336-5500
TDD/TTY: 202-336-6123
Website: www.apa.org

A-T (Ataxia-Telangiectasia) Children's Project
5300 W. Hillsboro Blvd.
Ste. 105
Coconut Creek, FL 33073
Toll-Free: 800-5-HELP-A-T
(800-543-5728)
Phone: 954-481-6611
Website: www.atcp.org
E-mail: info@atcp.org

Bachmann-Strauss Dystonia & Parkinson Foundation (BSDPF)
P.O. Box 38016
Albany, NY 12203
Phone: 212-509-0995
Website: www.dystonia-parkinsons.org

Benign Essential Blepharospasm Research Foundation (BEBRF)
P.O. Box 12468
755 N. 11th St., Ste. 211
Beaumont, TX 77726-2468
Phone: 409-832-0788
Fax: 409-832-0890
Website: www.blepharospasm.org
E-mail: bebrf@blepharospasm.org

Children's Hemiplegia & Stroke Association (CHASA)
4101 W. Green Oaks
Ste. 305-149
Arlington, TX 76016
Website: www.chasa.org

Christopher & Dana Reeve Foundation
636 Morris Tpke
Ste. 3A
Short Hills, NJ 07078
Toll-Free: 800-225-0292
Phone: 973-379-2690
Fax: 973-912-9433
Website: www.christopherreeve.org
E-mail: media@christopherreeve.org

Cleveland Clinic
9500 Euclid Ave.
Cleveland, OH 44195
Toll-Free: 800-223-2273
TTY: 216-444-0261
Website: my.clevelandclinic.org

CurePSP, Inc.
404 Fifth Ave.
Third Fl.
New York, NY 10018
Toll-Free: 800-457-4777
Phone: 347-294-2873
Fax: 410-785-7009
Website: www.psp.org
E-mail: info@curepsp.org

Disabled Sports USA
451 Hungerford Dr., Ste. 608
Rockville, MD 20850
Phone: 301-217-0960
Fax: 301-217-0968
Website: www.disabledsportsusa.org
E-mail: info@dsusa.org

Dystonia Medical Research Foundation (DMRF)
1 E. Wacker Dr., Ste. 1730
Chicago, IL 60601-1980
Toll-Free: 800-377-DYST (800-377-3978)
Phone: 312-755-0198
Fax: 312-803-0138
Website: www.dystonia-foundation.org
E-mail: dystonia@dystonia-foundation.org

The Dystonia Society
Camelford House
89 Albert Embankment
Second Fl.
Vauxhall London SE1 7TP
United Kingdom
Toll-Free: 020-7793-3650
Phone: 020-7793-3651
Website: www.dystonia.org.uk
E-mail: info@dystonia.org.uk

Easter Seals
230 W. Monroe St.
Ste. 1800
Chicago, IL 60606-4802
Toll-Free: 800-221-6827
Phone: 312-726-6200
TTY: 312-726-4258
Fax: 312-726-1494
Website: www.easterseals.com

*Facioscapulohumeral
Muscular Dystrophy (FSHD)
Society*
450 Bedford St.
Lexington, MA 0240
Phone: 781-301-6060
Website: www.fshsociety.org
E-mail: info@fshsociety.org

Family Caregiver Alliance
235 Montgomery St.
Ste. 950
San Francisco, CA 94104
Toll-Free: 800-445-8106
Phone: 415-434-3388
Website: www.caregiver.org
E-mail: info@caregiver.org

*Friedreich's Ataxia Research
Alliance (FARA)*
P.O. Box 1537
Springfield, VA 22151
Phone: 484-879-6160
Website: www.CureFA.org
E-mail: info@CureFA.org

*Hereditary Disease
Foundation (HDF)*
3960 Bdwy.
Sixth Fl.
New York, NY 10032
Phone: 212-928-2121
Fax: 212-928-2172
Website: www.hdfoundation.org
E-mail: cures@hdfoundation.org

*Huntington's Disease Society
of America (HDSA)*
505 Eighth Ave., Ste. 902
New York, NY 10018
Toll-Free: 800-345-HDSA
(800-345-4512)
Phone: 212-242-1968
Fax: 212-239-3430
Website: www.hdsa.org
E-mail: hdsainfo@hdsa.org

*International Essential
Tremor Foundation (IETF)*
11111 W. 95th St., Ste. 260
Overland Park, KS 66214
Toll-Free: 888-387-3667
Phone: 913-341-3880
Fax: 913-341-1296
Website: www.essentialtremor.
org
E-mail: info@essentialtremor.org

*International Joseph Disease
Foundation, Inc.*
P.O. Box 994268
Redding, CA 96099-4268
Phone: 530-246-4722
Fax: 530-232-2773
Website: www.rarediseases.org/
organizations/international-
joseph-disease-foundation-inc
E-mail: MJD@ijdf.net

*International Radiosurgery
Association*
P.O. Box 5186
Harrisburg, PA 17110
Website: www.irsa.org

*International Rett Syndrome
Foundation*
4600 Devitt Dr.
Cincinnati, OH 45246
Phone: 513-874-3020
Fax: 513-874-2520
Website: www.rettsyndrome.org
E-mail: admin@rettsyndrome.
org

Les Turner ALS Foundation
5550 W. Touhy Ave.
Ste. 302
Skokie, IL 60077-3254
Toll-Free: 888-ALS-1107
Phone: 847-679-3311
Fax: 847-679-9109
Website: www.lesturnerals.org
E-mail: info@lesturnerals.org

March of Dimes Foundation
1275 Mamaroneck Ave.
White Plains, NY 10605
Phone: 914-428-7100
Website: www.marchofdimes.
com

*Michael J. Fox Foundation
for Parkinson's Research*
Grand Central Station
P.O. Box 4777
New York, NY 10163-4777
Toll-Free: 800-708-7644
Website: www.michaeljfox.org

*Muscular Dystrophy
Association (MDA)*
3300 E. Sunrise Dr.
Tucson, AZ 85718
Toll-Free: 800-572-1717
Phone: 520-529-2000
Website: www.mda.org
E-mail: mda@mdausa.org

*Muscular Dystrophy Family
Foundation (MDFF)*
222 S. Riverside Plaza
Ste. 1500
Chicago, IL 60606
Website: www.mda.org

*Myasthenia Gravis
Foundation of America
(MGFA)*
355 Lexington Ave.
15th Fl.
New York, NY 10017
Toll-Free: 800-541-5454
Phone: 651-917-6256
Fax: 212-297-2159
Website: www.myasthenia.org

*Myotonic Dystrophy
Foundation (DM)*
1004-A O'Reilly Ave.
San Francisco, CA 94129
Toll-Free: 86-MYOTONIC
(866-968-6642)
Phone: 415-800-7777
Website: www.myotonic.org/
contact-us
E-mail: info@myotonic.org

National Alliance on Mental Illness (NAMI)
3803 N. Fairfax Dr.
Ste. 100
Arlington, VA 22203
Toll-Free: 800-950-NAMI
(800-950-6264)
Phone: 703-524-7600
Website: www.nami.org

National Ataxia Foundation (NAF)
600 Hwy 169 S.
Ste. 1725
Minneapolis, MN 55426
Phone: 763-553-0020
Fax: 763-553-0167
Website: www.ataxia.org
E-mail: naf@ataxia.org

National Dysautonomia Research Foundation (NDRF)
P.O. Box 301
Red Wing, MN 55066-0301
Phone: 651-267-0525
Fax: 651-267-0524
Website: www.ndrf.org
E-mail: ndrf@ndrf.org

National Multiple Sclerosis Society (NMSS)
Toll-Free: 800-344-4867
Website: www.nationalmssociety.org

National Organization for Rare Disorders (NORD)
55 Kenosia Ave.
Danbury, CT 06813
Toll-Free: 800-999-NORD
Phone: 203-744-0100
Fax: 203-263-9938
Website: www.rarediseases.org
E-mail: orphan@rarediseases.org

National Parkinson Foundation (NPF)
200 S.E. First St., Ste. 800
Miami, FL 33131
Toll-Free: 800-4PD-INFO
(800-473-4636)
Phone: 305-243-6666
Website: www.parkinson.org
E-mail: contact@parkinson.org

National Rehabilitation Information Center (NARIC)
8201 Corporate Dr.
Ste. 600
Landover, MD 20785
Toll-Free: 800-346-2742
Phone: 301-459-5900
TTY: 301-459-5984
Fax: 301-459-4263
Website: www.naric.com
E-mail: naricinfo@heitechservices.com

National Spinal Cord Injury Association (NSCIA)
120-34 Queens Blvd.
Ste. 320
Kew Gardens, NY 11415
Phone: 718-803-3782
Fax: 718-803-0414
Website: www.spinalcord.org

The Nemours Foundation (KidsHealth®)
1600 Rockland Rd.
Wilmington, DE 19803
Phone: 302-651-4000
Fax: 302-651-4055
Website: www.kidshealth.org
E-mail: info@KidsHealth.org

Paralyzed Veterans of America (PVA)
801 18th St. N.W.
Washington, DC 20006-3517
Toll-Free: 800-424-8200
Website: www.pva.org

Parent Project Muscular Dystrophy (PPMD)
401 Hackensack Ave.
Ninth Fl.
Hackensack, NJ 07601
Toll-Free: 800-714-5437
Phone: 201-250-8440
Fax: 201-250-8435
Website: www.parentprojectmd.org
E-mail: info@parentprojectmd.org

Parkinson Alliance
P.O. Box 308
Kingston, NJ 08528-0308
Toll-Free: 800-579-8440
Fax: 609-688-0875
Website: www.parkinsonalliance.org

Parkinson's Action Network (PAN)
P.O. Box 4777
New York, NY 10163-4777
Phone: 202-638-4101
Website: www.parkinsonsaction.org
E-mail: info@parkinsonsaction.org

Parkinson's Institute
675 Almanor Ave.
Sunnyvale, CA 94085
Phone: 408-734-2800
Fax: 408-734-9208
Website: www.thepi.org
E-mail: info@thepi.org

Parkinson's Resource Organization (PRO)
74-090 El Paseo Dr., Ste. 102
Palm Desert, CA 92260-4135
Toll-Free: 877-775-4111
Phone: 760-773-5628
Fax: 760-773-9803
Website: www.parkinsonsresource.org
E-mail: info@parkinsonsresource.org

Pathways Awareness Foundation
150 N. Michigan Ave., Ste. 100
Chicago, IL 60601
Toll-Free: 800-955-CHILD
(800-955-2445)
Phone: 312-893-6620
Website: www.pathwaysawareness.org
E-mail: friends@pathwaysawareness.org

Pediatric Brain Foundation
2144 E. Republic Rd., Bldg. B
Ste. 201
Springfield, MO 65804
Phone: 417-887-4242
Website: www.
pediatricbrainfoundation.org

Project ALS
801 Riverside Dr.
Ste. 6G
New York, NY 10032
Phone: 212-420-7382
Fax: 646 559 9290
Website: www.projectals.org
E-mail: info@projectals.org

Rehabilitation Institute of Chicago (RIC)
355 E. Erie
Chicago, IL 60611
Phone: 312-238-1000
Website: www.ric.org

Shy-Drager/Multiple System Atrophy Support Group, Inc.
9935-D Rea Rd.
Ste. 212
Charlotte, NC 28277
Toll-Free: 866-SDS-4999
(866-737-4999)
Website: www.shy-drager.org

Spasmodic Torticollis Dystonia/ST Dystonia
P.O. Box 28
Mukwonago, WI 53149
Toll-Free: 888-445-4588
Website: www.
spasmodictorticollis.org
E-mail: info@
spasmodictorticollis.org

Spastic Paraplegia Foundation (SPF)
7700 Leesburg Pike
Ste. 123
Fremont, CA 94539-7241
Toll-Free: 877-773-4483
Website: www.sp-foundation.org

Spina Bifida Association of America (SBAA)
1600 Wilson Blvd.
Ste. 800
Arlington, VA 22209
Toll-Free: 800-621-3141
Phone: 202-944-3285
Fax: 202-944-3295
Website: www.
spinabifidaassociation.org
E-mail: sbaa@sbaa.org

Tremor Action Network (TAN)
P.O. Box 5013
Pleasanton, CA 94566-5013
Phone: 510-681-6565
Fax: 925-369-0485
Website: www.tremoraction.org
E-mail: info@tremoraction.org

Tourette Syndrome Association (TAA)
42-40 Bell Bdwy.
Ste. 205
Bayside, NY 11361-2820
Toll-Free: 888-4-TOURET
(888-486-8738)
Phone: 718-224-2999
Fax: 718-279-9596
Website: tsa-usa.org
E-mail: ts@tsa-usa.org

United Cerebral Palsy (UCP)
1825 K St. N.W.
Ste. 600
Washington, DC 20006
Phone: 202-776-0406
Website: www.ucp.org
E-mail: info@ucp.org

WE MOVE (Worldwide Education & Awareness for Movement Disorders)
204 W. 84th St.
New York, NY 10024
Phone: 212-875-8312
Fax: 212-875-8389
Website: www.wemove.org
E-mail: wemove@wemove.org

Wilson Disease Association (WDA)
1732 First Ave.
#20043
New York, NY 10128
Toll-Free: 888-264-1450
Phone: 414-961-0533
Website: www.wilsonsdisease.org
E-mail: info@wilsonsdisease.org

Index

Index

Page numbers followed by 'n' indicate a footnote. Page numbers in *italics* indicate a table or illustration.

C